Practise Psychiatry

Practise Psychiatry

A Guide Through Vignettes and MCQs

Howard CH Khoe
National Psychiatry Residency Programme, Singapore

Cheryl WL Chang
National University Hospital, Singapore

Cyrus SH Ho
National University Hospital, Singapore

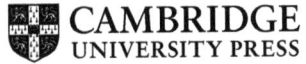
CAMBRIDGE
UNIVERSITY PRESS

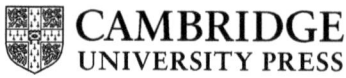

Shaftesbury Road, Cambridge CB2 8EA, United Kingdom

One Liberty Plaza, 20th Floor, New York, NY 10006, USA

477 Williamstown Road, Port Melbourne, VIC 3207, Australia

314–321, 3rd Floor, Plot 3, Splendor Forum, Jasola District Centre,
New Delhi – 110025, India

103 Penang Road, #05–06/07, Visioncrest Commercial, Singapore 238467

Cambridge University Press is part of Cambridge University Press & Assessment,
a department of the University of Cambridge.

We share the University's mission to contribute to society through the pursuit of
education, learning and research at the highest international levels of excellence.

www.cambridge.org
Information on this title: www.cambridge.org/9781009458665

DOI: 10.1017/9781009458634

First published 2025

A catalogue record for this publication is available from the British Library

A Cataloging-in-Publication data record for this book is available from the Library of Congress

ISBN 978-1-009-45866-5 Paperback

Cambridge University Press & Assessment has no responsibility for the persistence
or accuracy of URLs for external or third-party internet websites referred to in this
publication and does not guarantee that any content on such websites is, or will
remain, accurate or appropriate.

Every effort has been made in preparing this book to provide accurate and up-to-date
information that is in accord with accepted standards and practice at the time of publication.
Although case histories are drawn from actual cases, every effort has been made to disguise
the identities of the individuals involved. Nevertheless, the authors, editors, and publishers
can make no warranties that the information contained herein is totally free from error, not
least because clinical standards are constantly changing through research and regulation.
The authors, editors, and publishers therefore disclaim all liability for direct or consequential
damages resulting from the use of material contained in this book. Readers are strongly
advised to pay careful attention to information provided by the manufacturer of any drugs or
equipment that they plan to use.

Contents

v

Contents

Contents

Acknowledgements

In the writing of this textbook, we are grateful for the support, encouragement and inspiration provided by a range of individuals whose contributions extend beyond the academic realm.

We extend our sincere gratitude to the following individuals whose dedicated efforts have significantly enriched the content and depth of this textbook. We wish to thank Dr Grace Ho Cheng En (Singapore House Officer) for providing insights as a junior doctor which added a unique perspective to our material, playing a pivotal role in contributing to some chapters in this textbook. A special thanks to Dr Nicholas Lee Yew Wen (Singapore Psychiatry Resident Trainee) for his meticulous attention to detail and unwavering commitment to accuracy in proofreading and providing feedback which have left an indelible mark on this textbook. We are also deeply appreciative of our colleague Dr Stefanie Goh Wei Lynn for her creative contribution in designing the cover page of this textbook, which beautifully encapsulates the essence of our work. We are grateful to all for their commitment to academic excellence and for being an integral part of this endeavour.

To our patients, our deepest gratitude goes to you, whose life stories and resilience have formed the basis for these vignettes. Your trust in us has brought a human touch to this academic endeavour, reminding us daily of the profound impact our work can have on real lives.

To our mentors, your guidance and wisdom have been a guiding light throughout this undertaking, proving to be instrumental in the shaping of this textbook.

To our loved ones and families, who have been by our side with unwavering support, we express our deepest gratitude. Your encouragement during challenging times has been the bedrock upon which this project stands.

To the editorial team at Cambridge University Press, your editorial acumen has been indispensable in shaping the overall structure and coherence of this textbook. Your keen eye for detail has set the standard for the entire editorial process.

Thank you to each individual who has played a role in making this textbook possible.

With sincere appreciation,
Dr Howard Khoe, Dr Cheryl Chang, Dr Cyrus Ho

Part 1: Vignettes

Case 1: Schizophrenia

They told me so

Ryan is a 21-year-old male brought to the clinic by his parents after his teachers expressed concerns that he was failing his university examinations and had poor attendance. Over the past six months, Ryan had accused his classmate of inserting thoughts into his head and controlling his actions. He reported this as true because he heard 'the voices' warning him. His friends noticed that Ryan was more withdrawn, and he was seen talking to himself. Ryan denied taking recreational drugs, and a routine drug screen performed last month revealed no abnormalities.

- **Question 1: What are the diagnosis and differential diagnoses?**

Ryan accused his classmate of working for a sinister network of aliens called 'The Organisation.' They reference him on the radio whenever the radio uses a word that starts with 'R'. When these ideas were challenged, he rebuffed your assertions that perhaps he might be mistaken.

- **Question 2: What type of delusion is being demonstrated?**

You ask Ryan about the voices that he hears. He describes a male voice coming from outside his head, which talks to him throughout the day. The voices occasionally comment on his actions, for example 'Ryan is drinking the cup of coffee now' and at other times suggest that his classmate is going to hurt him 'They are coming to get you'. There had been times when he heard his thoughts spoken out loud, which bothered him greatly.

- **Question 3: How would you describe his hallucinations?**

With the constellation of symptoms presented, you diagnose Ryan with schizophrenia. Ryan's cousin (Jake) was also diagnosed with schizophrenia, but had a very different presentation. Jake was found to be increasingly quiet, and when he did speak, he was often incoherent. He refused to leave his room and did not appear to be excited over anything, often giving a blank stare with little emotion shown.

- **Question 4: How will you explain Jake's seemingly different presentation of schizophrenia?**

Ryan's parents suspect that he might have used recreational drugs in the past and wonder if that might have contributed to the development of his psychotic episode.

- **Question 5: Which illicit substance has a known association with the development of schizophrenia?**

Now that he has been diagnosed with psychosis, Ryan's parents want to know what investigations will be done.

- **Question 6: How will you investigate Ryan's first presentation of psychosis?**

Having heard his conspiracy theories, you ask Ryan if he feels safe currently. Ryan replies that he is worried "The Organisation" is plotting to abduct him and states that he would rather die than be abducted. He intends to hurt himself and shows you a kitchen knife he has hidden in his bag.

- **Question 7: What is the next step of management?**

Ryan is admitted, and investigations return as unremarkable. You explain to Ryan's parents that early intervention may improve cognition and will be in his best interest. His parents cautiously accept the treatment plan. However, his parents mention that Ryan was previously bullied for his heavy weight, and are worried about the side effects.

- **Question 8: Which antipsychotic medications would you avoid for Ryan?**

Ryan was started on haloperidol. Unfortunately, despite treatment with haloperidol and subsequently risperidone for six weeks each at a therapeutic dose, he remains symptomatic. He is diagnosed with treatment-resistant schizophrenia (TRS).

- **Question 9: What is the definition of TRS?**

Having diagnosed Ryan with TRS, clozapine is commenced.

- **Question 10: What are the potentially life-threatening side effects of clozapine ?**

Ryan's condition stabilises on clozapine and he reports compliance with his medications. While the risk of extrapyramidal side effects (EPSEs) with clozapine is low, he remains concerned about the side effects of antipsychotics.

- **Question 11: What are EPSEs and what are the different types?**

Answers to Case 1

Question 1
What are the diagnosis and differential diagnoses?

Answer
Schizophrenia

Apart from organic causes, the main differentials to consider for symptoms of psychosis without prominent affective symptoms would be:

- Acute and transient psychotic disorder
- Delusional disorder
- Schizotypal disorder

Explanation

Diagnosis of schizophrenia

At least two of the following symptoms must be present (by the individual's report or through observation by the clinician or other informants) most of the time for a period of 1 month or more. At least one of the qualifying symptoms should be from items (1) to (4) below:

1. Delusions
2. Hallucinations
3. Disorganised thinking
4. Passivity phenomenon
5. Negative symptoms
6. Grossly disorganised behaviour
7. Psychomotor disturbances (e.g., catatonia)

Specify if the first episode or multiple episodes, are continuous or in remission.

The onset of schizophrenia generally occurs in late adolescence or early adulthood. Auditory hallucinations are the most common form of hallucination, with an estimated prevalence of 40–80% [1, 2].

A diagnosis of delusional disorder is less likely as there is impairment in functioning with odd behaviour and prominent hallucinations. The history given in the vignette suggests an acute deterioration, which is not typically seen in personality disorders. Acute and transient psychotic disorder often lasts for a few days up to a month and does not exceed three months. Schizotypal disorder persists for at least two years and the individual must not have fulfilled the criteria for schizophrenia.

First-rank symptoms are commonly seen in schizophrenia:

First-rank symptoms in schizophrenia

- Hearing thoughts spoken aloud
- Third-person hallucinations
- Auditory hallucinations in the form of a 'running commentary'
- Somatic (bodily, tactile) hallucinations
- Thought withdrawal or insertion
- Thought broadcasting
- Delusional perception
- Passivity (feelings or actions felt as influenced by external forces)

 **Exam Essentials**

- Schneider's **first-rank symptoms** of schizophrenia – **ABCD**
  - **A**uditory hallucinations
  - **B**roadcasting, insertion, withdrawal
  - **C**ontrol, passivity
  - **D**elusional perception
- There are **two age peaks** of schizophrenia: early 20s and 40s
- **Late-onset schizophrenia**: aged 40 to 60 years

- **Very late-onset schizophrenia**: > 60 years
- Although first-rank symptoms are highly prevalent in patients with schizophrenia, they **should not be used as a sole diagnostic tool** due to their higher specificity but lower sensitivity

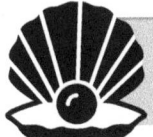

Clinical Pearls

- While auditory hallucinations are more common, visual hallucinations are also present in schizophrenia. The **visual hallucinations** experienced are **often unformed**, such as glowing orbs or flashes of colour

- If the patient presents with **predominant non-auditory hallucinations** (e.g., visual, olfactory, gustatory), it is important **to rule out organic causes** (e.g., epilepsy, encephalitis, brain tumours)

Question 2
What type of delusion is being demonstrated?

Answer
Delusions of reference

Explanation
A delusion is defined as a firmly maintained false belief contradicted by reality; idiosyncratic, incorrigible and preoccupying. Delusion of reference is characterised by the erroneous belief that innocuous events have strong personal significance, with complete conviction. Approximately 80% [2] of people with schizophrenia have delusions.

Impairment of insight is common and a delusional explanation for their hallucinations is often elicited. Bizarre delusions are implausible and absurd to same-culture peers and do not derive from ordinary life experiences (e.g., the belief that one's organ has been replaced entirely with another's, although there are no scars or evidence of such). A non-bizarre delusion is one that, while not true, can be derived from ordinary life experience with the possibility of it being true (e.g., believing that valuables have been stolen).

Exam Essentials

- Features of delusion can be remembered as three 'U's:

  ○ **Un**true
  ○ **Un**shared
  ○ **Un**shakeable

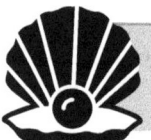

Clinical Pearls

- The differences between a delusion and an overvalued idea lie in the **degree of conviction and how it is being derived**

Question 3
How would you describe his hallucinations?

Answer
Second- and third-person auditory hallucinations in the form of a 'running commentary' with the presence of a thought echo.

Explanation
Perception is the organisation, identification and interpretation of sensory information to represent and understand the presented information or environment. Hallucinations are false perceptions that are not in any way distortions of a real perception but spring up on their own as something quite new and occur simultaneously with and alongside real perception. They may take the form of noises, music, single words, brief phrases, or whole conversations.

Approach to hallucinations should include:

1. Where?

   The first distinction is between hallucinations and pseudohallucinations. Ask where the voices are from and assess the degree of insight lost.

	Hallucination	Pseudohallucination
Space	External space	Inner subjective (not seeming to the patient to represent external reality, being located within the mind)
Insight	Impaired	Intact
Control	Cannot be willfully modified	Can be modified by will (initiated or interrupted) [3]

2. Who?
    Assess who the voice(s) have been identified as.

3. How?
    If it is an auditory hallucination, distinguish between the second person (voice speaking to the person addressing him as 'you') and the third person (voice talking about the person as 'he' or 'she'). Third-person auditory hallucinations are part of the first-rank symptoms in schizophrenia.

4. What?
    Examine the content of the hallucinations and determine if they are mood congruent or incongruent. Auditory hallucination may come in the form of a running commentary or voices arguing etc.

A thought echo refers to a form of auditory hallucination where the person hears his or her thoughts aloud after thinking them.

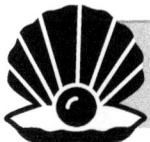

Clinical Pearls

- **Check for the presence of command hallucinations and passivity** as part of the risk assessment – higher risk if the patient has both

Question 4
How will you explain Jake's seemingly different presentation of schizophrenia?

Answer
Jake has predominantly negative symptoms of schizophrenia, whereas Ryan presents with predominantly positive symptoms of schizophrenia.

Explanation

Positive symptoms are characterised by delusions and hallucinations.

Negative symptoms are characterised by deficit symptoms leading to the absence or diminution of normal processes and functioning. They are often listed as the six 'A's: anhedonia (inability to feel pleasure), apathy (disinterest in daily activities), avolition (decreased motivation), alogia (decreased spontaneous speech), affective flattening (lack of emotional expressivity, but not depressed) and asociality (social withdrawal).

Patients may present in a varied manner, with features consisting of both positive and negative symptoms.

Exam Essentials

- **6 'A's** of negative symptoms:
  - **A**nhedonia
  - **A**pathy
  - **A**volition
  - **A**logia
  - **A**ffect flattening
  - **A**sociality

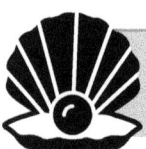

Clinical Pearls

- Differentials for apathy include:
  - Schizophrenia (negative symptoms)
  - Depression
  - Parkinsonism
  - Behavioural-variant frontotemporal neurocognitive disorder
  - Drug-induced (e.g., amotivation syndrome from chronic cannabis use)
  - Drug withdrawal (e.g., 'crash' from cocaine or stimulant use)

Question 5

Which illicit substance has a known association with the development of schizophrenia?

Answer
Cannabis

Explanation
Cannabis use has been associated with a two- to threefold increased prevalence of schizophrenia and schizophrenia spectrum disorders [4]. The reverse causation hypothesis also postulates that schizophrenia risk itself predicts the likelihood of cannabis initiation and a genetic predisposition for schizophrenia was associated with increased use of cannabis [5, 6].

While other drugs do not have as clear an association with the development of schizophrenia, their use can still precipitate an acute psychotic episode:

Recreational drugs	Alcohol Stimulants (e.g., amphetamine, cocaine, cannabis) Hallucinogens (e.g., phencyclidine, MDMA, LSD, ketamine) Inhalants
Medications	Steroids Anticholinergics Anti-Parkinson's disease drugs

 **Exam Essentials**

- Cannabis users who have **homozygous VAL/VAL alleles in the COMT genotype** have a higher risk of more severe psychosis [7]

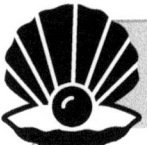 **Clinical Pearls**

- The lifetime prevalence of co-morbid substance use disorder in patients with schizophrenia is 74% [8]
- The risk of schizophrenia increases with the younger onset of cannabis use [9]

Question 6
How will you investigate Ryan's first presentation of psychosis?

11

Answer

Category	Investigations
Point-of-care test	Electrocardiogram
Biochemical	Electrolytes Liver panel Calcium Full blood count (FBC) Glucose Urine drug screen Urine microscopy and culture* HIV and syphilis screening* Thyroid function test* Parathyroid hormone* Cortisol* Urine and blood toxicology screen* Autoimmune workup including ANA, SLE panels, serum autoimmune encephalitis screens* Lumbar puncture*
Imaging	CT or MRI brain (in the presence of suggested neurological abnormality or persistent cognitive impairment)* Electroencephalogram (if there is a history of seizure or symptoms suggestive of temporal lobe epilepsy)*

* When suggested by history/examination.

Explanation

Psychosis can be a symptom of an underlying acute medical illness or chronic condition. Hence it would be prudent to rule out medical causes and medication and substance-related causes before considering primary psychiatric causes of the psychosis.

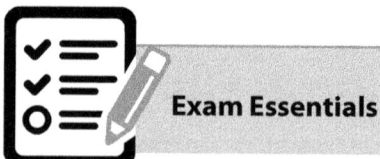

Exam Essentials

Symptoms suggestive of organic causes:

- Sudden onset

- Predominant non-auditory hallucinations (visual, gustatory, olfactory)

- Fluctuating altered mental status

- Autonomic instability

- Abnormal neurological examination

For very young and old patients, investigations should be done to rule out organic causes.

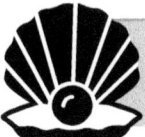

Clinical Pearls

- In individuals with an acute medical illness, **delirium is a common cause of psychosis**

- Consider urine and blood toxicology screen if high suspicion of drug-induced psychosis but the urine drug screen is negative

- New synthetic psychoactive substances may not be picked up by conventional drug screens

- Symptoms suggestive of drug-induced psychosis:

  ◦ Acute onset
  ◦ Temporal relationship to substance use
  ◦ Symptoms resolve suddenly
  ◦ Presence of autonomic instability
  ◦ Confusion

Question 7
What is the next step of management?

Answer
Inpatient admission and initiation of antipsychotic medications in the absence of an organic cause.

Explanation
The patient poses a high suicide risk and has demonstrated a concrete plan to hurt himself. His delusions severely impair insight into his condition, and one should not treat his threats lightly. The harm he poses to himself warrants an inpatient admission and early intervention for his psychosis. Antipsychotic drugs are the first-line treatment for schizophrenia.

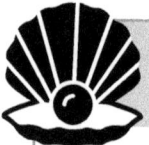

Clinical Pearls

- If the patient refuses to be admitted, doctors may base practices on the United Kingdom's **Mental Health Act** to mandate a review at a psychiatric institution

Question 8
Which antipsychotic medications would you avoid for Ryan?

Answer
Antipsychotics with a high propensity to cause weight gain, such as olanzapine, quetiapine, clozapine (although weighing of the risk–benefit ratio in patients with TRS is required).

Explanation
The side effects of each antipsychotic medication vary. As a rule of thumb, second-generation atypical antipsychotics are serotonin 2A/dopamine 2 antagonists with a lower risk of extrapyramidal side effects (EPSEs) and a higher risk of metabolic side effects (weight gain, insulin resistance, impairment of glucose tolerance, development of hyperlipidaemia, etc.).

Side effects of antipsychotic medications include:

- Metabolic (including weight gain and diabetes)
- Extrapyramidal (including akathisia, dyskinesia and dystonia)
- Cardiovascular (including prolonging the QT interval)
- Hormonal (including increasing plasma prolactin)
- Others (including unpleasant subjective experiences)

Below are different concerns which arise with antipsychotic use:

Concerns	Antipsychotic(s) to avoid	Preferred antipsychotic(s)
QTc prolongation (dose-dependent)	Typical antipsychotics (haloperidol, chlorpromazine)	Aripiprazole Lurasidone Brexpiprazole
EPSEs	Typical antipsychotics (e.g., haloperidol) Risperidone at high doses	Aripiprazole Olanzapine Risperidone Quetiapine Clozapine

Concerns	Antipsychotic(s) to avoid	Preferred antipsychotic(s)
Weight gain	Olanzapine Clozapine	Aripiprazole Lurasidone Brexpiprazole Haloperidol Trifluoperazine
Elevated prolactin levels	Risperidone Paliperidone Sulpiride Amisulpride	Aripiprazole Quetiapine Clozapine
Sedation	Quetiapine Olanzapine Clozapine	Aripiprazole
Seizure	Chlorpromazine Clozapine	Risperidone Aripiprazole Haloperidol Sulpiride/Amisulpride

Exam Essentials

- First- and second-generation antipsychotic medications are comparable in their clinical efficacy [10]
- The latter have a better effect on negative symptoms and have mood stabilisation properties [11]
- **Clozapine**, a second-generation antipsychotic, has proven superior efficacy in TRS (response rates between 40% and 54% [12, 13])

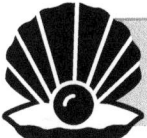

Clinical Pearls

- The NICE guidelines [14] suggest that the choice of antipsychotic medication should be jointly made by the patient and healthcare professional
- Irish guidelines [15] recommend the use of **metformin** as an adjunct in the treatment of antipsychotic-induced weight gain in adults with psychosis

Question 9

What is the definition of TRS?

Answer

Based on the 2017 Treatment Response and Resistance in Psychosis (TRRIP) Working Group [16] definition of TRS, there are two consensus-based criteria, minimal and optimal:

Minimal TRRIP criteria for TRS

- Diagnosis – DSM-5 diagnosis of schizophrenia [17]

- Symptom severity – at least moderate symptom severity (> 3 in psychotic symptom items) as rated using a standardised scale (e.g., Positive and Negative Syndrome Scale (PANSS) or Brief Psychiatric Rating Scale (BPRS))

- Functional impairment – at least moderate impairment measured using a validated scale (e.g., Social and Occupational Functioning Assessment Scale)

- Prior treatment – at least two trials of ≥ 6 weeks at a therapeutic dose (equivalent to ≥ 600 mg chlorpromazine) with adherence ≥ 80% of prescribed doses

Optimal TRRIP criteria for TRS

The minimal criteria (above) with the addition of:

- Prospective evaluation of symptom severity using a standardised scale (e.g., PANSS or BPRS) confirming < 20% symptom reduction over six weeks of treatment

- One of the two antipsychotic trials should be a long-acting injectable antipsychotic

- Antipsychotic adherence should be confirmed by ≥ 2 antipsychotic plasma levels

Explanation

There are varying definitions of TRS and the TRIPP working group was formed in 2017 to establish the consensus criteria to standardize the definition of TRS. The previous 2014 NICE guideline [14] definition of TRS was clinically defined as failure to respond to two trials of different antipsychotics, one usually an atypical antipsychotic, of adequate dose and duration.

Question 10
What are the potentially life-threatening side effects of clozapine?

Answer
Agranulocytosis, neutropenia
Myocarditis or cardiomyopathy
Pulmonary embolism
Seizures
Life-threatening gastrointestinal hypomotility

Explanation
Clozapine is initiated with close monitoring of the FBC for blood dyscrasias. Based on the NICE guidelines [14], the FBC must be repeated at weekly intervals for 18 weeks and then fortnightly until one year with a subsequent monthly FBC. Other side effects include:

System	Description of side effects [15]
Haematology	Agranulocytosis: leucopenia, eosinophilia, leucocytosis. The risk of fatal agranulocytosis is estimated to be 1:4,250 patients treated. The risk of fatal pulmonary embolism is estimated to be 1:4,500 patients treated. The mortality rate of a clotting complication while on clozapine was 44%
Cardiology	The risk of fatal myocarditis or cardiomyopathy is estimated to be up to 1:1,300 patients treated
Neurology	Associated with a dose-dependent seizure risk at a rate higher than that seen in most other antipsychotic drugs. Seen in 4.4% of patients prescribed with 600 mg/day or more. Caution required when used with lithium due to increased risk of neuroleptic malignant syndrome
Anticholinergic	Constipation Blurred vision Difficulty passing urine
Anti-adrenergic	Hypotension Sexual dysfunction
Others	Significant sedation Significant weight gain Insulin resistance and diabetes mellitus Nausea, vomiting ECG changes (dose-dependent prolongation of the QT interval) Headache, dizziness Tachycardia, hypertension Hypersalivation

Possible causes of TRS include non-compliance to treatment, misdiagnosis, ongoing psychosocial stressors, high EE, co-morbid affective disorder and organic causes.

Exam Essentials

- One important side effect of clozapine is **agranulocytosis**, which may worsen with co-prescription with other medications, such as valproate or carbamazepine. Lithium has been used to increase the neutrophil count and total white cell count in patients taking clozapine

- **High expressed emotion (EE)** is an adverse family environment and is one of the more robust predictors of relapse in schizophrenia. The construct of EE comprises of

  - Criticism
  - Hostility
  - Overinvolved emotionally

- Consider checking the clozapine level and review medications the patient may be on (e.g., fluoxetine) that may increase the clozapine level, if the patient develops side effects

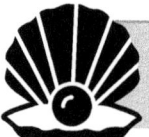

Clinical Pearls

- **Clozapine reduces mortality** in schizophrenia due to a lower risk of suicide [18]

- **Good** prognostic factors:

  - Female
  - Older age at the first episode
  - Rapid (versus insidious) symptom onset
  - Predominant positive (rather than negative) symptoms
  - Presence of mood symptoms
  - Good pre-morbid functioning

- **Poor** prognostic factors include (in addition to the reverse of positive factors above):
  - Positive family history of schizophrenia
  - Early illness onset
  - Structural brain abnormalities
  - Prominent cognitive symptoms

Question 11
What are EPSEs and what are the different types?

Answer
EPSEs consist of acute dystonia, akathisia, pseudoparkinsonism and tardive dyskinesia.

Explanation
Refer to the table on the next page for more elaboration.

Tardive dyskinesia has an insidious onset and is observed in 10 to 20% [19, 20] of patients who are treated for more than a year. It persists for at least a month after discontinuation of the offending agent and may be irreversible. Akinesia and rigidity develop more frequently than tremors.

Exam Essentials

- **Clozapine, quetiapine, aripiprazole, brexpriprazole and lurasidone** are antipsychotic medications that cause the fewest EPSEs

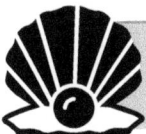

Clinical Pearls

- Patients starting an antipsychotic medication should be evaluated for the following EPSEs weekly until the medication dose has been stable for at least two weeks:

	Acute dystonia	Akathisia	Pseudoparkinsonism	Tardive dyskinesia
Incidence	10%	25 to 50%	20%	25 to 50% after chronic treatment
Risk factors	Young men Usage of high-potency antipsychotic Antipsychotic naïve patients	Rapid anti-psychotic dose increment	Older women, particularly those with neurological damage	Age > 55 years Chronic antipsychotic use Typical antipsychotic use
Onset	Few hours	Most commonly after the fifth day of initiation	Gradual	At least six months after initiation, usually seen after many years
Symptoms	Involuntary contractions of major muscle groups, characterised by: • Oculogyric crisis (fixed upward or lateral gaze) • Torsion dystonia • Torticollis • Spasms of lips, tongue, face, throat and muscles	• Irritability • Feeling unsettled • Restlessness (may complain of needing to go out or try to leave without any reason)	Mimics Parkinson's disease: • Mask-like facies • Resting tremor • Cogwheel rigidity • Shuffling gait • Psychomotor retardation (bradykinesia)	Oro-bucco-lingual and facial dyskinesia (e.g., 'Fly-catching', tongue protrusion) • Athetosis • Choreiform pill-rolling • Hand movements • Pelvic thrusting

	Acute dyskinesia (involuntary movements): • Grimacing • Exaggerated posturing • Twisting of head/neck/jaw • Trismus (dystonia affecting jaw muscles)		
Management	Intramuscular (IM) anticholinergic (e.g., IM benztropine) in oculogyric crisis and torsion dystonia Switch to atypical antipsychotic	Propranolol (best-established treatment) Anticholinergics, such as benztropine (acute akathisia) Benzodiazepines (chronic akathisia)	Gradual dose reduction Switch to atypical antipsychotic medications Anticholinergics (e.g., benzhexol)	Switch to atypical antipsychotic Maintain patients on the lowest effective dose of antipsychotic Valbenazine/Tetrabenazine Vitamin E may alleviate symptoms

Diving Deep ...

Over a lifetime, about 1% of the population will develop schizophrenia. Schizophrenia affects more than 24 million people worldwide, and more than two out of three people with psychosis in the world do not receive specialist mental healthcare for the disease [21].

The heritability of schizophrenia is between 60% and 80% [17]. Twins, family and adoption studies have consistently demonstrated familial aggregation of schizophrenia, largely attributed to genetic factors. The concordance rate for monozygotic twins is approximately 45%, and for dizygotic twins is approximately 10% [22].

Children of patients with schizophrenia have a 13% risk of developing schizophrenia:

- Children of BOTH patients with schizophrenia have a 46% risk of developing schizophrenia

- Grandchildren of patients with schizophrenia have a 4% risk of developing schizophrenia

- Parents of children with schizophrenia have a 6% risk of developing schizophrenia

- Siblings of patients with schizophrenia have a 17% risk of developing schizophrenia

The rate of suicide is higher in patients with schizophrenia than in the general population. Antipsychotic medications may decrease long-term suicide mortality with the risk of suicide attempts increasing fourfold with non-adherence to antipsychotics [23].

Inadequate response to clozapine alone is not uncommon and the augmentation of clozapine to treat TRS is increasingly common. If there are no clear benefits with augmentation, the medication should be discontinued after three to six months to reduce polypharmacy burden and adverse drug effects. Commonly used augmentation agents include antipsychotics for positive symptoms, antidepressants for negative symptoms and mood stabilisers for suicidal ideation or aggression. The Maudsley guidelines [23] have suggested the consideration of the following agents for augmentation of clozapine: amisulpride, aripirazole, haloperidol, lamotrigine, omega-3-triglycerides, risperidone, sulpiride, topiramate, valproate and ziprasidone.

The term 'at risk mental state' (ARMS) was first coined by Yung et al. [24, 25] and described patients in the prodromal phase before the onset of psychotic symptoms. These individuals have changes in well-being and psychosocial functioning, often associated with cognitive decline or subthreshold psychotic symptoms. Recognising individuals with ARMS allows the healthcare team the opportunity for early intervention, which could delay, ameliorate or even prevent the onset of frank psychosis. The Comprehensive Assessment of At-Risk Mental States (CAARMS) [26] is a widely used semi-structured assessment tool to identify patients with ARMS. The CAARMS includes the following subscales: disorders of thought content, perceptual abnormalities, conceptual disorganisation, motor changes, concentration and attention, emotion and affect, subjectively impaired energy and impaired tolerance to normal stress. Depending on the severity scale score under each subscale, patients are: Group 1, Attenuated psychosis group; Group 2, Brief limited intermittent psychotic symptoms; and Group 3, Vulnerability; or they are diagnosed with psychosis.

Management of patients with ARMS is dependent on the local healthcare systems in place but typically includes a form of early intervention in psychosis (EIP) services. Such EIP services may offer cognitive behavioural therapy (CBT)-focused interventions along with case management and treatment of psychiatric co-morbidities. More than half of patients with ARMS will not develop a psychotic illness and therefore antipsychotics, which are not without adverse effects, are not typically used as a first-line treatment as suggested by both the 2014 NICE guidelines [14] and the Early Psychosis Guidelines Writing Group [27].

References

1. Thomas P, Mathur P, Gottesman II, Nagpal R, Nimgaonkar VL, Deshpande SN. Correlates of hallucinations in schizophrenia: a cross-cultural evaluation. *Schizophr Res.* 2007 May;92(1–3):41–9.

2. Andreasen NC, Flaum M. Schizophrenia: the characteristic symptoms. *Schizophr Bull.* 1991;17(1):27–49.

3. Jaspers K, Jaspers K. *General psychopathology: volume two.* Baltimore: Johns Hopkins University Press; 1997. (A Johns Hopkins paperback.)

4. Gage SH, Hickman M, Zammit S. Association between cannabis and psychosis: epidemiologic evidence. *Biol Psychiatry.* 2016 Apr 1;79(7):549–56.

5. Gage SH, Jones HJ, Burgess S, Bowden J, Davey Smith G, Zammit S, et al. Assessing causality in associations between cannabis use and schizophrenia risk: a two-sample Mendelian randomization study. *Psychol Med.* 2017 Apr;47(5):971–80.

6. Power RA, Verweij KJH, Zuhair M, Montgomery GW, Henders AK, Heath AC, et al. Genetic predisposition to schizophrenia associated with increased use of cannabis. *Mol Psychiatry.* 2014 Nov;19(11):1201–4.

7. Nieman DH, Dragt S, van Duin EDA, Denneman N, Overbeek JM, de Haan L, et al. COMT Val(158)Met genotype and cannabis use in people with an At Risk Mental State for psychosis: exploring gene × environment interactions. *Schizophr Res.* 2016 Jul;174(1–3):24–8.

8. Boland RJ, Verduin ML, Ruiz P, Shah A, Sadock BJ, editors. *Kaplan & Sadock's synopsis of psychiatry,* 12th edition. Philadelphia: Wolters Kluwer; 2022.

9. Van Winkel R, Kuepper R. Epidemiological, neurobiological, and genetic clues to the mechanisms linking cannabis use to risk for nonaffective psychosis. *Annu Rev Clin Psychol.* 2014 Mar 28;10(1):767–91.

10. Jones PB, Barnes TRE, Davies L, Dunn G, Lloyd H, Hayhurst KP, et al. Randomized controlled trial of the effect on Quality of Life of second- vs first-generation antipsychotic drugs in schizophrenia: Cost Utility of the Latest Antipsychotic Drugs in Schizophrenia Study (CUtLASS 1). *Arch Gen Psychiatry*. 2006 Oct;63(10):1079–87.

11. Németh G, Laszlovszky I, Czobor P, Szalai E, Szatmári B, Harsányi J, et al. Cariprazine versus risperidone monotherapy for treatment of predominant negative symptoms in patients with schizophrenia: a randomised, double-blind, controlled trial. *Lancet*. 2017 Mar 18;389(10074):1103–13.

12. Siskind D, Siskind V, Kisely S. Clozapine response rates among people with treatment-resistant schizophrenia: data from a systematic review and meta-analysis. *Can J Psychiatry*. 2017 Nov;62(11):772–7.

13. Sanahan R, Sreeraj VS, Suhas S, Kumar V, Thirthalli J, Venkatasubramanian G. Response to clozapine and its predictors in treatment-resistant schizophrenia spectrum disorders: a retrospective chart review. *Schizophr Res*. 2025 Jan;275:179–88.

14. National Institute for Health and Care Excellence (NICE). Psychosis and schizophrenia in adults: prevention and management. Clinical guideline [CG178]. NICE; 2014. Available from: www.nice.org.uk/guidance/cg178

15. Fitzgerald I, O'Connell J, Keating D, Hynes C, McWilliams S, Crowley EK. Metformin in the management of antipsychotic-induced weight gain in adults with psychosis: development of the first evidence-based guideline using GRADE methodology. *Evid Based Ment Health*. 2022 Feb;25(1):15–22.

16. Howes OD, McCutcheon R, Agid O, de Bartolomeis A, van Beveren NJM, Birnbaum ML, et al. Treatment-resistant schizophrenia: Treatment Response and Resistance in Psychosis (TRRIP) Working Group Consensus Guidelines on Diagnosis and Terminology. *Am J Psychiatry*. 2017 Mar 1;174(3):216–29.

17. American Psychiatric Association. *Diagnostic and statistical manual of mental disorders*, 5th edition, text revision (DSM-5-TR). Washington, DC: American Psychiatric Association Publishing; 2022. Available from: www.psychiatry.org/psychiatrists/practice/dsm

18. Semple D, Smyth R. *Oxford handbook of psychiatry*, 4th edition. Oxford: Oxford University Press; 2019.

19. Meltzer HY, Alphs L, Green AI, Altamura AC, Anand R, Bertoldi A, et al. Clozapine treatment for suicidality in schizophrenia: International Suicide Prevention Trial (InterSePT). *Arch Gen Psychiatry*. 2003 Jan;60(1):82–91.

20. Novick D, Haro JM, Bertsch J, Haddad PM. Incidence of extrapyramidal symptoms and tardive dyskinesia in schizophrenia: thirty-six-month results from the European schizophrenia outpatient health outcomes study. *J Clin Psychopharmacol*. 2010 Oct;30(5):531–40.

21. Ortí-Pareja M, Jiménez-Jiménez FJ, Vázquez A, Catalán MJ, Zurdo M, Burguera JA, et al. Drug-induced tardive syndromes. *Parkinsonism Relat Disord*. 1999 Apr;5(1–2):59–65.

22. World Health Organization (WHO). Schizophrenia. 2022. Available from: www.who.int/news-room/fact-sheets/detail/schizophrenia

23. Puri BK, Hall AD, Ho R. *Revision notes in psychiatry*, 3rd edition. Boca Raton: CRC Press/Taylor & Francis Group; 2014.

24. Taylor DM, Barnes TRE, Young A. *The Maudsley prescribing guidelines in psychiatry*, 14th edition. Chichester Hoboken, NJ: Wiley Blackwell; 2021.

25. Yung AR, McGorry PD, McFarlane CA, Jackson HJ, Patton GC, Rakkar A. Monitoring and care of young people at incipient risk of psychosis. *Schizophr Bull.* 1996;22(2):283–303.

26. Yung AR, Yuen HP, McGorry PD, Phillips LJ, Kelly D, Dell'Olio M, et al. Mapping the onset of psychosis: the Comprehensive Assessment of At-Risk Mental States. *Aust N Z J Psychiatry.* 2005;39(11–12):964–71.

27. Orygen, The National Centre of Excellence, in Youth Mental Health. *Australian Clinical Guidelines for Early Psychosis*, 2nd edition. Parkville: Orygen; 2016.

Case 2: Delusional Disorder

Do not drink the poisoned water!

Tiffany is a 26-year-old sales assistant brought in by her concerned husband. In the past two months, Tiffany has been expressing strange concerns about things around her. She firmly believed her neighbour was trying to harm her by poisoning their water source and, hence, the tap water was no longer safe for consumption. The couple used only bottled water to shower, wash, drink and cook their food. She does not report any other first-rank symptoms. She continues to be employed at a nearby clinic as an assistant and her boss did not report any decline in her work performance.

- **Question 1: What is the diagnosis?**

Tiffany was started on oral risperidone and although her condition improved, she frequently forgot to take her medications in the outpatient setting, which led to multiple relapses.

- **Question 2: What pharmacological option is available for patients with poor adherence to prescribed oral medications?**

Tiffany was switched to intramuscular (IM) paliperidone and her condition stabilised. However, four months later, she started complaining of milky breast discharge and irregular menstruation.

- **Question 3: What conditions should one exclude?**

You changed Tiffany's medication to aripiprazole and her hyperprolactinaemia resolved. She remains stable on IM aripiprazole. Six months later, she informed you that she is 10 weeks pregnant.

- **Question 4: Does she need to change her antipsychotic after discovering she is pregnant?**

Tiffany has heard of post-partum psychosis and is concerned about it.

- **Question 5: What are the risk factors for post-partum psychosis?**

Answers to Case 2

Question 1
What is the diagnosis?

Answer
Delusional disorder (persecutory type)

Explanation

Diagnosis of delusional disorder [1]

1. The presence of one or more delusions for three months or longer

2. The delusions are variable in content across individuals, while showing remarkable stability within individuals, although they may evolve over time

3. Absence of clear and persistent hallucinations, severely disorganised thinking (formal thought disorder), experiences of influence, passivity or control or negative symptoms characteristic of schizophrenia are evident. However, in some cases, specific hallucinations typically related to the content of the delusions may be present

4. Apart from the actions and attitudes directly related to the delusional system, affect, speech and behaviour are typically unaffected

5. The symptoms are not a manifestation of another medical condition, substance, medication or another mental disorder

The different types of delusional disorders are

- Erotomanic type: also known as de Clérambault's syndrome, the central theme of delusion is that another person, more frequently someone of higher status, is in love with the patient

- Grandiose type: central theme of delusion is the conviction of having some great talent or insight or having made some important discovery

- Jealous type: also known as Othello syndrome, the central theme of delusion is that the patient's spouse is unfaithful

27

- Persecutory type: central theme of delusion is that the patient is being conspired against, cheated, spied on, followed, poisoned or drugged, maliciously maligned, harassed or obstructed

- Somatic type: central theme of delusion involves bodily function or sensations; the patient is convinced of the severity of the symptoms

- Mixed type: patient has two or more delusional themes

Exam Essentials

- In schizophrenia, there is a global functional decline seen, whereas the functional impairment seen in delusional disorder, if any, is predominantly due to the delusional theme

- A delusion is an unshakable belief that is usually unshared, not in keeping with the educational and social background of the person, with falsely drawn conclusions

- An over-valued idea is consistent with the person's background and may be amenable to change with persuasion

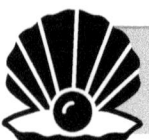

Clinical Pearls

- It is important to screen specifically for risks towards others (e.g., third parties whom the patient may be paranoid towards due to persecutory delusions, erotomania or delusions of jealousy) – does the patient know the identity and details of the third party?

- For elderly patients with delusions, always exclude organic causes (e.g., delirium, brain tumour) and a dementing process (e.g., behavioural and psychological symptoms of dementia)

Question 2
What pharmacological option is available in patients with poor adherence to prescribed oral medications?

Answer
Consider switching to long-acting injectable medications such as IM paliperidone.

Explanation
IM for therapeutic purposes is indicated for the following patients:

- Non-compliant

- Uncooperative and deemed to require immediate administration of a drug

Paliperidone (9-hydroxyrisperidone) is risperidone's active metabolite, making it a sensible option to consider switching to.

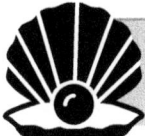

Clinical Pearls

- IM paliperidone is better than first-generation depot medications such as fluanxol in terms of side-effect profile. However, it may be costly – consider involving social services for subsidy support if required

Question 3
What conditions should one exclude?

Answer
Hyperprolactinaemia and pregnancy

Explanation
Assuming her pregnancy test is negative, Tiffany is likely to be suffering from drug-induced hyperprolactinaemia caused by antipsychotics acting via dopaminergic receptors in the hypothalamic tuberoinfundibular tract. Antipsychotics such as risperidone, paliperidone, sulpiride and amisulpride can significantly increase the level of serum prolactin, and the effects of antipsychotics are dose-dependent.

Hyperprolactinaemia can cause sexual dysfunction, infertility, galactorrhoea, decreased bone mineral density, osteoporosis and fractures. In serious cases, it may increase the risks of breast carcinomas.

Other causes can be divided into idiopathic, physiological causes (such as stress and pregnancy) and pathological causes (further divided into pituitary and non-pituitary causes).

Exam Essentials

- Symptomatic drug-induced hyperprolactinaemia is managed by **reducing the antipsychotic dose**, **switching** to an antipsychotic with a lesser propensity to cause hyperprolactinaemia, **adding on aripiprazole**, which lowers prolactin levels, or giving **dopamine agonists** (e.g., amantadine, cabergoline and bromocriptine)

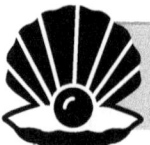

Clinical Pearls

- A full physical exam of the breast and eye fields should be performed to rule out other causes and complications of hyperprolactinaemia

Question 4
Does she need to change her antipsychotic after discovering she is pregnant?

Answer
At present, Tiffany does not need to change antipsychotics from IM aripiprazole.

Explanation
Aripiprazole, as with most antipsychotics, is United States Food and Drug Administration (FDA) pregnancy risk category C (refer to the Diving Deep section for more elaboration). However, untreated psychosis in the expectant mother is associated with greater risk than the risks associated with continued use of antipsychotics. Hence, most patients are encouraged to continue their medications during their pregnancy.

However, maternal weight gain in pregnancy and risk of increased birth weight may occur while on an atypical antipsychotic. Aripriazole, while a second-generation antipsychotic (SGA), may carry a lower risk of inducing gestational diabetes mellitus (GDM) compared to other SGAs such as olanzapine [2]. Nonetheless, it would be prudent to monitor weight and screen for GDM during Tiffany's obstetrician visits. Otherwise, another option will be to switch to typical antipsychotics such as haloperidol, but the higher risks of extrapyramidal side effects (EPSEs) should be counselled.

Third-trimester exposure to antipsychotics increases risks for neonatal extrapyramidal and withdrawal symptoms, including reports of agitation, hyper- or hypotonia, tremor, somnolence, respiratory distress and feeding problems. Close liaison with the obstetrician is advised.

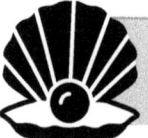

Clinical Pearls

- A patient already being treated should not be switched from one antipsychotic class to the other unless there are side effects or concerns about fetal exposure

Question 5

Tiffany has heard of post-partum psychosis and is concerned about it. What are the risk factors for post-partum psychosis?

Answer

A previous episode of post-partum psychosis

Personal history of bipolar or depressive disorder or schizophrenia

Family history of post-partum psychosis

Obstetric complications such as respiratory disorders in the neonate, severe birth asphyxia, preterm birth, perinatal death, small for gestational age infant and caesarean section

Explanation

Post-partum (puerperal) psychosis occurs in one to two out of every 1,000 live births [3, 4]. The risk of post-partum psychosis increases to one in seven births in women with a previous history of post-partum psychosis, one in four births in women with a history of bipolar disorder, and one in two births in women with a history of bipolar disorder and a family history of post-partum psychosis [5]. It appears more likely to occur in women with a history of major depressive disorder.

Exam Essentials

- Always screen for depression and psychosis in all post-partum cases

- Screen for disorientation (time and place) and affective symptoms in post-partum psychosis

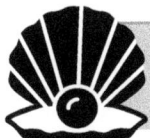

Clinical Pearls

- Always screen for **risks to children (infanticide)** and the partner

- Risk factors for post-partum psychosis are more biologically related while post-partum depression tends to be more psychosocial

Diving Deep ...

The lifetime prevalence of a delusional disorder is about 0.05–0.1% [6]. The prevalence of delusional disorder is much lower than that of other conditions like schizophrenia, bipolar disorder and other mood disorders; this may be in part due to underreporting of delusional disorder as those with delusional disorder may not seek mental health attention unless forced by family or friends.

The mean age of onset is about 40–49 years, but the range is from 18 to 90 years [7]. The persecutory and jealous type of delusion is more common in males, while the erotomanic type is more common in females.

Other delusional syndromes include:

- Capgras syndrome: the belief that a known person has been replaced by an impostor

- Frégoli syndrome: the belief that one or more familiar person(s) repeatedly changes their appearance

- Cotard syndrome: the belief that one has lost organs, blood or body parts and even insisting that one is dead

References

1. World Health Organization. *International classification of diseases*, 11th edition (ICD-11). Geneva: World Health Organization; 2024. Available from: https://icd.who.int/en

2. Taylor DM, Barnes TRE, Young A. *The Maudsley prescribing guidelines in psychiatry*, 14th edition. Chichester Hoboken, NJ: Wiley Blackwell; 2021.

3. Terp IM, Mortensen PB. Post-partum psychoses. Clinical diagnoses and relative risk of admission after parturition. *Br J Psychiatry*. 1998 Jun;172:521–6.

4. Videbech P, Gouliaev G. First admission with puerperal psychosis: 7–14 years of follow-up. *Acta Psychiatr Scand*. 1995 Mar;91(3):167–73.

5. Kendell RE, Chalmers JC, Platz C. Epidemiology of puerperal psychoses. *Br J Psychiatry*. 1987 May;150:662–73.

6. Kendler KS. Demography of paranoid psychosis (delusional disorder): a review and comparison with schizophrenia and affective illness. *Arch Gen Psychiatry*. 1982 Aug;39(8):890–902.

7. Semple D, Smyth R. *Oxford handbook of psychiatry*, 4th edition. Oxford: Oxford University Press; 2019.

Case 3: Major Depressive Disorder

In abyss

Claudia is a 22-year-old lady who comes in with reports of feeling down. She feels impatient and irritable more easily and is frequently in a 'foul mood'. She no longer finds interest or 'motivation' in exercising, and her weight has increased over the past three months from 54 kg to 60 kg due to an increased appetite. This was associated with poor sleep, poor concentration and feelings of 'paralysis'. She never felt 'over the top' with her emotions nor had racing thoughts. Her workload as an accountant had increased recently as well.

- **Question 1: What is the most likely diagnosis? Which differential diagnoses will you consider?**

- **Question 2: What will you expect her mental state to be like on examination?**

- **Question 3: What investigations will you order to confirm your diagnosis and guide management?**

- **Question 4: What are some risk factors for a depressive disorder?**

- **Question 5: Given her diagnosis of a depressive disorder, what are the common psychiatric co-morbidities you would like to screen for?**

Claudia is bothered by her weight gain and irritability and is keen on treatment.

- **Question 6: What are the broad principles of management?**

You plan to start Claudia on fluoxetine.

- **Question 7: What are the side effects that you will counsel her on before initiation?**

Claudia wants to know how long she has to be on antidepressants and has concerns over a possible 'addiction' to fluoxetine.

- **Question 8: How will you counsel her on antidepressants and the risk of dependence?**

Claudia wants to know if she will get better.

- **Question 9: What are the prognostic factors for a depressive disorder?**

After four weeks of treatment and up-titration of the fluoxetine dose, Claudia's depressive symptoms showed only a partial response to treatment.

- **Question 10: What are the principal considerations of management when patients do not initially respond to treatment?**

- **Question 11: Given the partial response to fluoxetine, what is the next step in the management of Claudia's depression?**

Claudia was subsequently given a trial of escitalopram and then venlafaxine but failed to respond to both.

- **Question 12: What is the revised diagnosis?**

- **Question 13: How would you manage Claudia's treatment-resistant depression?**

Answers to Case 3

Question 1
What is the most likely diagnosis? Which differential diagnoses will you consider?

Answer
In the absence of an organic cause, the most likely psychiatric diagnosis is a single-episode depressive disorder (ICD-10 atypical depression, which is not present in ICD-11) [1]. However, we must first rule out organic causes such as hypothyroidism and Cushing's

syndrome. Other differential diagnoses include dysthymia, grief, substance- or medication-induced depressive disorder, adjustment disorder with low mood, schizoaffective disorder and personality disorders such as borderline pattern specifier.

Explanation

Rule out organic causes of low mood and weight gain during the first presentation. Under organic causes, possibilities can be split into endocrine versus non-endocrine causes.

Endocrine causes	Non-endocrine causes
Hypothyroidism Cushing's syndrome Parathyroid dysfunction Hypopituitarism Addison's disease Menopausal symptoms	Systemic lupus erythematosus Syphilis HIV

Diagnosis of a depressive disorder

Five or more of the following symptoms over a two-week period. At least one symptom from the affective cluster must be present.

Affective cluster

- Low mood

- Anhedonia

Cognitive behavioural cluster

- Poor concentration

- Worthlessness or excessive or inappropriate guilt

- Hopelessness about the future

- Recurrent thoughts of death and suicidal ideations

Neurovegetative cluster

- Insomnia or hypersomnia

- Significant weight loss or poor appetite

- Psychomotor agitation or retardation

- Fatigue or low energy

Another way of categorising the symptoms is as follows:

Core features	Physical symptoms	Cognitive symptoms
Low mood Anhedonia	Change in weight/appetite Sleep disturbances Psychomotor changes Low energy	Guilt Cognition/concentration Suicidal ideations

In the absence of hypomanic or manic features, the most likely diagnosis for Claudia is a single-episode depressive disorder. Other ICD-11 specifiers of depressive disorder include severity, psychotic features (mood congruent or incongruent) and the presence of remission. Additional features include the presence of prominent anxiety symptoms, panic attacks, current depressive episode persistence, and melancholia, with seasonal pattern of mood episode onset or timing in relation to pregnancy (during pregnancy or six weeks following the delivery).

We need to differentiate between depression with psychotic features and schizoaffective disorder. In the former, psychosis generally occurs after depressive symptoms and is more likely to be mood congruent with common themes such as nihilism, poverty or guilt.

Exam Essentials

- For patients with low mood, you must screen for the presence or history of **hypomania and mania**

- Symptoms of depression – **DEPRESSION**

  - **D**epressed mood
  - **E**nergy low
  - **P**leasure loss (anhedonia)
  - **R**etardation (psychomotor)
  - **E**ating poorly
  - **S**leeping poorly
  - **S**uicide ideations
  - **I**'m worthless
  - **O**nly one to be blamed
  - **N**o concentration

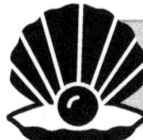

Clinical Pearls

- The first dichotomy should be psychiatric versus organic causes
- Depression does not always present with loss of appetite or weight. Watch for atypical features
- Symptoms of atypical features – **RAILS**
  - **R**eactive mood
  - **A**ppetite increase
  - **I**nterpersonal rejection sensitivity
  - **L**eaden paralysis
  - **S**leep increased
- Rating scales such as the clinician-administered Montgomery–Asberg Depression Rating Scale (MADRS) [2], and the self-administered Patient Health Questionnaire-9 (PHQ-9) [3], may help with diagnosis.

Question 2
What will you expect her mental state to be like on examination?

Answer

Appearance	Neglect in dressing and grooming Frowning, sullen-looking
Behaviour	Psychomotor agitation/retardation Poor eye contact
Speech	Latency: Increased latency in replies Rate: Slowed Volume: Soft Tone: Monotonous Quantity: Less spontaneous speech
Mood	Depressed, dysphoric
Affect	Restricted, constricted, blunted, flat

Thought process and content	Self-harm, suicide, homicide Fixed ideas/delusions, such as: • Guilt • Hypochondriasis • Nihilistic • Self-referential • Persecutory
Cognition	Poor concentration
Insight	Questions to assess for insight include: Does the patient believe that: • They are ill? • Their signs/symptoms are due to a psychiatric condition? • Psychiatric treatment can be helpful?

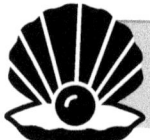

Clinical Pearls

• The presence of **psychomotor retardation** or agitation and psychotic symptoms are signs of severe depression

Question 3

What investigations will you order to confirm your diagnosis and guide management?

Answer

Category	Investigations
Point-of-care test	Electrocardiogram
Biochemistry	Full blood count Electrolytes – sodium, potassium, calcium, etc. Liver function test Thyroid function test Urine drug screen Vitamin B12/D/folate serum level
Imaging	CT or MRI of the brain if there are neurological symptoms, or if symptoms are atypical

Explanation

We need to balance the need for organic screening, but not advocate for over-investigating. Hence, it is advisable to do screening tests as stated above, before considering further investigations guided by abnormalities.

Exam Essentials

- Always categorise your investigations into, for example, point-of-care test, biochemistry and imaging
- Vitamin deficiencies (B12/D) and thyroid hormone deficiency are **reversible causes** of depression to screen for

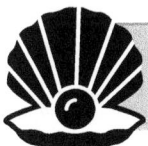

Clinical Pearls

- Investigations can be split into three main functions:
  - Looking for aetiological factors
  - Guiding management (e.g., choice of medications)
  - Complications which may arise from self-neglect in severely depressed patients
- Illicit substances, corticosteroids, sedative-hypnotics and anticonvulsants can also cause depressive symptoms

Question 4

What are some risk factors for depressive disorder?

Answer

Biological	Family history of psychiatric conditions (mood disorders in particular) Females (ratio of 2:1)
Psychological	Presence of cognitive errors (e.g., magnification, overgeneralisation, personalisation)

Social	Childhood traumatic experience
	Bereavement or grief
	Interpersonal conflict e.g., divorce
	Poor social support
	Medical illnesses which are chronic, severe or painful
	Financial difficulties
	Caregiver stress

Explanation

Patients with a first-degree family member who suffers from depression are 2.8 to 10 times more likely to develop depression themselves [4]. The presence of one or more chronic medical conditions raises the recent (six-month) and lifetime prevalence of mood disorders. Multiple adverse childhood experiences are a risk factor for later developing a depressive disorder. Studies have found that a lack of a confiding relationship was associated with an increased risk of depression [5].

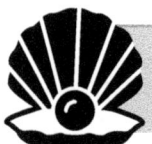

Clinical Pearls

- A positive family history is a significant risk factor for depression

Question 5

Given her diagnosis of a depressive disorder, what are the common psychiatric co-morbidities you would like to screen for?

Answer

The following disorders should be screened for [6–8]:

Anxiety disorder	Up to 60%
Other depressive disorders (e.g., dysthymia)	Up to 50%
Personality disorder	50%
Substance use disorder	Up to 33.3%

Explanation

The prevalence of co-morbid anxiety disorders and a major depressive disorder is as high as 60% [8]. One-third of patients with major depressive disorder also have substance use disorders, with a lifetime prevalence of 40% having an alcohol use disorder [9] and 17% having a drug use disorder, and the co-morbidity yields a higher risk of suicide and greater social and personal impairment as well as other psychiatric conditions.

Exam Essentials

- About two-thirds of patients will have a co-morbid psychiatric condition

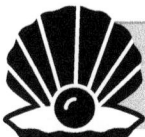

Clinical Pearls

- Anxiety is the most common co-morbid condition

Question 6
What are the broad principles of management?

Answer
Monotherapy medications, psychotherapy or combination therapy are acceptable options. If psychotherapy is offered, cognitive behavioural therapy (CBT) or interpersonal therapy (IPT) are preferred. If pharmacology is offered, a selective serotonin reuptake inhibitor (SSRI) is generally the first-line option.

Explanation
Based on the clinical vignette, she does not have suicidal ideations and most likely has mild to moderate depression.

CBT aims to change how one feels by changing the way one thinks. Therapists assist one in monitoring cognitions and associated emotions and behaviours. Psychoeducation, a thought diary, an activity diary, behavioural scheduling and behavioural experiments are some techniques used. Emotional disturbances tend to be associated with 'here and now' deficits in interpersonal functioning and IPT aims to improve interpersonal functioning and emotional symptoms. It focuses on four areas: role transitions, interpersonal disputes, grief and interpersonal deficits.

The Canadian Network for Mood and Anxiety Treatments (CANMAT) 2016 guidelines [10] recommend CBT or IPT as first-line psychological treatments and serotonin reuptake inhibitors (SSRIs) such as sertraline or escitalopram for pharmacological treatment. Other options include serotonin–noradrenaline (norepinephrine) reuptake inhibitors (SNRIs) such as venlafaxine, noradrenergic and specific serotonergic antidepressants (NaSSAs) such as mirtazapine, and noradrenaline–dopamine reuptake inhibitors (NDRIs) such as bupropion. The NICE guidelines [11] caution against using antidepressants as first-line treatment for mild to moderate depression in children; instead, psychotherapy should be the first-line treatment option.

You may want to look at the symptomatology of the patient to guide your choice of medications. Those with sleep problems may benefit from a more sedative agent such as mirtazapine or fluvoxamine. Those who lack energy may benefit from a more stimulating agent such as bupropion, fluoxetine or venlafaxine. Those with mixed symptoms such as anxiety may benefit from an SSRI such as sertraline and paroxetine.

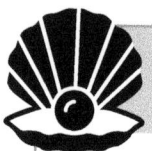

Clinical Pearls

- A shared decision should be reached after considering one's preference (e.g., some patients may be reluctant to start antidepressants due to personal concerns, or the presence of co-morbid medical conditions which may be affected by the antidepressants)

Question 7
What are the side effects that you will counsel her on before initiation?

Answer

Gastrointestinal	Nausea, abdominal pain, diarrhoea, constipation, weight changes
Autonomic	Agitation, sleep disturbances
Sexual dysfunction	Decreased libido, ejaculation problems (in males)
Electrolyte imbalances	Hyponatraemia (less likely in young patients with no major medical issues)
Discontinuation symptoms	If antidepressants are stopped abruptly, one may have short durations of headache, flu-like symptoms and insomnia. These symptoms usually get resolved with re-initiation of antidepressants
Black box warning	Increased risk of suicidal ideations (for children and adults up to 24 years of age)

Explanation

To reduce the risks of side effects, many clinicians take a 'start low, go slow' approach, starting with the lowest effective dose and up-titrating further as tolerated.

All antidepressants carry a United States Food and Drug Administration (FDA) black box warning [12, 13] of increased risk of suicidality in children and adults aged 18 to 24 years during initial treatment (first one to two months) of major depressive disorder and other psychiatric disorders.

If high doses of SSRIs are used or in combination with other sertonergic agents, patients should be counselled on the risk of serotonin syndrome as well.

Refer to the table below for a more detailed elaboration of the side effects of other antidepressants.

Symptoms or signs	Drug of choice
Insomnia	Fluvoxamine, agomelatine, mirtazapine, trazodone, tricyclic antidepressants
Lethargy	Bupropion, fluoxetine, venlafaxine
Loss of appetite	Mirtazapine
Pain	Duloxetine, venlafaxine, tricyclic antidepressants
Gastric problems	Mirtazapine
Liver problems	Sertraline, escitalopram
Risk of bleeding	Agomelatine, mirtazapine, bupropion
Prolonged QTc	Sertraline
High blood pressure	*Avoid* venlafaxine
Hyponatraemia	Agomelatine, bupropion, mirtazapine, vortioxetine, moclobemide
Sexual side effects	Agomelatine, bupropion, mirtazapine, vortioxetine
Epilepsy and those predisposed to epileptic risks (such as traumatic brain injury, anorexia nervosa, etc.)	*Avoid* bupropion and tricyclic antidepressants

Class	Example(s)	Mechanism of action	Common side effects
Serotonin–noradrenaline reuptake inhibitors (SNRIs)	Venlafaxine Duloxetine	SNRIs combine the robust serotonin transporter inhibition of the SSRIs with various degrees of inhibition of the noradrenaline transporter	Sustained hypertension Sexual dysfunction Headaches Nausea Dizziness Hyponatraemia
Serotonin antagonist and reuptake inhibitors (SARIs)	Trazodone Nefazodone	Block serotonin 2A and 2C (5HT2A and 5HT2C) receptors as well as serotonin reuptake	Priapism Orthostatic hypotension Headache Sedation Dry mouth Nausea
Noradrenergic specific serotonergic antidepressants (NaSSAs)	Mirtazapine Mianserin	Block alpha-2 receptors Potent antagonist actions upon 5HT2A receptors, 5HT2C receptors, 5HT3 receptors and histamine 1 receptors	Weight gain and increased appetite Agranulocytosis, neutropenia (rare) Dry mouth Drowsiness
Melatonergic antidepressant	Agomelatine	Agonist actions at melatonin 1 (MT1) and melatonin 2 (MT2) receptors and antagonist actions at 5HT2C receptors	Deranged liver enzymes Dizziness
Noradrenaline–dopamine reuptake inhibitors (NDRIs)	Bupropion	Inhibit the reuptake of both dopamine (i.e., dopamine transporter inhibitor) and noradrenaline (i.e., noradrenaline transporter inhibitor)	Minimal sexual dysfunction Seizure Weight loss Insomnia (stimulating) Dry mouth Nausea

Serotonin modulator and stimulator antidepressants (SMSAs)	Vortioxetine	Combination of five pharmacological actions: reuptake blocking mode (SERT), G-protein receptor mode (5HT1A and 5HT1B/D partial agonist, 5HT7 antagonist) and ion-channel mode (5HT3 antagonist)	Comparatively well tolerated GIT side effects: nausea, vomiting, constipation
Tricyclic antidepressants (TCAs)	Amitriptyline Desipramine Doxepin Imipramine Nortriptyline	Block the reuptake pumps for noradrenaline, or for both noradrenaline and serotonin transporters	Cardiotoxicity: QTc prolongation leading to arrhythmias Lower seizure threshold Hyponatraemia Anticholinergic: constipation, blurred vision, urinary retention, dry mouth, orthostatic hypotension Antihistaminergic: nausea, vomiting, weight gain, sedation
Monoamine oxidase inhibitors (MAOIs)	Moclobemide	Inhibitors of the enzyme monoamine oxidase (MAO) increasing circulating noradrenaline, serotonin, dopamine and tyramine	Risk of drug–food reaction leading to tyramine hypertensive crisis Higher risk of drug–drug reaction leading to serotonin syndrome Headache Dry mouth Gastrointestinal symptoms Orthostatic hypotension Liver enzyme elevation Weight gain

Exam Essentials

- An antidepressant with minimal side effects is **escitalopram**, which may be suitable for elderly patients
- However, escitalopram may cause **cardiac conduction issues** – do an ECG before starting, and prescribe with caution in patients with prolonged QTc

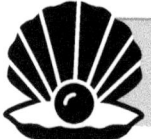

Clinical Pearls

- While SSRIs are generally the first-line choice of antidepressants, ultimately it depends on two main factors:
  - Matching of the patient's profile and side-effect profile of medication
  - The patient's perception of how well the medication works
- Before starting antidepressants, educate patients about the **risk of irritability** or **paradoxical anxiety symptoms** – if present, start at a lower dose, or change if symptoms persist

Question 8
How will you counsel her on antidepressants and the risk of dependence?

Answer
We recommend a treatment period of six to nine months after the resolution of symptoms. Antidepressants do not cause dependency and 'addiction'.

Explanation
As this is her first episode of depression, she will need to continue treatment for at least six to nine months after the resolution of symptoms. If there are multiple episodes or risk factors for recurrence, it would require a minimum duration of treatment of two years or more.

One may want to clarify with Claudia that fluoxetine is unlike a benzodiazepine, a sedative with the potential for dependence.

While antidepressants do not result in dependency, patients need to be counselled on the possibility of discontinuation symptoms. Discontinuation symptoms include anxiety, giddiness, flu-like symptoms, low mood, nausea and insomnia. This can be managed by tapering off antidepressants gradually over four weeks.

Exam Essentials

- Antidepressant discontinuation symptoms – **FINISH**
  - **F**lu-like symptoms
  - **I**nsomnia
  - **N**ausea
  - **I**mbalance
  - **S**ensory disturbance
  - **H**yperarousal

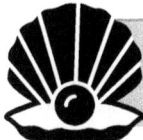

Clinical Pearls

- Antidepressants with a **short half-life** are more prone to **discontinuation symptoms** (e.g., venlafaxine and paroxetine)

Question 9
What are the prognostic factors for a depressive disorder?

Answer

Good prognostic factors	Poor prognostic factors
Acute onset of depression Endogenous depression with no clear inciting psychosocial stressors Earlier age of onset	Insidious onset of depression Elderly Residual symptoms despite treatment High neuroticism Psychiatric co-morbidity Poor social support

Explanation

Depressive episodes vary from 4 to 30 weeks for mild–moderate cases. An average of about six months for severe cases, with 25% lasting up to one year. Ten to twenty per cent of patients have episodes lasting more than two years. The risk of recurrence is approximately 30% at 10 years, and 60% at 20 years [14].

Question 10

What are the principal considerations of management when patients do not initially respond to treatment?

Answer

The following steps should be taken in the initial evaluation of a patient responding poorly to treatment:

1. Reassess the diagnosis

2. Assess for co-morbidity which needs to be treated

3. Assess adherence (assessing for side effects which may affect compliance is good practice)

4. Ensure adequate duration of the drug trial at a minimum effective dose

5. Consider environmental stressors perpetuating the symptoms

In this instance, assuming a diagnosis of depression with no co-morbidity and good compliance with fluoxetine for the past four weeks, a switch of antidepressants should be considered.

Explanation

All antidepressants show a pattern of response in which the rate of improvement is highest during the first to second weeks and lowest between the fourth and sixth weeks. In clinical practice, using simple observations, an antidepressant effect in an individual is usually seen by the second week. It follows that in individuals where no antidepressant effect is evident after approximately four weeks of treatment, a change in dose or medication should be considered.

Exam Essentials

- If the patient has **depression with psychotic features**, starting an **antipsychotic** medication in addition to an antidepressant is warranted

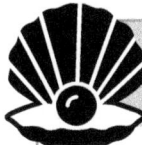

Clinical Pearls

- Be careful of the types of psychotropics that have a high risk of **lethality in an overdose**:

    ◦ **TCAs** and **lithium**

Question 11
Given only a partial response to fluoxetine, what is the next step in the management of Claudia's depression?

Answer
Switch to an SSRI or to a different class of antidepressant and titrate to a therapeutic dose. If a poor response remains, switch to another class of antidepressant.

Explanation
If there is no antidepressant effect after three to four weeks of treatment, a change in dose or medication should be considered. As fluoxetine has already been titrated to a therapeutic dose and remains non-effective, a switch in antidepressants is reasonable in this case. In cases of non-response, there is evidence that switching within a drug class could be effective. Alternatively, one could switch to a different drug class, such as an SNRI (e.g., venlafaxine), an atypical tetracyclic antidepressant (e.g. mirtazapine), or an SMSA (e.g., vortioxetine).

Question 12
What is the revised diagnosis?

Answer
Treatment-resistant depression

Explanation
'Treatment-resistant depression' as defined by the Sequenced Treatment Alternatives to Relieve Depression (STAR*D) study [15] refers to major depressive episodes that do not respond satisfactorily after two trials of antidepressant monotherapy. Each trial is typically defined as the use of antidepressants at an adequate dose (the maximum British National Formulary dose) and duration (at least four weeks).

The definition of treatment-resistant depression has not been standardised; in part, this is complicated by the lack of consensus in describing acute antidepressant responses. Generally, treatment response is classified based on the amount of improvement from baseline symptoms using a depression rating scale.

Category	Response rate
No response	Improvement < 25%
Partial response	Improvement 25% to 49%
Response	≥ Improvement of 50% but less than the threshold for remission
Remission	Depression rating scale score less than or equal to a specific cutoff that defines the normal range. For example, when using the 17-item Hamilton Rating Scale for Depression [2] or the Montgomery–Asberg Depression Rating Scale [2], remission is defined with a score ≤ 7

The term 'treatment-refractory depression' is similarly poorly defined with no stand-ardised definition and often there is no clear distinction between treatment-resistant depression and treatment-refractory depression.

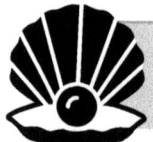

Clinical Pearls

- Some treatment-resistant unipolar depression may be bipolar-type depression, characterised by:

  - Increased irritability/lability/anxiety
  - Atypical features
  - Symptoms seemingly worsened by antidepressants

    * For such cases, adding mood-stabilising antipsychotics or mood stabilisers would be beneficial

- When patients are not responding to treatment, always review:

  - Therapy compliance
  - Any perpetuating factors

- Diagnosis (could it be something else?)

Question 13
How would you manage Claudia's treatment-resistant depression?

Answer
There are various ways one may choose to manage treatment-resistant depression:

- Add lithium to existing antidepressant

- Olanzapine and fluoxetine combination

- Add antipsychotic e.g., quetiapine, aripiprazole

- Mirtazapine and venlafaxine combination

- SSRI and bupropion combination

- Ketamine: intranasal (esketamine) or intravenous

- Add tri-iodothyronine

- Repetitive transcranial magnetic stimulation (rTMS)

- Electroconvulsive therapy (ECT)

General principals in the management of treatment-resistant depression

1. Change antidepressant – may consider changing to a different class

2. Combination antidepressants – two or more antidepressants

3. Augmentation – combining antidepressants with other psychotropics such as antipsychotics or mood stabilisers

4. Non-pharmacological methods (e.g., ECT) – refer to Case 36 for more information

Explanation

Apart from the Maudsley guidelines, other widely used guidelines in the treatment of depression include the NICE guidelines [16] and the CANMAT guidelines [10].

The addition of lithium is supported by the NICE guidelines, with a target plasma level of 0.4–0.8 mmol/L initially, which can be increased up to 1.0 mmol/L if there is suboptimal response. Olanzapine and fluoxetine combination is well researched and also used in the treatment of bipolar depression. Augmentation of antidepressive treatment with antipsychotics is common with quetiapine and aripiprazole carrying a good evidence base and tolerability. The SSRI and bupropion combination was supported by the STAR*D study. The mirtazapine and venlafaxine combination is also known as the 'California rocket fuel' and is well tolerated with a good evidence base.

The USA FDA has approved esketamine in nasal spray formulation for the management of treatment-resistant depression. It carries the risk of abuse and is usually given through restricted distribution systems. Tri-iodothyronine has reasonable literature support and requires clinical and biochemical thyroid function test monitoring. In patients who fail or are unable to tolerate two or more trials of antidepressants, ECT is an effective and safe option. ECT is elaborated further in Case 36.

Exam Essentials

- When combining antidepressants, beware of serotonin syndrome (refer to Case 37 for more information)
- ECT should be considered early in patients with severe depression and the following:
  - Actively suicidal
  - Refusing food intake
  - Catatonic
  - Non-response to antidepressants

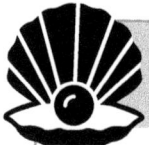

Clinical Pearls

- **Mood-stabilising antipsychotics** for depression augmentation include second-generation drugs such as risperidone, quetiapine, olanzapine, aripiprazole, lurasidone, cariprazine and brexpiprazole
- Mood stabilisers for depression augmentation include **lithium**. It has **anti-suicide properties**:
  - Patient needs to be compliant with medication and fluid intake
  - Patient should not be actively suicidal (as an overdose can be lethal)
- Lamotrigine can also be used for augmentation – good for those who are weight-conscious and prefer non-sedating medicine. However, the dose has to start low and titrate gradually due to the risk of rash and Stevens–Johnson syndrome
- rTMS may also be used as augmentation

Diving Deep ...

Globally, the lifetime rate of depression varies but is generally believed to lie between 10% and 20% [14]. Major depressive disorder is second only to hypertension as the most common chronic condition encountered in general medical practice and cause of disability [17]. By 2030, unipolar depression is predicted to be ranked as the number one cause of the global burden of diseases in terms of disability-adjusted life years (DALYs). The age of onset is most commonly between 18 to 34 years.

The 'monoamine theory' was an early theoretical model, which hypothesised diminished monoamine neurotransmission (decreased levels of serotonin, noradrenaline and dopamine) as the cause of depression. Current studies suggest that more complex dynamics, including intracellular cascades triggered by the monoamines, are involved in the onset of depression and the response to antidepressant medications. Imbalance in the levels of glutamate and gamma-aminobutyric acid (GABA) has been implicated in depression as well [18].

The STAR*D trial [15] was a landmark study which demonstrated that although medication switches were modestly helpful, switches within and outside a class were equally effective. In stage 1 of the STAR*D trial, subjects received citalopram and remission was seen in 28% of patients. The remaining patients were switched to either bupropion (21.3% remission), venlafaxine (24.8% remission) or sertraline (17.6% remission) or citalopram was augmented with bupropion (29.7% remission) or buspirone (30.1% remission). Those who failed to reach remission in stage 2 were then brought to stage 3 where existing antidepressants were switched to mirtazapine (12.3% remission), nortriptyline (19.8% remission) or augmented with lithium (15.9% remission) or tri-iodothyronine (24.7% remission). In stage 4, tranylcypromine (6.9%) was pitted against a mirtazapine and venlafaxine combination (13.7% remission) and tranylcypromine was less effective and less well tolerated. Worryingly, the rate of remission decreased with each stage of treatment, and the estimated cumulative remission rate over the four stages of treatment was 67%.

Short-term use of esketamine over one to four weeks is effective for treatment-resistant unipolar major depression without psychotic features. Intravenous ketamine in the form of one to two infusions per week over one to four weeks has also been used. The onset of action often occurs within hours of administration, including improved symptoms of suicidal ideation, and hence it can be used in the short term while waiting for the delayed effect of concomitant antidepressants. As esketamine/ketamine can produce psychotomimetic effects, it should not be used in patients with previous psychotic symptoms. Data on the long-term use and maintenance treatment with ketamine are limited but this is an exciting area of development.

References

1.   World Health Organization. *International classification of diseases*, 11th edition (ICD-11). Geneva: World Health Organization; 2024. Available from: https://icd.who.int/en

2.   Rush JA, First MB, Blacker D. *Handbook of psychiatric measures*, 2nd edition. Washington: American Psychiatric Publishing; 2008.

3. Kroenke K, Spitzer RL, Williams JB. The PHQ-9: validity of a brief depression severity measure. *J Gen Intern Med.* 2001 Sep;16(9):606–13.

4. Monroe SM, Slavich GM, Gotlib IH. Life stress and family history for depression: the moderating role of past depressive episodes. *J Psychiatr Res.* 2014 Feb;49:90–5.

5. Patten SB. Are the Brown and Harris "vulnerability factors" risk factors for depression? *J Psychiatry Neurosci.* 1991 Dec;16(5):267–71.

6. Friborg O, Martinsen EW, Martinussen M, Kaiser S, Overgård KT, Rosenvinge JH. Comorbidity of personality disorders in mood disorders: a meta-analytic review of 122 studies from 1988 to 2010. *J Affect Disord.* 2014 Jan;152–154:1–11.

7. Davis L, Uezato A, Newell JM, Frazier E. Major depression and comorbid substance use disorders. *Curr Opin Psychiatry.* 2008 Jan;21(1):14–8.

8. Calkins AW, Rogers AH, Campbell AA, Simon NM. Comorbidity of anxiety and depression. In Ressler KJ, Pine DS, Rothbaum BO, editors. *Anxiety disorders.* Oxford: Oxford University Press; 2015, 299–314. Available from: https://academic.oup.com/book/24459/chapter/187522352

9. Hasin DS, Goodwin RD, Stinson FS, Grant BF. Epidemiology of major depressive disorder: results from the National Epidemiologic Survey on Alcoholism and Related Conditions. *Arch Gen Psychiatry.* 2005 Oct;62(10):1097–106.

10. Kennedy SH, Lam RW, McIntyre RS, Tourjman SV, Bhat V, Blier P, et al. Canadian Network for Mood and Anxiety Treatments (CANMAT) 2016 clinical guidelines for the management of adults with major depressive disorder: Section 3. Pharmacological treatments. *Can J Psychiatry.* 2016 Sep;61(9):540–60.

11. National Institute for Health and Care Excellence (NICE). Depression in children and young people: identification and management. NICE guideline [NG134]. NICE; 2019. Available from: www.nice.org.uk/guidance/ng134

12. Medicines and Healthcare products Regulatory Agency (MHRA) Committee on the Safety of Medicine. Report of the CSM expert working group on the safety of selective serotonin reuptake inhibitor antidepressants. MHRA; 2014. Available from: www.gov.uk/government/publications/ssris-and-snris-use-and-safety

13. US Food and Drug Administration (FDA). Suicidality in children and adolescents being treated with antidepressant medications. FDA; 2018. Available from: www.fda.gov/drugs/postmarket-drug-safety-information-patients-and-providers/suicidality-children-and-adolescents-being-treated-antidepressant-medications

14. Semple D, Smyth R. *Oxford handbook of psychiatry*, 4th edition. Oxford: Oxford University Press; 2019.

15. Rush AJ, Trivedi MH, Wisniewski SR, Nierenberg AA, Stewart JW, Warden D, et al. Acute and longer-term outcomes in depressed outpatients requiring one or several treatment steps: a STAR*D report. *Am J Psychiatry.* 2006 Nov;163(11):1905–17.

16. NICE. Depression in adults: treatment and management. NICE guideline [NG222]. NICE; 2022. Available from: www.nice.org.uk/guidance/ng222

17. Ferrari AJ, Charlson FJ, Norman RE, Patten SB, Freedman G, Murray CJL, et al. Burden of depressive disorders by country, sex, age, and year: findings from the global burden of disease study 2010. *PLoS Med.* 2013 Nov;10(11):e1001547.

18. Boland RJ, Verduin ML, Ruiz P, Shah A, Sadock BJ, editors. *Kaplan & Sadock's synopsis of psychiatry*, 12th edition. Philadelphia: Wolters Kluwer; 2022.

Case 4: Dysthymic Disorder and Premenstrual Dysphoric Disorder

A long dark road

Sandra is a 22-year-old lady who presented with complaints of low mood, lethargy, poor sleep and an inability to enjoy her hobbies as she used to. These feelings started gradually three years ago, with recent acute worsening of her mood over the past week. In addition, she reports feelings of hopelessness and states, 'I often wonder if I'm better off dead. What is the point of it all anyway?' However, she does not have any active suicidal ideations and has no plans to hurt herself.

- **Question 1: What is the most likely initial diagnosis?**

Having diagnosed Sandra with dysthymic disorder, you counselled her on the initiation of psychotropics, but she was keen on psychotherapy instead. You referred her to a psychologist for cognitive behavioural therapy and her symptoms began to remit.

Three years later Sandra returns with complaints of mood lability around the time of her menstrual period. Symptoms are most severe in the week before the onset of menses and resolve quickly after. Over the past six months, her mood swings have been worse than before and this has led to increased irritability. She reports difficulties in concentration, lack of energy, overeating, oversleeping and abdominal bloating each menstrual cycle. While she has had symptoms of premenstrual syndrome (PMS) in the past, her recent symptoms are worse than before and have resulted in increased conflicts and strain in her relationship with her boyfriend. While her symptoms fully resolve in the days to a week after her menses, she worries about the cyclical recurrence of symptoms.

- **Question 2: What is the secondary diagnosis now?**

- **Question 3: How is PMS different from premenstrual dysphoric disorder (PMDD)?**

- **Question 4: How would you manage Sandra's PMDD?**

Answers to Case 4

Question 1
What is the most likely initial diagnosis?

Answer

Dysthymic disorder with a current depressive episode

Explanation

Diagnosis of dysthymic disorder [1]

Persistent depressed mood for at least two years for most of the day, for more days than not:

1. Anhedonia

2. Poor concentration

3. Low self-worth, or excessive or inappropriate guilt

4. Hopelessness about the future

5. Disturbed sleep or increased sleep

6. Diminished or increased appetite

7. Low energy or fatigue

In children and adolescents, mood can be irritable with a duration of more than year.

Dysthymic disorder shares overlapping features with a depressive disorder. Distinguishing features include a more chronic course (lasting more than two years) and symptoms tend to be milder. If full criteria for a depressive episode have been met after the preceding two-year period, both dysthymic disorder and either single-episode depressive disorder or recurrent depressive disorder may be diagnosed.

While comparatively less acute in its course, dysthymia still causes significant distress or psychosocial impairment. Twenty-five per cent of all patients with dysthymia never attain complete recovery [2].

Exam Essentials

- Dysthymic disorder = 2Ds
  - **2** years
  - **2** listed criteria
  - Never asymptomatic for > **2** months
- Patients with a depressive episode on top of underlying dysthymia are known as having 'double depression'. The symptoms are usually worse, and the prognosis is poorer.

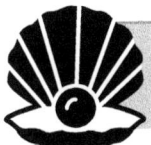

Clinical Pearls

- Children and adolescents require only one year of symptoms
- Single-episode/recurrent depressive disorder is episodic while dysthymia is more pervasive

Question 2
What is the secondary diagnosis now?

Answer
PMDD

Explanation

Diagnosis of PMDD [1]

During a majority of menstrual cycles within the past year, a pattern of mood, somatic or cognitive symptoms is present that begins several days before the onset of menses, starts to improve within a few days after the onset of menses, and then becomes minimal or absent within approximately one week following the onset of menses.

The temporal relationship of the symptoms and luteal and menstrual phases of the cycle should ideally be confirmed by a prospective symptom diary over at least two symptomatic menstrual cycles:

At least one affective symptom:

- Mood lability
- Irritability
- Depressed mood
- Anxiety

Additional somatic or cognitive symptoms:

- Lethargy
- Joint pain
- Overeating
- Hypersomnia
- Breast tenderness
- Swelling of extremities
- Concentration difficulties or forgetfulness

Prospective daily ratings during at least two symptomatic cycles should be performed.

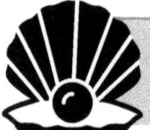 **Clinical Pearls**

- Onset of PMS symptoms can occur any time after menarche, but usually by one's early 20s

It is unlikely to be a recurrence of her existing persistent depressive disorder as her symptoms are cyclical and remit in the follicular phase after her menstrual period begins.

Question 3
How is PMS different from PMDD?

Answer
PMS is less severe than PMDD and does not require a minimum of five symptoms or mood-related symptomology.

Explanation

Clinically significant PMS is also more common with a prevalence of around 3–8% of women while the rate of PMDD is closer to 2% [3, 4]. PMS symptoms start with the onset of menses whereas symptoms of PMDD start in the week before the onset of menses and start to improve in the days after the onset of menses.

Question 4

How would you manage Sandra's PMDD?

Answer

Mild PMS can be treated with lifestyle changes and supplements while PMDD is likely to require psychotherapy or pharmacological treatment:

- Lifestyle changes: aerobic exercise, dietary changes (decreasing caffeine and sodium intake), alcohol and smoking cessation

- Supplements: vitamin B6, vitamin E, calcium carbonate, evening primrose oil, chaste tree berry

- Psychotherapy: cognitive behavioural therapy (CBT)

- Pharmacological therapy: serotonin reuptake inhibitors (SSRIs), hormonal therapies (e.g. combined oestrogen–progestin contraception or gonadotropin-releasing hormone (GnRH) agonist therapy)

Explanation

Decreasing caffeine intake can abate anxiety and irritability, and reducing sodium decreases oedema and bloating.

Evidence for supplements is variable, with some studies [5, 6] showing modest efficacy for each of the above-mentioned supplements. Vitamin B6 (100 mg per day) and calcium supplementation (1,200 to 1,600 mg per day) is likely to benefit patients with premenstrual symptoms. Vitamin E seems to reduce the affective and physical symptoms of PMS. Evening primrose oil is thought to assist in the synthesis of anti-inflammatory prostaglandins E1, while chaste tree berry may reduce prolactin levels and help with symptoms of breast engorgement [7].

A meta-analysis [8] comparing CBT to other interventions has shown a reduction in symptoms of anxiety and depression in PMDD.

SSRIs are a safe first-line therapy, which increases central serotonergic transmission and reduces symptoms effectively. Commonly used SSRI agents include fluoxetine, sertraline and citalopram. Venlafaxine, a serotonin–noradrenaline reuptake inhibitor, is also effective but carries the risk of discontinuation symptoms.

With the cyclical nature of PMDD, studies [2, 9] have shown that both continuous and intermittent dosing of SSRIs are equally effective in symptom reduction. Under an intermittent dosing regimen, there are two main forms. In luteal-phase therapy, patients take the medication only during the luteal phase, which typically begins 14 days after menses,

59

and continue taking the medication until menses begin. In symptom-onset therapy, medication is started at the point of symptom onset until the first few days of menses. Both types of intermittent dosing regimens carry the benefit of reduced long-term side effects, discontinuation syndrome and cost of care. If patients have symptoms throughout the menstrual cycle with premenstrual worsening, longer unpredictable intermenstrual intervals or have stated a preference for simplicity, a continuous daily dosing regimen can be chosen instead. If patients have predictable symptoms, a luteal-phase regimen is sufficient. If patients have symptoms lasting for a week or less with easily recognisable symptom onset, symptom-onset therapy is suitable.

Refer to diving deep for the mechanism of action of hormonal therapy.

Diving Deep …

The aetiology of PMDD is multifactorial and involves biological, psychological and environmental factors. The concordance rate in monozygotic twins is 93%, compared with 44% of dizygotic twins [9]. The environmental factors associated with PMDD include stress, history of interpersonal trauma, seasonal changes, female gender roles and sociocultural aspects of female sexual behaviour.

Hormonal therapy in PMDD works by inducing anovulation and amenorrhoea, which helps with PMS symptoms but does not help with mood symptoms experienced in PMDD. Therefore, hormonal therapy is useful in patients who do not have impairing depressive symptoms and who desire contraception. If depressive symptoms are present and contraception desired, SSRIs and hormonal therapy can be given together. Drospirenone-containing combined oral contraceptives (COCs) are an effective first-line hormonal therapy, which suppresses the hypothalamic–pituitary–ovarian axis and ovulation and relieves symptoms of PMS. In patients with severe symptoms not responding to COCs, GnRH agonist therapy with low-dose oestrogen-progesterone 'add-back' therapy can be considered. If add-back therapy is omitted, there is a risk of menopausal symptoms (e.g., hot flashes and loss of bone mineral density).

References

1. World Health Organization. *International classification of diseases*, 11th edition (ICD-11). Geneva: World Health Organization; 2024. Available from: https://icd.who.int/en

2. Boland RJ, Verduin ML, Ruiz P, Shah A, Sadock BJ, editors. *Kaplan & Sadock's synopsis of psychiatry*, 12th edition. Philadelphia: Wolters Kluwer; 2022.

3. Deuster PA, Adera T, South-Paul J. Biological, social, and behavioral factors associated with premenstrual syndrome. *Arch Fam Med.* 1999;8(2):122–8.

4. Borenstein J, Chiou CF, Dean B, Wong J, Wade S. Estimating direct and indirect costs of premenstrual syndrome. *J Occup Environ Med.* 2005 Jan;47(1):26–33.

5. Johnson WG, Carr-Nangle RE, Bergeron KC. Macronutrient intake, eating habits, and exercise as moderators of menstrual distress in healthy women. *Psychosom Med.* 1995;57(4):324–30.

6. Wyatt KM, Dimmock PW, Jones PW, Shaughn O'Brien PM. Efficacy of vitamin B-6 in the treatment of premenstrual syndrome: systematic review. *BMJ.* 1999 May 22;318(7195):1375–81.

7. van Die MD, Burger HG, Teede HJ, Bone KM. *Vitex agnus-castus* extracts for female reproductive disorders: a systematic review of clinical trials. *Planta Med.* 2013 May;79(7):562–75.

8. Busse JW, Montori VM, Krasnik C, Patelis-Siotis I, Guyatt GH. Psychological intervention for premenstrual syndrome: a meta-analysis of randomized controlled trials. *Psychother Psychosom.* 2009;78(1):6–15.

9. Bhatia SC, Bhatia SK. Diagnosis and treatment of premenstrual dysphoric disorder. *Am Fam Physician.* 2002 Oct 1;66(7):1239–48.

Case 5: Grief

I still miss her ...

Rick is a 58-year-old gentleman who comes in with complaints of low mood. His wife passed away from cancer one month ago. He reports low mood, poor appetite and guilt over having not spent more time with her. He feels drawn to things associated with her (e.g., hair comb) and, at times, even hears her voice speaking to him. He told you 'I know she's gone, but sometimes I feel like she is still around watching over me. That gives me comfort'. He reports fleeting thoughts of death, to be with his wife, but at the same time recognises that his wife would have wanted him to move on and 'be strong for the kids'.

- **Question 1: What is Rick's diagnosis?**

- **Question 2: What are the differences between grief and single-episode depressive disorder?**

Two years on, Rick continues to experience pervasive and intense symptoms of grief. He has left his wife's room untouched since her passing and even prepares meals for her at times. He was let go from his work after he repeatedly failed to show up and spent most of his time cooped up at home. You diagnosed him with prolonged grief disorder.

- **Question 3: What is prolonged grief disorder?**

- **Question 4: How does the management of normal grief differ from that of prolonged grief disorder?**

Answers to Case 5

Question 1
What is Rick's diagnosis?

Answer
Normal grief

Explanation
Grief is a response to a significant loss. Examples of losses can include bereavement, financial ruin, damages from natural disasters or disability. In this case, the grief is in response to bereavement (the death of someone close) and is a natural response with a focus on thoughts and memories of the deceased person, accompanied by sadness and yearning. In normal grief, the feelings of sadness are commonly intermingled with periods of positive feelings and reminiscing.

Exam Essentials

- The five stages of grief noted by Elisabeth Kübler-Ross are:

    I. Denial

    II. Anger

    III. Bargaining

    IV. Depression

    V. Acceptance

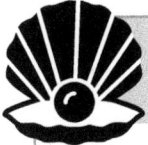

Clinical Pearls

- Individuals respond to grief differently – the stages of grief and duration may vary. **Cultural factors may also influence the grief presentation**

Question 2

What are the differences between grief and single-episode depressive disorder?

Answer

Feature	Normal grief	Depressive disorder
Timing	Symptoms occur in the context of the significant loss	Depressive symptoms are pervasive across various situations and do not solely relate to the loss
Duration	Adaptation to the loss is usually within six months to a year. Dysphoria in grief occurs in waves and is likely to decrease in intensity over days to weeks	Lasts more than two weeks to fulfil criteria, but is usually more persistent
Mood	May have positive emotions intermingling	Pervasive unhappiness and misery
Affect	Feelings of emptiness and loss	Persistent depressed mood and inability to anticipate happiness or pleasure
Guilt and cognition	Self-esteem usually preserved. Transient guilt related to the significant loss	Guilt is self-critical and rooted in a pervasive sense of failure and worthlessness
Hallucinations	Hallucinations of the deceased with retained insight	Hallucinations other than the image and voice of the deceased
Suicidality	Fleeting wish they had died with their loved one or instead of that person	Persistent and strong, unrelated to the deceased

Explanation

There are multiple overlapping features between grief and depressive disorder, with grief not being an exclusion criterion in diagnosing depressive disorder.

Exam Essentials

- Risk factors for depression after bereavement include:
    - History of depression
    - Intense early grief/depressive symptoms
    - Lack of social support
    - Traumatic/unexpected death

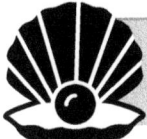

Clinical Pearls

- **Strong suicidal ideation or excessive guilt are not features of normal grief**
- Hallucinations other than the image and voice of the deceased should raise suspicion of other psychopathologies (e.g., major depressive disorder or psychotic disorders)
- Psychomotor retardation or agitation is also not seen in normal grief

Question 3
What is prolonged grief disorder?

Answer

The presence of prolonged grief disorder is suggested by thoughts, feelings and behaviours that are present in bereavement, but are intense, disabling, inconsistent with cultural and religious norms and persist for at least six months to a year.

Explanation

Prolonged grief disorder is a separate diagnosis from depressive disorder. It is distinguished from normal grief primarily in its persistence over a period beyond that which is expected by the bereaved person's social group and the presence of clinically significant distress or impaired functioning. Prolonged grief disorder is believed to affect approximately 7% of bereaved people [1].

Other diagnostic clues are as follows [2, 3]:

- Evidence of persistent psychic pain
    - Separation distress
    - Inhibited exploration of the world
    - Traumatic distress

65

- Persistence of early grief defensive processes

  - Disbelief and/or protest
  - Counterfactual thinking
  - Caregiver self-blame or anger
  - Intense emotional and/or physiological reactions to reminders of the loss
  - Maladaptive behaviours (excessive avoidance of reminders of the loss or seeking closeness to the deceased through sensory stimulation)
  - Difficulty regulating emotions

Exam Essentials

- 'Mummification' occurs when the grieving person acts as if the deceased is alive and will return later, preserving the deceased's belongings and, in extreme cases, his or her corpse (e.g., keeping the deceased's room the same for years after)

- Pathological grief includes:

  - Inhibited grief
  - Delayed grief
  - Prolonged grief

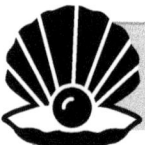

Clinical Pearls

- The current consensus is generally a **limit of one year for normal grief.** Symptoms should get better with time. However, if symptoms are not subsiding or are worsening over the months, one needs to be cautious of pathological grief or prolonged grief disorder

- Risk factors for pathological grief include:

  - Multiple losses
  - Psychiatric illness
  - Traumatic/unnatural death
  - Lack of closure
  - Enmeshed relationship with deceased
  - No avenue to grieve
  - Poor social support

Question 4
How does the management of normal grief differ from that of prolonged grief disorder?

Answer
Individuals with normal grief generally do not require specific treatment but can benefit from social support, while those who suffer from prolonged grief disorder require psychotherapy (e.g., prolonged grief disorder therapy).

Explanation
Normal grief does not require specific treatment, although benzodiazepines may be used to reduce severe autonomic arousal or treat problematic sleep disturbances in the short term. The role of grief counselling, other psychotherapies or pharmacotherapy is limited in normal grief.

Prolonged grief disorder is treated by facilitating the integration of the loss by addressing impediments to adaptation. The best treatments are prolonged grief disorder therapy and cognitive behavioural therapy (CBT) modified for prolonged grief disorder.

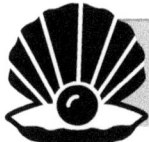

Clinical Pearls

- Suicidal ideations may occur in patients with prolonged grief disorder. Hence, it is prudent to screen for suicide risks during the assessment and management of the condition

Diving Deep ...

There have never been any adequately controlled clinical studies showing that major depressive syndromes following bereavement differ in nature, course or outcome from depression of equal severity in any other context – or from depressive disorder appearing 'out of the blue'.

Depressive disorder episodes occurring after an episode of bereavement are comparable with depressive disorder unrelated to bereavement, concerning risk factors (e.g., genetic influences and history of depression), symptoms (including guilt, psychomotor retardation and suicidal ideation), impaired functioning, co-morbidities, course of illness and response to treatment.

Other types of grief include:

- Anticipatory grief: sorrow and anxiety experienced by someone who expects a loved one to die within a short period

67

- Disenfranchised grief: grief that is not acknowledged by society. Examples include the death of a friend, the death of a celebrity, pregnancy loss, loss of a job, etc.

Suicidal ideation and behaviour occur in approximately 40–60% of patients with prolonged grief disorder [4]. There are reports of overt suicide attempts in 9% of such patients [5, 6].

The theoretical foundation for prolonged grief disorder therapy is based on an attachment theory model. The model hypothesises that people are biologically motivated to form close relationships with other people, and that adaptation to losing a close relationship requires acknowledging the finality and consequences of the loss, revising the internalised representation of the deceased and re-envisioning life plans and goals. Prolonged grief disorder therapy facilitates adaptation to bereavement by focusing on two key areas:

- Loss – accepting the reality of the death, including its finality and consequences, a changed relationship with the deceased and the permanence of grief

- Restoration – restoring the capacity to thrive in a world without a loved one, including a sense of purpose and meaning, and possibilities for happiness

References

1. Kersting A, Brähler E, Glaesmer H, Wagner B. Prevalence of complicated grief in a representative population-based sample. *J Affect Disord.* 2011 Jun;131(1–3):339–43.
2. Friedman MJ. Seeking the best bereavement-related diagnostic criteria. *Am J Psychiatry.* 2016 Sep 1;173(9):864–5.
3. Boelen PA, Smid GE. Disturbed grief: prolonged grief disorder and persistent complex bereavement disorder. *BMJ.* 2017 May 18;357:j2016.
4. Szanto K, Prigerson H, Houck P, Ehrenpreis L, Reynolds CF. Suicidal ideation in elderly bereaved: the role of complicated grief. *Suicide Life Threat Behav.* 1997;27(2):194–207.
5. Latham AE, Prigerson HG. Suicidality and bereavement: complicated grief as psychiatric disorder presenting greatest risk for suicidality. *Suicide Life Threat Behav.* 2004;34(4):350–62.
6. Szanto K, Shear MK, Houck PR, Reynolds CF, Frank E, Caroff K, et al. Indirect self-destructive behavior and overt suicidality in patients with complicated grief. *J Clin Psychiatry.* 2006 Feb;67(2):233–9.

Case 6: Bipolar Disorder

Life is a roller coaster

Samantha is a 25-year-old lady brought in by her parents for 'irritability'. Over the past two weeks, her parents noted that Samantha seems to have 'boundless energy' with little need for sleep (one to two hours a night). She has been going to multiple tennis classes in a single day. She speaks rapidly and is hard to interrupt, frequently claiming that 'no one is a match for her' and that she can beat the best players in the world. Her parents noted that she always seemed to be in a 'good mood' until her tennis skills were questioned, at which she became agitated and verbally abusive. They decided to bring her in after she interrupted an ongoing tennis competition and started challenging contestants to a match, refusing to leave until the police had to be called in. Samantha says she is quitting her job as a cashier as she will become a billionaire from all the 'tennis championship money'. She proclaims, 'Money is of no issue. I will have a new Rolls Royce delivered to all my friends and family'.

- **Question 1: What is her diagnosis?**

- **Question 2: What investigations and differential causes of mania would you consider?**

Initial investigations came back unremarkable.

- **Question 3: What are the principles in the management of her acute episode of mania?**

You start Samantha on quetiapine and there is only a partial response to it. Given the inadequate response and persistent symptoms of mania, you plan to add on a mood stabiliser.

- **Question 4: Which mood stabiliser would you start her on?**

Following the initiation of lithium, you plan to check her lithium level seven days after starting and seven days after each change of dose. Blood samples are to be taken 12 hours post-dose. Samantha expresses concerns over the need for such close monitoring and wants to know the side effects of lithium.

- **Question 5: How would you counsel Samantha on the side effects of lithium?**

Four years later, Samantha presented to the emergency department for drowsiness. She has become increasingly drowsy over the past few days, is nauseous and thirsty and has significantly increased urine output (more than three litres a day). Samantha was recently prescribed a new medication for the control of her newly diagnosed hypertension. On examination, her blood pressure is 88/58 mmHg and her pulse is 110 beats per minute. Preliminary investigations show raised serum urea and creatinine.

- **Question 6: Which class of antihypertensive medications is most likely to cause lithium toxicity?**

Samantha was treated for lithium toxicity and the hydrochlorothiazide antihypertensives were changed. Samantha remained well for three years and she was keen for lithium to be discontinued. She was gradually taken off lithium over two months. Unfortunately, she presented to the clinic one year later with symptoms of low mood, poor appetite, poor sleep, lethargy and poor concentration. These symptoms came on quickly and have been ongoing for three weeks. You diagnose her with bipolar depression.

- **Question 7: How would you treat Samantha's episode of bipolar depression?**

Answers to Case 6

Question 1
What is her diagnosis?

Answer
Bipolar disorder – currently in a manic episode

Explanation
Bipolar disorder is characterised by episodes of mania, hypomania and major depression. Patients with bipolar I disorder have at least one manic episode and nearly always experience hypomanic and major depressive episodes. Bipolar II disorder has absence

of manic episodes, at least one hypomanic episode and at least one major depressive episode.

Diagnostic criteria for bipolar disorder [1]

Persistently elevated, expansive, or irritable mood with persistently increased activity or energy lasting at least one week or if the patient is hospitalised earlier.

Several of the following symptoms are present, representing a significant change from the individual's usual behaviour or subjective state:

1. Talkative or pressured speech

2. Flight of ideas or racing thoughts

3. Grandiosity

4. Decreased need for sleep

5. Distractibility

6. Impulsive reckless behaviour

7. Increase in sexual drive, sociability or goal-directed activity

---

In Samantha's case, the duration of symptoms, presence of delusions of grandiosity and degree of functional impairment suggest mania over hypomania:

	Mania	Hypomania
Duration	≥ 7 days	≥ 4 days (based on DSM-5-TR [2])
Functional impairment	The mood disturbance is sufficiently severe to cause marked impairment in social or occupational functioning Hospitalisation = mania	Not severe enough to cause marked impairment in social or occupational functioning or to necessitate hospitalisation
Psychotic features	Present	NOT present

A mixed state occurs when the patient has symptoms of mania and depression, and usually presents with labile mood and irritability.

One should observe the presence of rapid cycling, which is seen in patients who present with at least four mood episodes in the previous 12 months that meet the criteria for manic, hypomanic or major depressive episodes. Rapid cycling is also associated with hypothyroidism, the use of antidepressants that can induce switching, excessive use of stimulants including caffeine, non-compliance with medications and the presence of temporal lobe disturbances.

Differentials for mania/hypomania include cyclothymia. However, cyclothymia requires symptoms for at least two years with hypomanic symptoms that do not meet criteria for a hypomanic episode, and numerous periods of depressive symptoms that do not meet the criteria for a major depressive episode.

To differentiate mood symptoms in bipolar disorder from personality disorder with borderline pattern, the following are more commonly seen in bipolar disorder:

- Symptoms are more consistent and last for weeks rather than hours/days

- Symptoms are not reactive to environmental factors

- Decreased need for sleep without being tired

- No existential issues, sense of chronic emptiness, abandonment

However, do note that bipolar disorder and borderline personality disorder can co-exist in a patient.

Exam Essentials

- Symptoms of mania – **A-MANIAC**

    ◦ **A** lot of talk
    ◦ **M**any racing thoughts
    ◦ **A** lot of thoughts
    ◦ **N**o sleep needed
    ◦ **I**mpulsive behaviours
    ◦ **A**ttention distracted
    ◦ **C**onfidence inflated

- A manic episode must be diagnosed (instead of hypomania) if the patient

    ◦ Presents with psychotic features
    ◦ Is hospitalised due to the symptoms
    ◦ Reports significant functional impairment

- In patients presenting with low mood, always ask for current or previous episodes of hypomania or mania!

- Rapid cycling = at least four mood episodes per year

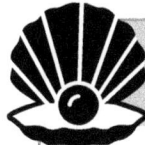

Clinical Pearls

- Suspiciousness in mania can develop into well-formed persecutory delusions
- Paranoia does not always mean a diagnosis of primary psychotic disorder. Features pointing towards schizoaffective disorder instead of bipolar disorder:
  - More disorganised speech
  - More disorganised behaviour
  - Negative symptoms
- Symptoms suggesting a depressed patient on an antidepressant could have bipolarity:
  - Not improving with treatment (e.g., more irritability, anxiety, insomnia)
  - Became hypomanic or manic after treatment
  - Depressed episodes are cyclical and without trigger

Question 2

What investigations and differential causes of mania would you consider?

Answer

Category	Investigations
Point-of-care test	Capillary blood glucose ECG
Biochemical	Full blood count, erythrocyte sedimentation rate, glucose, electrolytes, serum calcium, thyroid function test, liver panel, drug screen, renal panel Urinary 24-hour copper/serum caeruloplasmin (to exclude Wilson's disease)* Anti-nuclear antibodies (systemic lupus erythematosus)* Infection screen (venereal disease research laboratory test, HIV test)*
Imaging	EEG CT/MRI brain (to exclude tumour, infarction, haemorrhage and multiple sclerosis)

*When suggested by history/examination.

Differentials of mania	
Psychiatric causes	Bipolar disorder Schizoaffective disorder
Substance/medication-induced bipolar disorder	Illicit substances (e.g., amphetamine, cannabis, cocaine) Medications (e.g., antidepressants, anticholinergic drugs, dopamine agonists such as levodopa, corticosteroids or anabolic steroids, withdrawal from baclofen, clonidine, etc.)
Neurological causes	Right-sided cerebral vascular accident lesions/head injury/cerebral tumour Lesions in the frontal and temporal lobes Dementia Epilepsy Acquired immunodeficiency syndrome Multiple sclerosis
Endocrine	Thyrotoxicosis Cushing's syndrome Fahr's disease

Explanation

Mania can be a symptom of an underlying acute medical illness or chronic condition. Mania can also be caused by many organic causes (HIV, stroke, brain tumour, systemic lupus erythematosus, drugs, etc.). Hence it would be prudent to rule out medical causes and medication- and substance-related causes before considering primary psychiatric causes of mania, especially in acute presentations.

Exam Essentials

- Medications that may cause mania – **BAAD MACS**

  - **B**ronchodilators
  - **A**ntidepressants
  - **A**nticholinergics
  - **D**opamine agonist (levodopa)
  - **M**DMA
  - **A**mphetamines
  - **C**ocaine
  - **S**teroids

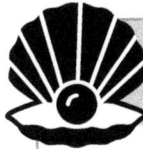

Clinical Pearls

- Always perform a urine/blood pregnancy test before starting medications
- Wilson's disease should be excluded in a relatively young patient presenting with unusual mood and/or psychotic symptoms, especially in those with motor or speech problems

Question 3
What are the principles in the management of her acute episode of mania?

Answer
Admit Samantha as an inpatient

Start her on an antipsychotic (e.g., quetiapine)

If the response is inadequate, combine the antipsychotic with a mood stabiliser (e.g., lithium)

A short-term trial of a benzodiazepine is also useful in the treatment of agitation

Explanation
Patients with mania/hypomania often have impaired insight into their condition and need for treatment, interfering with their ability to make rational treatment decisions. Inpatient admission to initiate effective treatment is often required.

The Maudsley guidelines [3] suggest that drug treatment is the mainstay of therapy for mania and hypomania. Any antidepressants that the patient is on should be discontinued. If the patient is already on anti-manic medications, compliance and plasma levels should be checked. If the patient is not on any anti-manic medications, an antipsychotic can be initiated first.

Certain antipsychotics are preferred as they possess sedative, anxiolytic and mood-stabilising properties, for example quetiapine and olanzapine. If still ineffective, combining lithium or valproate with an antipsychotic has been proven to be more efficacious than monotherapy.

A short-term benzodiazepine such as lorazepam or clonazepam can be used as adjunctive therapy to treat insomnia, agitation or anxiety in patients with mania.

Exam Essentials

- The first step in the management of mania is to **ensure that antidepressants** (if prescribed) **are suspended**

- Valproate should NOT be given to women of child bearing age unless there are no other options (due to the risk of polycystic ovary syndrome and teratogenicity in pregnancy)

- **Males under age 55** looking to be fathers should NOT be prescribed valproate either! Refer to Diving Deep for more elaboration

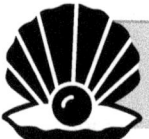

Clinical Pearls

- Antipsychotics help in the rapid tranquilisation and management of an agitated patient with mania

- Mood stabilisers will take several days to a week to work, and thus antipsychotics and benzodiazepine can help with symptoms in the acute phase

Question 4
Which mood stabiliser would you start her on?

Answer
Lithium

Explanation
Lithium is effective for the treatment of mania, at a plasma level of 0.8–1.0 mmol/L, and is recommended by the NICE guidelines [4] as the first-line long-term pharmacological treatment for bipolar disorder.

While valproate is a suitable alternative first-line mood stabiliser, the NICE guidelines recommend that valproate be avoided in women of childbearing potential because of its teratogenic nature. Patients are likely to be sexually disinhibited when experiencing a manic/hypomanic relapse, and there is a risk of an unplanned pregnancy. Valproate is associated with a 10% risk of fetal malformation including neural tube defects, and a 40% risk of long-term cognitive difficulties in children exposed to it during pregnancy [3].

Carbamazepine has a similar causal link with an increased risk of fetal abnormalities, particularly neural tube defects including spina bifida. Prior to starting carbamazepine, clinicians need to screen patients for the presence of the HLA-B*1502 allele.

Lamotrigine has better evidence in the treatment of bipolar depression and should not be used solely in the treatment of mania. Clinicians must monitor the risk of rashes and Stevens–Johnson syndrome (SJS) when on lamotrigine, by starting slowly and increasing doses every two weeks. Be very cautious when giving lamotrigine with valproate (which will increase lamotrigine levels and the risk of SJS).

Exam Essentials

- **Lithium reduces the risk of** both attempted and completed **suicide** by 80% [5] of patients with bipolar illness
- Lithium can also be used as an augmentation agent for unipolar depression
- Side effects of valproate – **VALPROATE**
    - **V**omiting
    - **A**ppetite increase
    - **L**iver toxicity
    - **P**ancytopenia/pancreatitis
    - **R**etained fats
    - **O**edema
    - **A**lopecia
    - **T**hrombocytopenia
    - **E**nzyme inducer

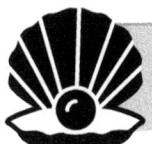

Clinical Pearls

- For pregnant women, mood stabilisers should be avoided due to the risk of teratogenicity. If there is a clear indication to start, consider starting only after the first trimester
- NICE guidelines [4] recommend the use of mood-stabilising antipsychotics as a preferable alternative to continuation with a mood stabiliser in pregnant women

- Lethality is high in lithium overdose. Patients need to be compliant with lithium intake (increased risk of suicide/relapse if premature stopping), fluid status and medication intake (e.g., non-steroidal anti-inflammatory drugs (NSAIDs) increase blood lithium levels)

Question 5

How would you counsel Samantha on the side effects of lithium?

Answer

System	Complications [6]
Renal	Decreased renal function Polyuria and polydipsia (70%)
Cardiac	Cardiac dysrhythmias ECG changes (e.g., T-wave changes, widening of QRS)
Endocrine	Thyroid: goitre, hypothyroidism, chronic autoimmune thyroiditis, rarely hyperthyroidism Hyperparathyroidism Weight gain
Neurological	Tremors (25%) Cognitive impairment
Gastrointestinal	Nausea, diarrhoea
Dermatology	Acne, alopecia, worsening psoriasis
Reproductive	Sexual dysfunction (e.g., arousal, sexual drive and penile erection/vaginal lubrication) (37%) Increased risks of fetal cardiac defects (e.g., Ebstein's anomaly) when taken during pregnancy

Explanation

System	Complications [7]
Renal	Extended lithium exposure reduced the estimated glomerular filtration rate by approximately 30% more than that associated with ageing alone
Cardiac	Contraindicated in heart failure, sick sinus syndrome

System	Complications [7]
Endocrine	Thyroid: 5–35%, more frequent in women, tends to appear after 6–18 months of treatment, and may be associated with rapid cycling Patients with lithium-induced hypercalcaemia and hyperparathyroidism are generally asymptomatic Clinically significant weight gain occurred in nearly twice as many treated with lithium than placebo
Neurological	Higher lithium doses and serum levels result in more coarse tremors
Gastrointestinal	Nausea is seen in 10% to 20% of patients Diarrhoea is seen in up to 10% of patients
Dermatology	Lithium-related skin conditions range from 3% to 45%
Reproductive	20-fold relative increased risk of Ebstein's abnormality. While the overall risk of congenital malformations was twice as great in exposure, the increase in absolute risk of congenital abnormalities (7 per 1,000) is considered small

Exam Essentials

- Symptoms of lithium toxicity – **A LITHIUM**
    - **A**cne/**A**lopecia
    - **L**eucocytosis
    - **I**nsipidus
    - **T**remors
    - **H**ypothyroidism
    - **I**ncreased **U**rine
    - **M**alformation/**M**etallic taste

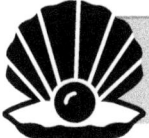

Clinical Pearls

- Patients on steady doses of lithium should have their levels checked every 6–12 months, along with renal and thyroid panel testing to monitor for complications

Question 6
Which class of antihypertensive medications is most likely to cause lithium toxicity?

Answer
Thiazides

Explanation
Thiazides (e.g., hydrochlorothiazide) carry the greatest risk of lithium toxicity. There is a 25–40% increase in lithium concentration after initiation due to a marked reduction in lithium excretion [8].

Drugs that increase lithium serum levels	Drugs that decrease lithium serum levels	Drugs that may increase or decrease lithium serum levels
Thiazides Angiotensin converting enzyme inhibitors NSAIDs (except aspirin) Antibiotics (tetracyclines, metronidazole)	Potassium-sparing diuretics Theophylline	Loop diuretics Calcium channel blockers

Important lithium serum levels to remember:

	Unit mmol/L
Acute mania	0.8–1.2
Maintenance	0.6–1.0
Mild–moderate toxicity	1.5–2.0
Moderate–severe toxicity	> 2.0

Lithium poisoning can occur when there is an increase in the quantity of lithium consumed, or a decrease in lithium clearance (reduced renal function) or volume of distribution (dehydration, fluid loss). Severe lithium toxicity will warrant an urgent referral to the nephrologist for emergent dialysis.

Mild–moderate (1.5–2.0 mmol/L)	Moderate–severe (2.0–2.5 mmol/L)	Severe (> 2.5 mmol/L)
Vomiting Abdominal pain Dryness of mouth Ataxia Dizziness Slurred speech Nystagmus Lethargy or excitement Muscle weakness	Persistent vomiting Anorexia Blurred vision Muscle fasciculations Clonic limb movements Hyperactive reflexes Seizures Delirium Circulatory failure (hypotension, cardiac arrhythmias)	Generalised convulsions Oliguria Renal failure Death

Exam Essentials

- For serum lithium level > 4.0 mmol/L, emergent haemodialysis is usually required

- Lithium levels can inform us if:
  - The patient is compliant with medication (though they may be fast or slow metabolisers)
  - The therapeutic dose is reached
  - Toxic levels are present

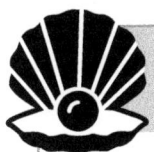

Clinical Pearls

- Early signs and symptoms of lithium toxicity: marked tremors, anorexia, nausea/vomiting, diarrhoea (sometimes bloody), with dehydration and lethargy

- If a patient on lithium comes to the accident and emergency department with severe gastroenteritis, check the lithium level to exclude toxicity

- Continuous cardiac monitoring is required because of possible fatal cardiac arrhythmias

Question 7

How would you treat Samantha's episode of bipolar depression?

Answer

Psychological therapies: cognitive behavioural therapy (CBT), interpersonal therapy (IPT)

Olanzapine and fluoxetine combination

Quetiapine

Lurasidone

Lamotrigine

Lithium

Electroconvulsive therapy (ECT)

Explanation

In patients not on any psychotropics, the NICE guidelines recommend the initial use of fluoxetine combined with olanzapine or quetiapine on its own. While olanzapine alone is effective, its combination with fluoxetine is more effective with reasonable prophylactic effects. Quetiapine alone also prevents relapse into depression and mania. First-line treatments recommended by the Canadian Network for Mood and Anxiety Treatments (CANMAT) [9] and International Society for Bipolar Disorders (ISBD) guidelines [10] include quetiapine, lurasidone (with or without a mood stabiliser), lamotrigine and lithium. Lamotrigine as a mood stabiliser is effective in both treatment for bipolar depression and prophylaxis against further episodes. Lamotrigine does not induce switching or rapid cycling.

Diving Deep ...

Sixty-one per cent of patients with bipolar disorder have at least one psychotic symptom in their lifetime and delusions are more common than hallucinations [11].

Bipolar disorder confers the highest genetic relative risk for first-degree relatives compared to other psychiatric conditions [12]. Risk factors for bipolar disorder include a significant family history of bipolar disorder and advancing paternal age, which is associated with increased genetic mutations during spermatogenesis, increasing the risk of bipolar disorder in one's offspring.

First manic episodes are often precipitated by life events such as bereavement, personal separation, work-related problems or loss of role. High-expressed emotions and sleep deprivation are common triggers for relapse.

The kindling hypothesis states that, throughout recurrent affective disorders, there is a weakening temporal relationship between major life stress and episode initiation that could reflect either a progressive sensitisation or progressive autonomy to life stress [13].

The estimated 12-month prevalence of bipolar disorder with rapid cycling in the general population is 0.3% [14, 15]. Rapid cycling occurs in 5–15% of bipolar patients at some point in their life. It is more common in women, and in those with bipolar II disorder and a positive family history. Among rapid-cycling individuals, bipolar disorder occurred at a younger age compared with non-rapid-cycling individuals. Other risk factors for rapid cycling include neglect during childhood and parental divorce, which is more common in rapid-cycling individuals in the general population compared with non-rapid-cycling individuals. 'Ultra-rapid cycling' refers to rapid shifts between mood states alternating between periods of mania/hypomania, depression and euthymia, with each mood state lasting approximately 24 hours.

In January 2024, the United Kingdom's Medicines and Healthcare products Regulatory Agency (MHRA) introduced a warning that given the risk of impaired fertility and increased risk of neurodevelopmental disorders in children whose fathers took valproate in the three months before conception, males younger than 55 years should not be started on valproate unless two specialists independently consider and document that there is no other effective or tolerated treatment, or there are compelling reasons that the reproductive risks do not apply [16]. These recommendations came after a study found that 5 children in 100 born to fathers treated with valproate around conception were diagnosed with a neurodevelopmental disorder compared to 3 in 100 children whose fathers were taking lamotrigine or levetiracetam around conception [17].

References

1. World Health Organization. *International classification of diseases*, 11th edition (ICD-11). Geneva: World Health Organization; 2024. Available from: https://icd.who.int/en

2. American Psychiatric Association. *Diagnostic and statistical manual of mental disorders*, 5th edition, text revision (DSM-5-TR). Washington, DC: American Psychiatric Association Publishing; 2022. Available from: www.psychiatry.org/psychiatrists/practice/dsm.

3. Taylor DM, Barnes TRE, Young A. *The Maudsley prescribing guidelines in psychiatry*, 14th edition. Chichester Hoboken, NJ: Wiley Blackwell; 2021.

4. National Institute for Health and Care Excellence (NICE). Bipolar disorder: assessment and management. Clinical guideline [CG185]. NICE; 2014. Available from: www.nice.org.uk/guidance/cg185

5. Baldessarini RJ, Tondo L, Davis P, Pompili M, Goodwin FK, Hennen J. Decreased risk of suicides and attempts during long-term lithium treatment: a meta-analytic review. *Bipolar Disord*. 2006 Oct;8(5 Pt 2):625–39.

6. Semple D, Smyth R. *Oxford handbook of psychiatry*, 4th edition. Oxford: Oxford University Press; 2019.

7. Boland RJ, Verduin ML, Ruiz P, Shah A, Sadock BJ, editors. *Kaplan & Sadock's synopsis of psychiatry*, 12th edition. Philadelphia: Wolters Kluwer; 2022.

8. Finley PR, Warner MD, Peabody CA. Clinical relevance of drug interactions with lithium. *Clin Pharmacokinet*. 1995 Sep;29(3):172–91.

9. Kennedy SH, Lam RW, McIntyre RS, Tourjman SV, Bhat V, Blier P, et al. Canadian Network for Mood and Anxiety Treatments (CANMAT) 2016 clinical guidelines for the management of adults with major depressive disorder: Section 3. Pharmacological treatments. *Can J Psychiatry*. 2016 Sep;61(9):540–60.

10. Yatham LN, Kennedy SH, Parikh SV, Schaffer A, Bond DJ, Frey BN, et al. Canadian Network for Mood and Anxiety Treatments (CANMAT) and International Society for Bipolar Disorders (ISBD) 2018 guidelines for the management of patients with bipolar disorder. *Bipolar Disord*. 2018 Mar;20(2):97–170.

11. Goodwin FK, Jamison KR. *Manic-depressive illness: bipolar disorders and recurrent depression*, 2nd edition. New York: Oxford University Press; 2007.

12. Lichtenstein P, Yip BH, Björk C, Pawitan Y, Cannon TD, Sullivan PF, et al. Common genetic determinants of schizophrenia and bipolar disorder in Swedish families: a population-based study. *Lancet*. 2009 Jan 17;373(9659):234–9.

13. Post RM. Kindling and sensitization as models for affective episode recurrence, cyclicity, and tolerance phenomena. *Neurosci Biobehav Rev*. 2007;31(6):858–73.

14. Kupka RW, Luckenbaugh DA, Post RM, Leverich GS, Nolen WA. Rapid and non-rapid cycling bipolar disorder: a meta-analysis of clinical studies. *J Clin Psychiatry*. 2003 Dec;64(12):1483–94.

15. Lee S, Tsang A, Kessler RC, Jin R, Sampson N, Andrade L, et al. Rapid-cycling bipolar disorder: cross-national community study. *Br J Psychiatry*. 2010 Mar;196(3):217–25.

16. Medicines and Healthcare products Regulatory Agency. Valproate (Belvo, Convulex, Depakote, Dyzantil, Epilim, Epilim Chrono or Chronosphere, Episenta, Epival, and Syonell): new safety and educational materials to support regulatory measures in men and women under 55 years of age. *Drug Safety Update*. 2024 Jan;17(6):1). Available from: www.gov.uk/drug-safety-update/valproate-belvo-convulex-depakote-dyzantil-epilim-epilim-chrono-or-chronosphere-episenta-epival-and-syonellv-new-safety-and-educational-materials-to-support-regulatory-measures-in-men-and-women-under-55-years-of-age

17. Florent Richy. A post-authorization safety study (PASS) to evaluate the paternal exposure to valproate and the risk of neurodevelopmental disorders including autism spectrum disorders as well as congenital abnormalities in offspring – a population-based retrospective study. Study protocol EUPAS34201. European Network of Centres for Pharmacoepidemiology and Pharmacovigilance (ENCEPP); 2020. Available from: https://catalogues.ema.europa.eu/node/3611/administrative-details

Case 7: Generalised Anxiety Disorder

Why do I keep worrying?

Jamie is a 40-year-old female who comes in for insomnia. She is currently a teacher with two children of school-going age. For the past eight months, she has had difficulty falling asleep and is waking up earlier than planned. She sleeps only four hours a day. In addition, she experiences stiff shoulders and headaches and feels fatigued most of the day. She feels on edge throughout the day, with her mind constantly worrying about everyday events, from her children to work to finances, etc. She worries whether they will get to school safely and cope well. She has difficulties controlling her worries, which occur throughout the day. Her concentration at work has been affected, and her superiors recently gave her a warning letter.

- **Question 1: What is the most likely diagnosis? Which differential diagnoses would you consider?**

- **Question 2: What investigations would you order to confirm your diagnosis and guide management?**

You diagnosed Jamie with generalised anxiety disorder.

- **Question 3: What are the risk factors for generalised anxiety disorder?**

- **Question 4: What other psychiatric co-morbidities would you screen for?**

- **Question 5: Jamie is keen for treatment, how would you manage her generalised anxiety disorder?**

Jamie was started on a trial of sertraline. However, despite an adequate trial of sertraline over four weeks her symptoms failed to remit.

- **Question 6: When first-line treatment has failed, what other pharmacological treatments can be considered?**

Answers to Case 7

Question 1
What is the most likely diagnosis? Which differential diagnoses would you consider?

Answer
Generalised anxiety disorder is the most likely diagnosis. Other differential diagnoses to rule out include hyperthyroidism, phaeochromocytoma and other anxiety spectrum disorders including panic disorder, etc.

Explanation

Diagnosis of generalised anxiety disorder

Marked symptoms of anxiety are required for diagnosis, manifested in either [1]:

1. General apprehensiveness that is not restricted to any particular environmental circumstance (i.e., 'free-floating anxiety'); or

2. Excessive worry (apprehensive expectation) about negative events occurring in several different aspects of everyday life (e.g., work, finances, health, family)

Anxiety and general apprehensiveness or worry are accompanied by additional:

- Muscle tension or motor restlessness

- Sympathetic autonomic overactivity as evidenced by frequent gastrointestinal symptoms such as nausea and/or abdominal distress, heart palpitations, sweating, trembling, shaking and/or dry mouth

- Nervousness, restlessness or being 'on edge'

- Difficulty concentrating

- Irritability

- Sleep disturbances

Anxiety spectrum disorders are a good masquerade of one another. Some of the defining features include:

Condition	Defining feature(s)
Panic disorder	Anticipatory anxiety of the next panic attack
Agoraphobia	The individual fears or avoids certain situations because of thoughts that escape might be difficult or help might not be available in the event of developing panic-like symptoms or other incapacitating or embarrassing symptoms
Social phobia	Specific to social situations where the individual might come under the scrutiny of others
Post-traumatic stress disorder (PTSD)	Follows a traumatic event (actual or threatened death, serious injury or sexual violence). The main features are hyperarousal, avoidance, intrusion symptoms and dissociation

Generalised anxiety disorder tends to present with free-floating anxiety while the other anxiety spectrum disorders have a waxing and waning anxiety pattern.

Exam Essentials

- Symptoms of generalised anxiety disorder – **MR TICS**

  ○ **M**uscle tension
  ○ **R**estlessness
  ○ **T**ired
  ○ **I**rritability
  ○ **C**oncentration
  ○ **S**leep difficulties

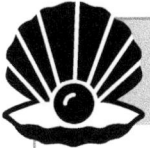

Clinical Pearls

- Rating scales such as the clinician-administered Hamilton Anxiety (HAM-A) rating scale and, more specifically, self-administered GAD-7, may help with the assessment and monitoring of symptoms

- Consider caffeine use as a contributor to anxiety

Question 2

What investigations would you order to confirm your diagnosis and guide management?

Answer

Category	Investigations
Point-of-care test	ECG Blood pressure reading
Biochemistry	Full blood count Renal panel Liver function test Thyroid function test Urine 24-hour catecholamines Urine drug screen (for suspected cases or unusual presentation – e.g., sudden onset)
Imaging	MRI adrenals (only if history and if biochemical tests are suggestive of phaeochromocytoma)

Explanation

We need to have high levels of suspicion for organic causes if Jamie presents with high blood pressure, tachycardia, diarrhoea, weight loss, extreme diaphoresis and throbbing headache, which do not go away with symptomatic treatment. Imaging such as MRI adrenals should only be ordered if biochemical tests are suggestive of phaeochromocytoma.

Other prescribed medications can cause anxiety symptoms as well (refer to the Diving Deep section).

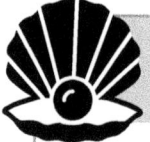

Clinical Pearls

- Always take a history and potentially **screen for illicit substance use**, as anxiety symptoms may be part of the withdrawal or intoxication syndrome

Question 3

What are the risk factors for generalised anxiety disorder?

Answer

Modifiable risk factors: lower economic resources, unemployment, divorced/ widowed

Non-modifiable risk factors: age, female gender, family history of psychiatric disorders, history of sexual abuse

Explanation

Age is known to be a risk factor up to the age of 65. Early-onset generalised anxiety disorder is associated with childhood fears and marital or sexual disturbances, while cases with a later onset often occur after a stressful event.

Question 4

What other psychiatric co-morbidities would you screen for?

Answer

The following are common co-morbidities of generalised anxiety disorder [1]:

- Mood disorders: major depressive disorder (62%) [2], bipolar disorder (18%) [3]

- Anxiety spectrum disorders: obsessive–compulsive disorder (OCD) (33.5%) [4], panic disorder (24%) [5]

- Alcohol and other substance use disorders (20–40%) [6]

Explanation

Anxiety disorders are independent risk factors for suicide attempts [7].

Question 5

Jamie is keen for treatment, how would you manage her generalised anxiety disorder?

Answer

Pharmacology: selective serotonin reuptake inhibitors (SSRIs)

Psychotherapy: CBT

Self-help/psychoeducational groups

Explanation

The NICE guidelines [8] suggest a step-based approach. Education and active monitoring are the first steps. The second step requires psychological interventions (CBT, self-help, psychoeducational groups). The third step involves the pharmacological use of an SSRI such as sertraline, or more intensive psychological intervention.

The Canadian Network for Mood and Anxiety Treatments (CANMAT) guidelines [9] for the management of anxiety, PTSD and OCD suggest that psychotherapy and pharmacotherapy have equivalent efficacy for the treatment of most anxiety and related disorders. While CBT is traditionally delivered as an individual or group therapy for most anxiety and related disorders, recent studies have shown that self-directed or minimal intervention formats (e.g., bibliotherapy/self-help books, or internet/computer-based programs with or without minimal therapist contact) are effective [10, 11]. There are different areas that CBT focuses on. In exposure, the patient faces their fears in a graded manner. In safety response inhibition, patients are taught to restrict anxiety-reducing behaviours (e.g., the need for reassurance), which decreases negative reinforcement and breaks the cycle of anxiety. Cognitive strategies include cognitive restructuring and behavioural experiments. Arousal management uses relaxation and breath control techniques. Safety-signal learning refers to the conditioning of distinct stimuli in one's environment to the absence of aversive events. In surrendering safety signals, self-efficacy beliefs are adopted and safety signals relinquished.

Exam Essentials

- Refer to Case 3 for further reading on SSRIs

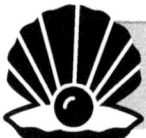

Clinical Pearls

- Do not offer benzodiazepines except for short-term use in breakthrough anxiety

- Risks of benzodiazepines include:
  - Dependence
  - Cognitive impairment
  - Fall risks
  - Respiratory depression (especially in patients with lung diseases)

Question 5
When first-line treatment has failed, what other pharmacological treatments can be considered?

Answer
Benzodiazepines as an adjunct therapy

Other antidepressants (e.g., imipramine, bupropion extended release (XL), vortioxetine)

Antipsychotics (e.g., quetiapine)

Buspirone

Explanation
Based on the CANMAT guidelines [9], the above medications are second-line treatment options.

While benzodiazepines have level 1 evidence, they are usually only prescribed for short-term use because of their side effects and risk of dependence.

Imipramine has a similar level 1 evidence for generalised anxiety disorder but because of its side effects and potential lethality in overdose, it is used as a second-line treatment. There are fewer data on both bupropion XL and vortioxetine, but they are deemed to be effective treatment options. Quetiapine, while effective, carries side effects of weight gain and sedation with accompanying higher dropout rates. Buspirone has limited clinical effectiveness in practice and is hence considered a second-line treatment option.

Diving Deep …

Generalised anxiety disorder is more common in high-income countries and has a lifetime prevalence of around 5.7% [12].

Medications can also cause anxiety-like symptoms, and these include:

- Cardiovascular: antihypertensives, antiarrhythmics

- Respiratory: bronchodilators, alpha-1- or beta-adrenergic agonists

- Central nervous system: anticonvulsants, withdrawal from a benzodiazepine or alcohol, reaction from disulfiram

- Others: levothyroxine, chemotherapy, non-steroidal anti-inflammatory drugs

Generalised anxiety disorder can be a chronic and disabling disorder, with low remission rates, and up to 68% of patients continue to have residual symptoms even after years of treatment [12].

Citation/References

1. World Health Organization. *International classification of diseases*, 11th edition (ICD-11). Geneva: World Health Organization; 2024. Available from: https://icd.who.int/en

2. Wittchen HU, Jacobi F, Rehm J, Gustavsson A, Svensson M, Jönsson B, et al. The size and burden of mental disorders and other disorders of the brain in Europe 2010. *Eur Neuropsychopharmacol*. 2011 Sep;21(9):655–79.

3. Simon NM. Generalized anxiety disorder and psychiatric comorbidities such as depression, bipolar disorder, and substance abuse. *J Clin Psychiatry*. 2009 Apr;70(Suppl 2):10–4.

4. Sharma P, Rosário MC, Ferrão YA, Albertella L, Miguel EC, Fontenelle LF. The impact of generalized anxiety disorder in obsessive–compulsive disorder patients. *Psychiatry Res*. 2021 Jun;300:113898.

5. Brawman-Mintzer O, Lydiard RB, Emmanuel N, Payeur R, Johnson M, Roberts J, et al. Psychiatric comorbidity in patients with generalized anxiety disorder. *Am J Psychiatry*. 1993 Aug;150(8):1216–8.

6. Boland RJ, Verduin ML, Ruiz P, Shah A, Sadock BJ, editors. *Kaplan & Sadock's synopsis of psychiatry*, 12th edition. Philadelphia: Wolters Kluwer; 2022.

7. Bolton JM, Cox BJ, Afifi TO, Enns MW, Bienvenu OJ, Sareen J. Anxiety disorders and risk for suicide attempts: findings from the Baltimore Epidemiologic Catchment area follow-up study. *Depress Anxiety*. 2008 Jun 1;25(6):477–81.

8. National Institute for Health and Care Excellence (NICE). Generalised anxiety disorder and panic disorder in adults: management. Clinical guideline [CG113]. NICE; 2011. Available from: www.nice.org.uk/guidance/cg113

9. Kennedy SH, Lam RW, McIntyre RS, Tourjman SV, Bhat V, Blier P, et al. Canadian Network for Mood and Anxiety Treatments (CANMAT) 2016 clinical guidelines for the management of adults with major depressive disorder: Section 3. Pharmacological Treatments. *Can J Psychiatry*. 2016 Sep;61(9):540–60.

10. Bandelow B, Seidler-Brandler U, Becker A, Wedekind D, Rüther E. Meta-analysis of randomized controlled comparisons of psychopharmacological and psychological treatments for anxiety disorders. *World J Biol Psychiatry*. 2007;8(3):175–87.

11. Roshanaei-Moghaddam B, Pauly MC, Atkins DC, Baldwin SA, Stein MB, Roy-Byrne P. Relative effects of CBT and pharmacotherapy in depression versus anxiety: is medication somewhat better for depression, and CBT somewhat better for anxiety? *Depress Anxiety*. 2011 Jul;28(7):560–7.

12. Semple D, Smyth R. *Oxford handbook of psychiatry*, 4th edition. Oxford: Oxford University Press; 2019.

Case 8: Panic Disorder and Agoraphobia

Am I having a heart attack?

Leah is a 50-year-old lady who was referred to the psychiatry clinic after presenting to the emergency department for recurrent episodes of chest pain. She has been having symptoms for the past six months, but in the past three weeks, she has had worsening daily episodes of chest pain and has since visited the emergency department four times. During each emergency department visit, she was told that the investigations were unremarkable. Each episode begins abruptly within minutes and resolves spontaneously within an hour. She experiences chest tightness, hyperventilates and feels as if 'there is not enough air filling my lungs'. She frequently gets light-headed and has the sensation that her heart is pounding rapidly against her chest. These symptoms are usually accompanied by hot flashes and the feeling that 'something bad is going to happen'. Because of these frequent episodes, Leah constantly worries about when the next episode will happen. Leah has stopped exercising as she is worried that it may stress her heart further.

- **Question 1: What is Leah's diagnosis?**

During these episodes of hyperventilation, Leah complains of peri-oral numbness. This is accompanied by acral numbness and cramping of her hands and legs. On physical examination, you note forced adduction of the thumb, flexion of the metacarpophalangeal joints and wrists and extension of the fingers on bilateral hands.

- **Question 2: What phenomenon is being described?**

You ask Leah how these panic attacks have affected her life. The symptoms have been present for more than six months and often there is no clear trigger for the attacks. This leads her to worry greatly about the next attack, which in turn affects her ability to leave her house. She worries about having a panic attack and being 'trapped' in open places like parking lots or in areas with large crowds of people and the embarrassment that comes with it. Lately, she has been relying more on delivery services to get her groceries and, when she leaves her house, she does so with the company of one of her children and avoids public transportation.

- **Question 3: What co-morbid condition does she have?**

You explain the diagnosis of panic disorder and agoraphobia to Leah and how it relates to the symptoms she experiences. She is keen for treatment.

- **Question 4: How would you manage Leah's panic disorder and agoraphobia?**

Question 1
What is Leah's diagnosis?

Answer
Panic disorder

Explanation

Diagnosis of panic disorder [1]

1. Recurrent panic attacks, which are discrete episodes of intense fear or apprehension characterised by the rapid and concurrent onset of several characteristic symptoms, are required for diagnosis. These symptoms may include, but are not limited to, the following:

    - Palpitations

    - Sweating

    - Trembling or shaking

    - Shortness of breath

    - Sensation of choking

    - Chest pain or discomfort

    - Nausea or abdominal discomfort

    - Giddiness or light-headedness

    - Hot or cold sensations

    - Paraesthesia

- Derealisation or depersonalisation
- Fear of losing control or 'going crazy'
- Fear of dying

2. At least some of the panic attacks are unexpected – that is, they are not restricted to particular stimuli or situations but rather seem to arise 'out of the blue'

3. Following a panic attack, for several weeks or more, one or both of the following occurs:
   - There is a persistent concern about additional panic attacks or their consequences
   - There is a significant maladaptive change in behaviour related to the attacks

Exam Essentials

- An important feature of panic disorder is the **presence of some panic attacks which are not triggered** or expected
- A panic attack is characterised by sudden, discrete episodes of severe anxiety, in a crescendo–decrescendo manner
- Explore other anxiety disorders such as generalised anxiety disorder, social phobia and agoraphobia as they are common co-morbidities

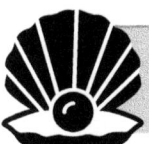

Clinical Pearls

- Hyperventilation is a diagnosis of exclusion
- Rule out medical causes for anxiety symptoms, such as hyperthyroidism, phaeochromocytoma, medications or drugs (refer to the Diving Deep section in Case 7)

Question 2
What phenomenon is being described?

Answer
Carpopedal spasms

Explanation
Carpopedal spasm constitutes 9% of the somatic complaints as part of hyperventilation syndrome [2]. Proposed mechanisms for carpopedal spasms from hyperventilation include a reduction in cerebral blood flow due to decreasing partial pressure of carbon dioxide ($PaCO_2$) levels resulting in cerebral vasoconstriction. Respiratory alkalosis from hyperventilation results in acute changes in ionised serum calcium levels, affecting the binding of calcium to albumin and consequently paraesthesia and tetany.

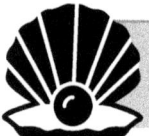

Clinical Pearls

- The use of **rebreathing techniques** (e.g., breathing into a paper bag) **is no longer recommended** due to significant hypoxia and risk of death. Carbon dioxide in itself is a chemical trigger for anxiety

Question 3
What co-morbid condition does she have?

Answer
Agoraphobia

Explanation
Agoraphobia is a common co-morbid condition of panic disorder.

Explanation

Diagnosis of agoraphobia [1]

1. Marked and excessive fear or anxiety that occurs in, or in anticipation of, multiple situations where escape might be difficult or help might not be available is required for diagnosis. Examples include using public transportation, being in crowds, outside the home alone, in shops or theatres or standing in line

2. The individual is consistently fearful or anxious about these situations due to a fear of specific negative outcomes such as panic attacks, symptoms of panic,

or other incapacitating (e.g., falling) or embarrassing physical symptoms (e.g., incontinence)

3.   The situations are actively avoided, are entered only under specific circumstances (e.g., in the presence of a companion), or else are endured with intense fear or anxiety

4.   The symptoms are not transient – that is, they persist for an extended period of time (e.g., at least several months)

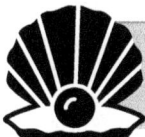

Exam Essentials

- If an individual's presentation meets the criteria for panic disorder and agoraphobia, both diagnoses should be assigned

Question 4
How would you manage Leah's panic disorder and agoraphobia?

Answer
Pharmacological: antidepressants (e.g., selective serotonin reuptake inhibitors (SSRIs) and judicious limited use of benzodiazepines)

Psychological: cognitive behavioural therapy (CBT)

Explanation
As per the NICE guidelines [3], CBT or SSRIs are first-line treatment options. Based on the Canadian Network for Mood and Anxiety Treatments (CANMAT) guidelines [4] for the management of anxiety, post-traumatic stress and obsessive–compulsive disorders, the specific SSRIs recommended with level 1 evidence include citalopram, fluoxetine, fluvoxamine, paroxetine and sertraline. Escitalopram and paroxetine controlled release are level 2-evidence recommended. Other medication classes such as mirtazapine, serotonin–noradrenaline reuptake inhibitors (SNRIs) and tricyclic antidepressants are also effective. Venlafaxine, in particular, is an SNRI with level 1 evidence useful in reducing the severity of panic disorder symptoms. Although benzodiazepines may have a role in rapid anti-panic effects, they are prone to abuse and dependence. Hence, benzodiazepine prescription should be judicious and limited to two weeks until the effects of a co-administered antidepressant are seen. Side effects of long-term benzodiazepines include:

- Dependency

- Cognitive impairment

- Motor incoordination

- Fall risk

- Respiratory problems (especially in the elderly or those with pre-existing respiratory conditions)

In the management of moderate to severe panic disorder, the choice of an SSRI versus CBT is largely dependent on the patient's preference and treatment availability [5, 6]. However, in patients treated for panic disorder who have suicidality or co-occurring disorders, consideration can be made to treat with both medications and CBT.

In CBT, behavioural methods help by treating phobic avoidance by exposure, use of relaxation and control of hyperventilation. Cognitive methods teach about bodily responses associated with anxiety, educate patients about panic attacks and modify thinking errors.

The 1997 Panic Disorder Severity Scale [7] was developed by Shaer et al. and is a brief seven-item clinician rating scale that measures the severity of panic attacks and panic disorder symptoms, which helps in assessing baseline severity and monitoring treatment response. The 1995 Panic and Agoraphobia Scale [8] developed by Bandelow is available in both self-rated and clinician-rated versions and measures the severity of agoraphobia with or without panic attacks over the past week.

Exam Essentials

- The NICE guidelines suggest that sedating antihistamines and beta-blockers have limited efficacy

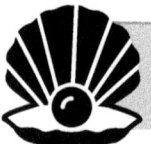

Clinical Pearls

- There is good evidence for the benefit of maintenance treatment for at least six months [9]

- 'Go-low, go-slow' approach in prescribing antidepressants should be adopted given the potential side effects of increasing panic symptoms

- Pregabalin may be used to alleviate anxiety symptoms. Risks however include possible dependence, sedation and cognitive impairment

Diving Deep …

Women are two to three times more likely to be affected than men with panic disorder [10]. Age of onset has a bimodal distribution with the highest peak incidence at age 15–24 and a second peak at age 45–54 [11, 12]. The condition is rare after age 65 (0.1%). Other risk factors include: being widowed, divorced or separated; living in a city; limited education; early parental loss; and physical or sexual abuse.

In deciding the choice of SSRI, there is no evidence for superior efficacy in panic disorder of some SSRIs over others [9]. Therefore, the choice of SSRI should be dependent on the side-effect profiles of each SSRI.

Antipsychotics should not be prescribed for the treatment of panic disorder. A clinical trial [13] has shown their lack of efficacy both as monotherapy and in augmentation of SSRIs with no difference in panic-symptom reduction between both groups.

Functional recovery is seen in 25–75% of patients with panic disorder after two years, falling to 10–30% after five years. In the long term, around 50% of individuals will experience only mild symptoms [12].

References

1. World Health Organization. *International classification of diseases*, 11th edition (ICD-11). Geneva: World Health Organization; 2024. Available from: https://icd.who.int/en

2. Saisch SG, Wessely S, Gardner WN. Patients with acute hyperventilation presenting to an inner-city emergency department. *Chest*. 1996 Oct;110(4):952–7.

3. National Institute for Health and Care Excellence (NICE). Generalised anxiety disorder and panic disorder in adults: management. Clinical guideline [CG113]. NICE; 2011. Available from: www.nice.org.uk/guidance/cg113

4. Kennedy SH, Lam RW, McIntyre RS, Tourjman SV, Bhat V, Blier P, et al. Canadian Network for Mood and Anxiety Treatments (CANMAT) 2016 clinical guidelines for the management of adults with major depressive disorder: Section 3. Pharmacological Treatments. *Can J Psychiatry*. 2016 Sep;61(9):540–60.

5. Furukawa TA, Watanabe N, Churchill R. Combined psychotherapy plus antidepressants for panic disorder with or without agoraphobia. *Cochrane Database Syst Rev*. 2007 Jan 24;2007(1):CD004364.

6. Hofmann SG, Smits JAJ. Cognitive–behavioral therapy for adult anxiety disorders: a meta-analysis of randomized placebo-controlled trials. *J Clin Psychiatry*. 2008 Apr;69(4):621–32.

7. Shear MK, Brown TA, Barlow DH, Money R, Sholomskas DE, Woods SW, et al. Multicenter collaborative panic disorder severity scale. *Am J Psychiatry*. 1997 Nov;154(11):1571–5.

8. Bandelow B. Assessing the efficacy of treatments for panic disorder and agoraphobia. II. The Panic and Agoraphobia Scale. *Int Clin Psychopharmacol*. 1995 Jun;10(2):73–81.

9. Taylor DM, Barnes TRE, Young A. *The Maudsley prescribing guidelines in psychiatry*, 14th edition. Chichester Hoboken, NJ: Wiley Blackwell; 2021.

10. American Psychiatric Association. *Diagnostic and statistical manual of mental disorders*, 5th edition, text revision (DSM-5-TR). Washington, DC: American Psychiatric Association Publishing; 2022. Available from: www.psychiatry.org/psychiatrists/practice/dsm

11. Kessler RC, Chiu WT, Demler O, Merikangas KR, Walters EE. Prevalence, severity, and comorbidity of 12-month DSM-IV disorders in the National Comorbidity Survey Replication. *Arch Gen Psychiatry*. 2005 Jun;62(6):617–27.

12. Semple D, Smyth R. *Oxford handbook of psychiatry*, 4th edition. Oxford: Oxford University Press; 2019.

13. Goddard AW, Mahmud W, Medlock C, Shin YW, Shekhar A. A controlled trial of quetiapine XR coadministration treatment of SSRI-resistant panic disorder. *Ann Gen Psychiatry*. 2015;14:26.

Case 9: Social Anxiety Disorder

They are probably judging me

Taylor is a 19-year-old girl who presented to your clinic for a consultation. She reports that, since the age of 14, she has been worried about how others in school and the public view her. Her mother reports that she used to be a cheerful and talkative girl until the age of 14. From age 14, she constantly worries that others are judging her negatively. She has avoided all family gatherings since her symptoms started. She struggles with group work, finds it difficult to express herself, and often shies away from group discussions. As her current curriculum heavily relies on her performance in group work, she failed her semester and had to repeat the school year.

- **Question 1: What is Taylor most likely suffering from?**

- **Question 2: What are the other phobias you are aware of?**

Taylor is also concerned that she may have an avoidant personality disorder.

- **Question 3: What are the differences between avoidant personality disorder and social anxiety disorder?**

Taylor is interested in exploring treatment options for her social anxiety disorder.

- **Question 4: What is the treatment for social anxiety disorder?**

Answers to Case 9

Question 1
What is Taylor most likely suffering from?

Answer
Social anxiety disorder (social phobia)

Explanation

Diagnosis of social anxiety disorder [1]

1. Marked and excessive fear or anxiety that occurs consistently in one or more social situations such as social interactions (e.g., having a conversation), doing something while feeling observed (e.g., eating or drinking in the presence of others) or performing in front of others (e.g., giving a speech) is required for diagnosis

2. The individual is concerned that they will act in a way, or show anxiety symptoms, that will be negatively evaluated by others (i.e., be humiliating, be embarrassing, lead to rejection or be offensive)

3. Relevant social situations are consistently avoided or endured with intense fear or anxiety

4. The symptoms are not transient – that is, they persist for an extended period of time (e.g., at least several months)

Exam Essentials

- Always assess for other anxiety co-morbidities and differentials:
  - Generalised anxiety disorder
  - Panic disorder
  - Agoraphobia
  - Specific phobias
  - Psychotic disorders
  - Obsessive–compulsive disorder

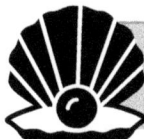

Clinical Pearls

- Rating scales such as the self-rated Social Phobia Inventory may be helpful

- Always check for co-morbid mood disorders and substance use

- For patients with poor scholastic achievement and coping, and/or school refusal, do screen for social phobia

Question 2
What are the other phobias you are aware of?

Answer
Specific phobias
Social phobia, performance only

Explanation
Other forms of phobia include animal phobia (e.g., spiders, insects, dogs), natural environment (e.g., heights, storms, water), blood–injection–injury (e.g., needles, invasive medical procedures) and situational (e.g., aeroplanes, elevators, enclosed places). If the fear is restricted to speaking or performing in public, it should be diagnosed as social phobia, performance only.

The lifetime prevalence of specific phobias around the world ranges from 3% to 15%, with fears and phobias concerning heights and animals being the most common [2].

Question 3
What are the differences between avoidant personality disorder and social anxiety disorder?

Answer
Although they share similar social-based anxiety, there are some differences which may help differentiate between them:

	Social anxiety disorder	**Avoidant personality disorder**
Classification	Anxiety disorder	Personality disorder
Duration	Shorter, usually after childhood	Longer, since childhood
Onset	May be more acute	Insidious
Insight	Frustrated by their anxiety, and hence have insight that their fears are irrational	Believe that they deserve such anxiety, and hence genuinely believe they are inferior

Explanation

Avoidant personality disorder is characterised by a pervasive pattern of social inhibition, feelings of inadequacy and hypersensitivity to negative evaluation, with avoidance of activities due to fear of criticism, disapproval or rejection. Individuals with avoidant personality disorder usually are unwilling to get involved with others unless they are certain that they are liked, and view themselves as socially inept, personally unappealing or inferior to others. They are rather preoccupied with being criticised or rejected, and show restraint within intimate relationships due to fear of being shamed or ridiculed.

In clinical practice, it is not uncommon to see patients with both social anxiety disorder and avoidant personality disorder, with 32–50% of people with avoidant personality disorder also suffering from social anxiety disorder [3].

Exam Essentials

- Symptoms of avoidant personality disorder – **CRINGES**
  - **C**riticism preoccupies thought
  - **R**estraint in a relationship due to shame
  - **I**nhibited in new relationships
  - **N**eeds to be sure of being liked
  - **G**ets around activities needing interpersonal contact
  - **E**mbarrassment prevents risk-taking
  - **S**elf-view: unappealing and inadequate

Question 4
What is the treatment for social anxiety disorder?

Answer

Psychological management with cognitive behavioural therapy (CBT) and pharmacological management with selective serotonin reuptake inhibitors (SSRIs) or serotonin–noradrenaline reuptake inhibitors (SNRIs).

Explanation

CBT in a group or individual format is considered to be the gold-standard non-pharmacological treatment for social anxiety disorder. The cognitive techniques employed involve restructuring and challenging maladaptive thoughts, while the behavioural component typically uses exposure therapy.

Based on the Canadian Network for Mood and Anxiety Treatments (CANMAT) guidelines [4] for the management of anxiety disorders, SSRIs such as escitalopram, fluvoxamine, fluvoxamine controlled release, paroxetine, sertraline and SNRIs such as venlafaxine have level 1 evidence and are considered first-line treatment options for social anxiety disorder. Pregabalin is effective in treating social anxiety disorder at higher doses (e.g., 600 mg/day).

> **Diving Deep …**
>
> The CANMAT guidelines recommend therapy for specific phobias such as exposure-based therapy, virtual reality therapy and applied muscle tension therapy. While both in vivo exposure and virtual-reality exposure are effective, in vivo exposure is superior to alternative types (e.g., imaginal, virtual reality, etc.) at post-treatment but not at follow-up.
>
> As many as 90% of patients with social anxiety disorder have co-morbidity with another psychiatric disorder [5], with the highest rates for major depressive disorder and other anxiety disorders. Avoidant personality disorder, body dysmorhpic disorder and schizophrenia are also common co-morbid psychiatric disorders. Between half and two-thirds of patients respond to efficacious treatments for social anxiety disorder in clinical trials, while medication should be continued for 6–12 months to reduce the risk of relapse [6, 7].

References

1. World Health Organization. *International classification of diseases*, 11th edition (ICD-11). Geneva: World Health Organization; 2024. Available from: https://icd.who.int/en

2. Eaton WW, Bienvenu OJ, Miloyan B. Specific phobias. *Lancet Psychiatry*. 2018 Aug;5(8):678–86.

3. Baljé A, Greeven A, Van Giezen A, Korrelboom K, Arntz A, Spinhoven P. Group schema therapy versus group cognitive behavioral therapy for social anxiety disorder with comorbid avoidant personality disorder: study protocol for a randomized controlled trial. *Trials*. 2016 Dec;17(1):487.

4. Kennedy SH, Lam RW, McIntyre RS, Tourjman SV, Bhat V, Blier P, et al. Canadian Network for Mood and Anxiety Treatments (CANMAT) 2016 clinical guidelines for the management of adults with major depressive disorder: Section 3. Pharmacological Treatments. *Can J Psychiatry*. 2016 Sep;61(9):540–60.

5. Koyuncu A, İnce E, Ertekin E, Tükel R. Comorbidity in social anxiety disorder: diagnostic and therapeutic challenges. *Drugs Context*. 2019;8:212573.

6. Taylor DM, Barnes TRE, Young A. *The Maudsley prescribing guidelines in psychiatry*, 14th edition. Chichester Hoboken, NJ: Wiley Blackwell; 2021.

7. Ipser JC, Kariuki CM, Stein DJ. Pharmacotherapy for social anxiety disorder: a systematic review. *Expert Rev Neurother*. 2008 Feb;8(2):235–57.

Case 10: Separation Anxiety and Selective Mutism

A silent struggle

Charlotte is a seven-year-old girl who has refused school for the past four weeks. When the topic of leaving home for school comes up, she becomes visibly distressed and states her desire to stay at home with her mum. Each morning, she cries and complains of having abdominal pain when it is time to go to school. She also has an increased frequency of nightmares, dreaming of scenarios where she is alone and apart from her family.

- **Question 1: What is Charlotte's diagnosis?**

- **Question 2: What are the aetiological factors of separation anxiety disorder?**

- **Question 3: What is the treatment for separation anxiety?**

Following a course of cognitive behavioural therapy (CBT), Charlotte experienced a remission of her separation anxiety disorder and she was able to return to school. Two years later, her teachers called her mother to report that Charlotte had been quiet during classes for the past month. Even when directly spoken to or amongst her peers, she remains silent. This has caused the teachers to be worried about her academic performance. This surprised her mother as she was noted to be speaking fine at home and her mood appeared to be fine.

- **Question 4: What is the new diagnosis?**

- **Question 5: Apart from selective mutism, what differentials should one consider in a child presenting with mutism?**

Answers to Case 10

Question 1
What is Charlotte's diagnosis?

Answer
Separation anxiety disorder

Explanation

Diagnosis of separation anxiety disorder [1]

1.   Marked and excessive fear or anxiety about separation from those individuals to whom the person is attached (i.e., with whom the individual has a deep emotional bond) is required for diagnosis.

     Manifestations of fear or anxiety related to separation depend on the individual's developmental level, but may include:

     •   Persistent thoughts that harm or some other untoward event (e.g., being kidnapped) will lead to separation
     •   Reluctance or refusal to go to school or work
     •   Recurrent excessive distress (e.g., tantrums, social withdrawal) related to being separated from the attachment figure
     •   Reluctance or refusal to go to sleep without being near the attachment figure
     •   Recurrent nightmares about separation
     •   Physical symptoms such as nausea, vomiting, stomach pain or headache on occasions that involve separation from the attachment figure, such as leaving home to go to school or work

2.   The symptoms are not transient – that is, they persist for an extended period of time (e.g., at least several months)

Developmentally, appropriate separation anxiety manifests from six months of age till three years old typically. It becomes a disorder when it persists and interferes with functioning. Separation anxiety disorder usually remits spontaneously in adulthood. It may be episodic, with periods of impairing anxiety that remit and may reoccur.

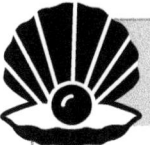

Clinical Pearls

•   Compared to other anxiety disorders, the onset of separation anxiety disorder is much earlier, occurring before the age of 18

Question 2
What are the aetiological factors of separation anxiety disorder?

Answer
Genetic vulnerability
Anxious, inconsistent or overinvolved parenting styles
Regression during periods of stress, illness or abandonment

Explanation
Co-morbidities of separation anxiety disorder include depression, anxiety disorders (panic with agoraphobia in older children), attention deficit hyperactivity disorder, oppositional disorders, learning disorders and developmental disorders.

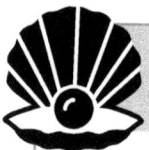

Clinical Pearls

- Having asthma confers a risk for separation anxiety disorder

Question 3
What is the treatment for separation anxiety?

Answer
Psychoeducation
Psychotherapy: CBT
Pharmacological options: selective serotonin reuptake inhibitors (SSRIs)

Explanation
CBT replaces negative beliefs with realistic and neutral thoughts. Children are encouraged to confront their fears and this reduces the element of avoidance; this can be done through a systematic programme of graded exposure to feared situations. Parental involvement is important in psychotherapy for children. SSRIs are effective in paediatric anxiety disorders. Combination treatment with SSRIs and CBT is superior to either monotherapy.

Question 4
What is the new diagnosis?

Answer
Selective mutism

Explanation

Diagnosis of selective mutism [1]

1. Consistent selectivity in speaking, such that a child demonstrates adequate language competence in specific social situations (typically at home) but consistently fails to speak in others (typically at school) is required for diagnosis

2. The duration of the disturbance is at least one month, not limited to the first month of school

3. The disturbance is not due to a lack of knowledge of, or comfort with, the spoken language demanded in the social situation

4. The symptoms are not better accounted for by another mental disorder (e.g., a neurodevelopmental disorder such as autism spectrum disorder or developmental language disorder)

5. Selectivity of speech is sufficiently severe to interfere with educational achievement or with social communication, or is associated with significant impairment in other important areas of functioning

Treatment aims to lower the anxiety that a child has when speaking in certain situations and to increase the contexts in which the child may speak comfortably. The first-line treatment options include behavioural treatments, CBT and/or play therapy. Family and parents should be involved in the treatment process.

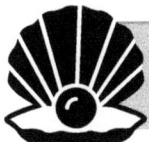

Clinical Pearls

- **Check if the child can speak in a different setting**, which suggests that language impairment cannot fully account for the child's reticence to speak

Question 5
Apart from selective mutism, what differentials should one consider in a child presenting with mutism?

Answer
Autism
Intellectual disability
Paediatric catatonia
Dissociative stupor
Negative symptoms of psychosis

Explanation

Children with autism and intellectual disability may present with delayed language acquisition and appear mute. Paediatric catatonia, while less common in children, may also present with mutism accompanied by other motor features. Organic causes of catatonia may include anti-NMDA-receptor encephalitis, paediatric autoimmune neuropsychiatric disorders associated with streptococcal infections (PANDAS) or metabolic and genetic conditions (e.g., Wilson's disease). Children who experience a dissociative stupor may present with mutism and immobility. Patients suffering from negative symptoms of psychosis may present with alogia.

Diving Deep ...

Approximately 4% of children and 1.6% of adolescents suffer from separation anxiety disorder [2]. Separation anxiety disorder may even develop in children and adolescents who, previously, had no concerns about separation.

Most children with selective mutism also meet the criteria for social phobia. Prevalence ranges from 0.11% in clinical settings to 2.0% in population surveys [3]. It is slightly more common in girls. Many children with selective mutism have pre-morbid speech and language problems. Co-morbidities include developmental delay/disorder, communication disorder, elimination disorders and anxiety disorders.

References

1. World Health Organization. *International classification of diseases*, 11th edition (ICD-11). Geneva: World Health Organization; 2024. Available from: https://icd.who.int/en

2. American Psychiatric Association. *Diagnostic and statistical manual of mental disorders*, 5th edition, text revision (DSM-5-TR). Washington, DC: American Psychiatric Association Publishing; 2022. Available from: www.psychiatry.org/psychiatrists/practice/dsm

3. Thapar A. *Rutter's child and adolescent psychiatry*, 6th edition. Chichester: Wiley; 2015.

Case 11: Obsessive–Compulsive Disorder

The thoughts keep coming

Faith is a 24-year-old lady who has had pervasive thoughts that 'something bad is going to happen' for the past year. These intrusive thoughts usually come in the form of doubts. Whenever she leaves a room, she checks the door lock repeatedly. She recognises that such thoughts are irrational but struggles to ignore them. She has since developed a routine of locking the door which involves counting four counts of eight. She is unable to explain why she has to carry out this ritual but describes a sense of discomfort if it is not adhered to, having to repeat her routine if interrupted. These routines were formed to assuage her anxiety, giving her a sense of relief. However, it is time-consuming, and she is often late for her work. Her family is also worried about the perceived oddness of her behaviours.

- **Question 1: Does she fulfil the criteria for obsessive–compulsive disorder (OCD)? What other differential diagnoses will you consider?**

- **Question 2: What physical health investigations would you order to confirm your diagnosis and guide management?**

- **Question 3: What are the common co-morbidities associated with OCD?**

- **Question 4: At the point of Faith's presentation, what is her prognosis like?**

- **Question 5: How would you treat Faith's OCD symptoms?**

Faith was started on a course of fluoxetine for her OCD but, unfortunately, her symptoms did not remit. She was switched over to clomipramine but did not respond either.

- **Question 6: What other management options are there for treatment-resistant OCD?**

Answers to Case 11

Question 1
Does she fulfil the criteria for OCD? What other differential diagnoses will you consider?

Answer
Faith's symptoms are consistent with a diagnosis of OCD. Differentials include specific phobias, obsessive–compulsive personality disorder (OCPD) and psychotic disorders.

Explanation
Faith fulfils the diagnosis of OCD, as she experiences obsessions and compulsions which are time-consuming and ego-dystonic, causing her significant distress.

Diagnosis of OCD [1]

The presence of persistent obsessions and/or compulsions is required for diagnosis.

Obsessions are defined as:

- Repetitive and persistent thoughts (e.g., of contamination), images (e.g., of violent scenes) or impulses/urges (e.g., to stab someone) that are experienced as intrusive, unwanted, senseless, originate from one's own thoughts and are commonly associated with anxiety

- The individual typically attempts to ignore or suppress obsessions or to neutralize them by performing compulsions

Compulsions are defined as:

- Repetitive behaviours or rituals, including repetitive mental acts, that the individual feels driven to perform in response to an obsession, according to rigid rules, or to achieve a sense of 'completeness'

- Examples of overt behaviours include repetitive washing, checking and ordering of objects

- Examples of analogous mental acts include mentally repeating specific phrases in order to prevent negative outcomes, reviewing a memory to make sure that one has caused no harm and mentally counting objects

- Compulsions are either not connected in a realistic way to the feared event (e.g., arranging items symmetrically to prevent harm to a loved one) or are clearly excessive (e.g., showering daily for hours to prevent illness)

An obsession can exist as a doubt, image, or rumination. The patient attempts to ignore or suppress such obsession. Common obsessions include symmetry (31%) and fear of contamination (45%) [2].

A compulsion is usually thematically related to the obsession, and it is aimed to reduce distress or anxiety. A compulsion is usually not pleasurable to an individual and is excessive. It is also not usually connected realistically with what it is designed to neutralise. Common compulsions include checking (63%), and handwashing (50%) [2].

In specific phobias, fears are often managed through avoidance only (there are no compulsions). OCPD is characterised by excessive perfectionism, orderliness and control, associated with compulsivity in performing tasks in a 'correct' manner. OCPD as a diagnosis is less likely as the obsessive–compulsive symptoms are ego-dystonic and the onset of the symptoms is acute. Some patients with the psychotic symptom of thought insertion may describe their symptoms as an 'obsession' and other symptoms of psychosis should be screened for as well.

Exam Essentials

- Other themes of obsession include violence, sex, religion and doubts

- In OCD, there may be more than one obsession or compulsion. Hence, it is important to screen for other themes of obsession or compulsive behaviours

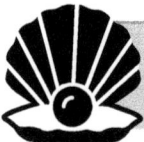

Clinical Pearls

- Assess the level of insight (how much they believe their obsessions to be true)
- The Yale–Brown Obsessive Compulsive Scale (Y-BOCS) [3] can be used to guide diagnosis and monitor the improvement of symptoms
- For psychotic patients with intrusive thoughts, you need to differentiate between thought insertion and OCD

Question 2

What physical health investigations would you order to confirm your diagnosis and guide management?

Answer

Category	Investigations
Point-of-care test	ECG Urine drug screen
Biochemistry	Full blood count Electrolytes: sodium Liver function test Thyroid function test

Explanation

We need to be judicious in balancing the organic workup and over-investigating. Hence, it is advisable to do only the screening tests as stated above, and have further investigations guided by abnormalities. ECG is important as prolonged QTc might preclude the patient from medications such as clomipramine.

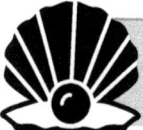

Clinical Pearls

- OCD usually presents in adolescence and early adulthood. **If symptoms present suddenly in later years, it is important to rule out organic causes**

Question 3
What are the common co-morbidities associated with OCD?

Answer
The following are common co-morbidities [4–7]:

- Anxiety disorders (76%)

- Suicidality (46%)

- Major depressive disorder (41%)

- Eating disorders such as anorexia nervosa or bulimia nervosa (40%)

- Substance use disorder (39%)

- Tic disorder (30%)

- OCPD (23–32%)

- Bipolar disorder (22%)

Explanation
Patients with co-morbidities were often associated with earlier age of onset, severe symptomatology as well as treatment resistance. Suicide risk was noted to be an independent risk in a study. Hence it is important to screen for suicide risk, especially in patients with OCD.

Exam Essentials

- Paediatric autoimmune neuropsychiatric disorders associated with streptococcal infections (PANDAS) is a risk factor for OCD in childhood and adolescence. A child may be diagnosed with PANDAS when OCD, a tic disorder or both suddenly appear following a Group A streptococcus infection, such as strep throat or scarlet fever

Question 4
At the point of Faith's presentation, what is her prognosis like?

Answer
Faith has a good prognosis because she has a relatively short duration of symptoms, good insight and displays help-seeking behaviour.

Explanation
OCD has a high treatment gap (57%) [8] among mental health disorders worldwide. The gap is attributed to poor public awareness and other social factors such as cost and mental health stigmatisation.

Prognostic factors in OCD affecting outcomes	
Favourable	Good pre-morbid social and occupation status Episodic symptoms Fewer avoidant symptoms
Poor	Male Early onset Bizarre compulsions Co-morbid depression Longer duration of untreated illness Presence of tics Poor insight

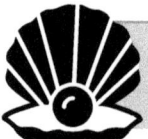

Clinical Pearls

- OCD symptoms usually wax and wane, triggered by stress.
- The type of obsessions and compulsions can also change with time

Question 5
How would you treat Faith's OCD symptoms?

Answer
Medications: selective serotonin reuptake inhibitors (SSRIs such as fluoxetine)
Psychotherapy: exposure response prevention (ERP) therapy; danger ideation reduction therapy (DIRT) for contamination themes

Explanation
OCD should be treated early as a longer duration of untreated disease portends a poorer prognostic. SSRIs are the first line of pharmacological options and are highly recommended. For example, fluoxetine can be titrated to a high dose of 60–80 mg. Clomipramine is just as efficacious as SSRIs but has adverse anticholinergic effects and can reduce the seizure threshold, making it a second-line choice. The Canadian Network for Mood and Anxiety Treatments (CANMAT) guidelines [9] and the Maudsley guidelines [10] both recommend clomipramine as a choice of treatment should SSRIs be ineffective.

ERP is a type of cognitive behavioural therapy (CBT) that has the focus of confronting the subject of anxiety through a graded and prolonged exposure, and for the anxiety to subside without the use of compulsions. It aims to break the obsession–compulsion cycle. DIRT is also recommended by the CANMAT guideline for contamination themes.

With treatment, 20–30% significantly improve, 40–50% show moderate improvement, but 20–40% have chronic or worsening symptoms after treatment [11]. Relapse rates are high after stopping medications.

Exam Essentials

- Treatment:
  - First-line: SSRIs
  - Second-line: clomipramine

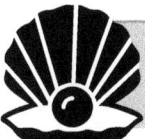

Clinical Pearls

- The antidepressant dosage used to treat OCD is usually higher than that in mood disorder management.

Question 6
What other management options are there for treatment-resistant OCD?

Answer
Other second-line treatment options: mirtazapine, venlafaxine, citalopram
Adjunctive therapy: atypical antipsychotics (e.g. aripiprazole, risperidone)
Third-line treatment options: intravenous clomipramine, intravenous citalopram, duloxetine, phenelzine, tramadol, tranylcypromine, acetylcysteine
Last-line treatment options: surgical interventions (e.g. capsulotomy or cingulotomy)

Explanation
Third-line agents in the treatment of OCD may be useful in patients who have failed first- and second-line monotherapies or in whom adjunct therapies have been ineffective. Adjunctive medication may improve response rates by approximately twice that of a placebo with the most evidence for the addition of risperidone, aripiprazole and quetiapine [12, 13]. Haloperidol as a typical antipsychotic is effective but less well tolerated. However, the addition of antipsychotics carries an additional pharmacological burden and possible adverse effects, which reduces tolerability.

Surgical interventions such as capsulotomy or cingulotomy may be effective in reducing symptoms in patients with severe treatment-refractory OCD; however, its invasive nature relegates surgery to the last line of treatment.

Areas of increasing interest and promise include repetitive transcranial magnetic stimulation (rTMS), which has conflicting results but may improve co-morbid depressive symptoms in patients with OCD. Deep brain stimulation has also been shown to improve symptoms and functionality in up to two-thirds of patients with highly treatment-refractory OCD [9, 14, 15].

Exam Essentials

- Response rates of SSRIs are generally twice that of placebo, with 40–60% responding compared to < 20% with placebo [16]

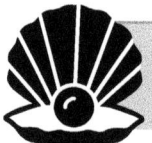

Clinical Pearls

- Atypical antipsychotics can be used for augmentation (e.g., aripiprazole, risperidone, quetiapine)

Diving Deep …

The lifetime prevalence of OCD worldwide is estimated at 2% [17]. The mean age of onset is young at 20 years of age.

Sydenham's chorea (up to 70% of cases) [18], Tourette's syndrome and post-encephalitis parkinsonism are associated with OCD.

Possible aetiological factors of OCD include neurochemical dysregulation of the serotonin system, cell-mediated autoimmune factors (such as that seen in Sydenham's chorea), neuroimaging changes (bilateral reduction in caudate size, hypermetabolism in the orbitofrontal gyrus, basal ganglia and cingulum), genetic factors (3–7% of first-degree relatives affected) [11], psychological factors (defective arousal system or inability to control unpleasant internal states) and psychoanalytical factors ('obsessional neurosis' coined by Freud is described to be the result of regression from the oedipal stage to the pre-genital anal-erotic stage of development as a defence against aggressive or sexual impulses). Defence mechanisms such as isolation, undoing and reaction formation may be seen in patients with OCD.

References

1. World Health Organization. *International classification of diseases*, 11th edition (ICD-11). Geneva: World Health Organization; 2024. Available from: https://icd.who.int/en

2. Boland RJ, Verduin ML, Ruiz P, Shah A, Sadock BJ, editors. *Kaplan & Sadock's synopsis of psychiatry*, 12th edition. Philadelphia: Wolters Kluwer; 2022.

3. Goodman WK, Price LH, Rasmussen SA, Mazure C, Fleischmann RL, Hill CL, et al. The Yale–Brown Obsessive Compulsive Scale. I. Development, use, and reliability. *Arch Gen Psychiatry*. 1989 Nov;46(11):1006–11.

4. Pallanti S, Grassi G, Sarrecchia ED, Cantisani A, Pellegrini M. Obsessive–compulsive disorder comorbidity: clinical assessment and therapeutic implications. *Front Psychiatry*. 2011;2:70.

5. American Psychiatric Association. *Diagnostic and statistical manual of mental disorders*, 5th edition, text revision (DSM-5-TR). Washington, DC: American Psychiatric Association Publishing; 2022. Available from: www.psychiatry.org/psychiatrists/practice/dsm

6. Kaye WH, Bulik CM, Thornton L, Barbarich N, Masters K. Comorbidity of anxiety disorders with anorexia and bulimia nervosa. *Am J Psychiatry*. 2004 Dec;161(12):2215–21.

7. Angelakis I, Gooding P, Tarrier N, Panagioti M. Suicidality in obsessive compulsive disorder (OCD): a systematic review and meta-analysis. *Clin Psychol Rev*. 2015 Jul;39:1–15.

8. Kohn R, Saxena S, Levav I, Saraceno B. The treatment gap in mental health care. *Bull World Health Organ*. 2004 Nov;82(11):858–66.

9. Kennedy SH, Lam RW, McIntyre RS, Tourjman SV, Bhat V, Blier P, et al. Canadian Network for Mood and Anxiety Treatments (CANMAT) 2016 clinical guidelines for the management of adults with major depressive disorder: Section 3. Pharmacological Treatments. *Can J Psychiatry*. 2016 Sep;61(9):540–60.

10. Taylor DM, Barnes TRE, Young A. *The Maudsley prescribing guidelines in psychiatry*, 14th edition. Chichester Hoboken, NJ: Wiley Blackwell; 2021.

11. Semple D, Smyth R. *Oxford handbook of psychiatry*, 4th edition. Oxford: Oxford University Press; 2019.

12. Ipser JC, Carey P, Dhansay Y, Fakier N, Seedat S, Stein DJ. Pharmacotherapy augmentation strategies in treatment-resistant anxiety disorders. *Cochrane Database Syst Rev*. 2006 Oct 18; 2006(4): CD005473. Available from: https://doi.wiley.com/10.1002/14651858.CD005473.pub2

13. Katzman MA, Bleau P, Blier P, Chokka P, Kjernisted K, Van Ameringen M, et al. Canadian clinical practice guidelines for the management of anxiety, posttraumatic stress and obsessive–compulsive disorders. *BMC Psychiatry*. 2014;14(Suppl 1):S1.

14. Greenberg BD, Gabriels LA, Malone DA, Rezai AR, Friehs GM, Okun MS, et al. Deep brain stimulation of the ventral internal capsule/ventral striatum for obsessive-compulsive disorder: worldwide experience. *Mol Psychiatry*. 2010 Jan;15(1):64–79.

15. Goodman WK, Foote KD, Greenberg BD, Ricciuti N, Bauer R, Ward H, et al. Deep brain stimulation for intractable obsessive compulsive disorder: pilot study using a blinded, staggered-onset design. *Biol Psychiatry*. 2010 Mar 15;67(6):535–42.

16. Soomro GM, Altman D, Rajagopal S, Oakley-Browne M. Selective serotonin re-uptake inhibitors (SSRIs) versus placebo for obsessive compulsive disorder (OCD). *Cochrane Database Syst Rev*. 2008 Jan 23;2008(1):CD001765.

17. Sasson Y, Zohar J, Chopra M, Lustig M, Iancu I, Hendler T. Epidemiology of obsessive–compulsive disorder: a world view. *J Clin Psychiatry*. 1997;58(Suppl 12):7–10.

18. Asbahr FR, Negrão AB, Gentil V, Zanetta DM, da Paz JA, Marques-Dias MJ, et al. Obsessive–compulsive and related symptoms in children and adolescents with rheumatic fever with and without chorea: a prospective 6-month study. *Am J Psychiatry*. 1998 Aug;155(8):1122–4.

Case 12: Body Dysmorphic Disorder

The mirror's deception

Harry is a 25-year-old gentleman who is disturbed by how his nose looks in the mirror. He mentions that he is only here for a psychiatric review because his plastic surgeon told him it is a mandatory review before any operation. He claims his nose is crooked after a ball hit his face three years ago during a basketball game. Despite having multiple doctors and friends reassure him that his nose looks normal, he remains distressed. He spends many hours each day checking his nose in the mirror. When his partner tells him that his nose looks fine, it relieves Harry's concerns for only a short while before the doubts recur. Previous imaging of his nose did not reveal any abnormality of his nasal cavity, cartilage or bony structure in his face.

- **Question 1: What is Harry's diagnosis?**

- **Question 2: What are some differential diagnoses that are important to rule out?**

- **Question 3: What are the common psychiatric co-morbidities of body dysmorphic disorder?**

- **Question 4: What are some important points to enquire about during history taking to complete your assessment of Harry's body dysmorphic disorder?**

- **Question 5: How would you manage Harry's body dysmorphic disorder?**

Answers to Case 12

Question 1
What is Harry's diagnosis?

Answer

Body dysmorphic disorder

Diagnosis of body dysmorphic disorder [1]

1. Persistent preoccupation with one or more perceived defects or flaws in appearance, or ugliness in general, that is either unnoticeable or only slightly noticeable to others, is required for diagnosis

2. The presentation is characterised by excessive self-consciousness about the perceived defects or flaws, often including ideas of self-reference (the conviction that people are taking notice, judging or talking about the perceived defects or flaws)

3. The preoccupation or self-consciousness is accompanied by any of the following:

   - Repetitive and excessive behaviours, such as repeated examination of the appearance or severity of the perceived defects or flaws (e.g., by checking in reflective surfaces) or comparison of the relevant features with those of others

   - Excessive attempts to camouflage or alter the perceived defects or flaws (e.g., specific and elaborate forms of dress, undergoing ill-advised cosmetic surgical procedures)

   - Marked avoidance of social or other situations or stimuli that increase distress about the perceived defects or flaws (e.g., reflective surfaces, changing rooms, swimming pools)

Explanation

Harry presents with a preoccupation that a particular aspect of his physical appearance is abnormal. Such belief has the characteristics of an overvalued idea and is usually not amenable to reassurance. At times, even if there is an abnormality, it should only be deemed as slight to everyone else. There is repetitive behaviour of checking the mirror in response to his concerns but, in this case, there is no evidence that his nose is deformed.

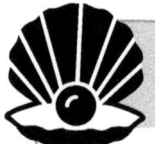

Clinical Pearls

- Rating scales such as the clinician-administered body dysmorphic disorder Yale–Brown Obsessive Compulsive Scale [2] and the self-administered Body Dysmorphic Disorder Questionnaire (BDDQ) [3] may help with diagnosis

Question 2
What are some differential diagnoses that are important to rule out?

Answer
Delusional disorder, somatic type
Obsessive–compulsive disorder (OCD)
Somatic symptom disorder and illness anxiety disorder
Eating disorders such as anorexia nervosa and bulimia nervosa

Explanation
Patients with body dysmorphic disorder report an over-valued idea of their physical aspect(s), which preoccupies and dominates their thinking without complete conviction, whereas those with delusional disorder report the complete conviction of their concern which is false and unshakable.

While OCD is closely related to body dysmorphic disorder, those with OCD are more likely to report irrationality about their obsessions, whereas those with body dysmorphic disorder will have physical concern(s) with poorer insight.

In somatic symptom disorder, patients are preoccupied with a somatic complaint (such as pain) rather than a body deformity, and in illness anxiety disorder, patients are preoccupied with having a terminal illness rather than the deformity itself.

Patients with anorexia nervosa and bulimia nervosa present with disturbances in the way in which one's body weight or shape is experienced. This is different from those with body dysmorphic disorder where the preoccupation is about the particular aspect(s) of the physical appearance, such as one's face, or arm or thigh only.

Exam Essentials

- It is important to distinguish between an over-valued idea and a delusion. Questions to ask include:
  - What is the degree of conviction?
  - Can it be challenged?
  - Is it in keeping with sociocultural beliefs and background?

Question 3
What are the common psychiatric co-morbidities of body dysmorphic disorder?

Answer
The following are the more common co-morbidities [4–8]:

- Unipolar major depression (75%)

- Personality disorders (40–100%)

- Social anxiety disorder (40%), agoraphobia and other anxiety disorders such as panic disorders (13–20%)

- Substance use disorder (30–50%)

- OCD (33%)

- Eating disorders (33%)

Explanation

In patients with body dysmorphic disorder, the mean number of lifetime co-morbid mental conditions is approximately 2.5 [6, 9].

Question 4

What are some important points to enquire about during history taking to complete your assessment of Harry's body dysmorphic disorder?

Answer

Risk assessment is vital, including suicidality and psychotic symptoms, which may be present due to co-morbid depression. A history of dermatological or cosmetic procedures, and their desire to perform procedures on their own ('self-surgery'), are important to elicit. Always assess for co-morbid psychiatric conditions.

Explanation

It is important to screen for co-morbidities and complete the history taking by doing a risk assessment as well. Suicidality and possible command hallucinations place him at risk to himself and others. Enquire about his personality and the presence of body image/self-esteem issues. A history of procedures done is also an indication of the severity of preoccupations and should prompt the physician to ask about further plans for procedures which may not be medically indicated.

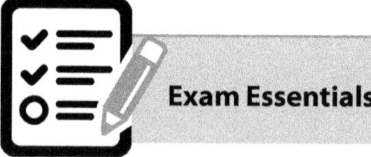

Exam Essentials

- Always ask if the patient has concerns about other body parts

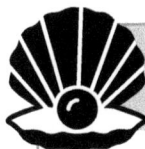

Clinical Pearls

- A unique risk associated with body dysmorphic disorder includes **self-surgery** to alter the perceived flaws
- It is important to check for any index incident that led to the preoccupation (e.g., bullying or comments on the patient's appearance)

Question 5
How would you manage Harry's body dysmorphic disorder?

Answer
Selective serotonin reuptake inhibitors (SSRIs), cognitive behavioural therapy (CBT) or a combination of both.

Explanation
SSRIs are known to reduce symptoms in at least 50% of patients with body dysmorphic disorder [10]. Typically, higher doses of antidepressants are required. If SSRIs do not work, clomipramine may be another option. Augmentation with antipsychotics may improve response in more resistant cases. There is also evidence of CBT or a combination of CBT and medications for such patients. Unfortunately, body dysmorphic disorder is usually associated with a chronic course with fluctuating symptom severity. Partial rather than full remission is usually seen.

Diving Deep …

The prevalence of body dysmorphic disorder is estimated to be approximately 1% in the general population with equal sex incidence [11]. Prevalence may be higher in college student populations, at approximately 5%, and in clinical populations [12].

The areas of the body most commonly affected in body dysmorphic disorder are: skin (e.g., acne, scarring, blemishes, color or wrinkles), hair (e.g., balding or too much facial or body hair), nose (e.g., size or shape), stomach, breasts/chest and eyes [5, 13, 14]. Ideas or delusions of reference, where patients with body dysmorphic disorder believe that other people take special notice of the 'defective' body areas and speak ill about the patient occurs in 60% of patients [15].

Muscle dysmorphia is a subtype where the affected individual is preoccupied with the idea that his or her body build is too small or insufficiently muscular. These individuals may look normal or even very muscular if they abuse androgenic steroids or work out excessively.

References

1. World Health Organization. *International classification of diseases*, 11th edition (ICD-11). Geneva: World Health Organization; 2024. Available from: https://icd.who.int/en

2. Phillips KA, Hollander E, Rasmussen SA, Aronowitz BR, DeCaria C, Goodman WK. A severity rating scale for body dysmorphic disorder: development, reliability, and validity of a modified version of the Yale–Brown Obsessive Compulsive Scale. *Psychopharmacol Bull.* 1997;33(1):17–22.

3. Phillips KA, Atala KD, Pope HG. Diagnostic instruments for body dysmorphic disorder. New Research Program and Abstracts, American Psychiatric Association 148th Annual Meeting, Miami; 1995, p. 157.

4. American Psychiatric Association. *Diagnostic and statistical manual of mental disorders*, 5th edition, text revision (DSM-5-TR). Washington, DC: American Psychiatric Association Publishing; 2022. Available from: www.psychiatry.org/psychiatrists/practice/dsm

5. Phillips KA, Menard W, Fay C, Weisberg R. Demographic characteristics, phenomenology, comorbidity, and family history in 200 individuals with body dysmorphic disorder. *Psychosomatics.* 2005;46(4):317–25.

6. Gunstad J, Phillips KA. Axis I comorbidity in body dysmorphic disorder. *Compr Psychiatry.* 2003;44(4):270–6.

7. Grant JE, Menard W, Pagano ME, Fay C, Phillips KA. Substance use disorders in individuals with body dysmorphic disorder. *J Clin Psychiatry.* 2005 Mar;66(3):309–16; quiz 404–5.

8. Phillips KA, McElroy SL. Personality disorders and traits in patients with body dysmorphic disorder. *Compr Psychiatry.* 2000;41(4):229–36.

9. Zimmerman M, Mattia JI. Body dysmorphic disorder in psychiatric outpatients: recognition, prevalence, comorbidity, demographic, and clinical correlates. *Compr Psychiatry.* 1998;39(5):265–70.

10. Varma A, Rastogi R. Recognizing body dysmorphic disorder (dysmorphophobia). *J Cutan Aesthet Surg.* 2015;8(3):165–8.

11. Semple D, Smyth R. *Oxford handbook of psychiatry*, 4th edition. Oxford: Oxford University Press; 2019.

12. Bohne A, Wilhelm S, Keuthen NJ, Florin I, Baer L, Jenike MA. Prevalence of body dysmorphic disorder in a German college student sample. *Psychiatry Res.* 2002 Jan 31;109(1):101–4.

13. Koran LM, Abujaoude E, Large MD, Serpe RT. The prevalence of body dysmorphic disorder in the United States adult population. *CNS Spectr.* 2008 Apr;13(4):316–22.

14. Buhlmann U, Glaesmer H, Mewes R, Fama JM, Wilhelm S, Brähler E, et al. Updates on the prevalence of body dysmorphic disorder: a population-based survey. *Psychiatry Res.* 2010 Jun 30;178(1):171–5.

15. Phillips KA. Psychosis in body dysmorphic disorder. *J Psychiatr Res.* 2004 Jan;38(1):63–72.

Case 13: Trichotillomania and Excoriation Disorder

Pulling and picking

Monica is a 14-year-old girl who presented to the hospital with generalised abdominal pain, vomiting and constipation for the past three days. Abdominal X-ray revealed small bowel dilation at the ileocaecal junction. The post-operative diagnosis was revealed to be a small bowel obstruction secondary to a trichobezoar (hairball). Further examination of the patient revealed patchy hair loss; the bedside hair pull test was negative. After further prompting, Monica admits to pulling out her hair whenever she is under stress. This is typically triggered by nasty comments made by her peers or during the school examination period. Despite the awareness of such habits, she reports being unable to stop herself, especially when her emotions are intensely felt.

- **Question 1: What is the diagnosis?**

You diagnosed Monica with trichotillomania.

- **Question 2: Which other co-morbid conditions would you screen for?**

Monica's sister, Stella, has been seen by a dermatologist for recurrent skin infections requiring multiple courses of tetracycline ointments. The dermatologist who reviewed her was unable to find an underlying organic cause for the skin lesions and made a psychiatric referral. On further history, she mentions that during exam periods, she tends to peel off calluses over her palms, and also pick the skin on her forearm. Because of the multiple scars on her arm, she feels ashamed of them and tends to go out in long-sleeved apparel.

- **Question 3: What is your diagnosis?**

- **Question 4: Noting that both trichotillomania and excoriation disorder are of the same spectrum, how would you manage the condition of both sisters?**

Answers to Case 13

Question 1
What is the diagnosis?

Answer
Trichotillomania

Explanation

Diagnosis of trichotillomania (hair-pulling disorder) [1]

1. Recurrent pulling of the individual's hair
2. Unsuccessful attempts to stop or decrease hair-pulling
3. Significant hair loss results from pulling behaviour

Ensure the hair loss is not due to another medical condition (e.g., dermatological condition) or part of another mental disorder (e.g., pulling out hair in response to perceived body defect in body dysmorphic disorder).

Exam Essentials

- Rule out hair loss secondary to alopecia areata, which affects the same gender and age group

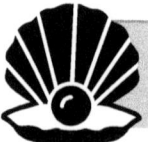

Clinical Pearls

- Dermoscopy in trichotillomania will reveal decreased hair density, short vellus hair and broken hairs with different shaft lengths

Question 2
Which other co-morbid conditions would you screen for?

Answer

Co-morbidities of trichotillomania	
Psychiatric related [2, 3]	Major depressive disorder Anxiety disorders Excoriation disorder (skin picking) Obsessive–compulsive disorder (OCD)
Non-psychiatric related	Musculoskeletal injury (e.g., muscle strains, carpal tunnel syndrome) Intestinal obstruction and associated perforation

Explanation

It is known that patients suffering from trichotillomania often have other repetitive body-focused symptoms that range from skin picking, to nail biting, to lip chewing. OCD is another psychiatric condition to look out for as it is a risk factor for developing trichotillomania. Major depressive disorder and anxiety disorders are noted to be common psychiatric co-morbid conditions.

Musculoskeletal injury can result from the patient's repetitive motion and awkward positioning during the hair-pulling behaviours.

Trichophagia occurs in a subset of patients. It can lead to the formation of trichobezoars as in our case above, and lead to intestinal obstruction and even perforation if intestinal obstruction is complete.

Exam Essentials

- Screen for any underlying causes or stressors that lead to the development of trichotillomania

Question 3
What is your diagnosis?

Answer
Excoriation (skin picking) disorder

Explanation

Diagnosis of excoriation (skin-picking) disorder [1]

1. Recurrent picking of the individual's skin

2. Unsuccessful attempts to stop or decrease skin picking

3. Significant skin lesions resulting from picking behaviour

Ensure the skin picking is not due to another medical condition (e.g., dermatological condition) or part of another mental disorder (e.g., picking at skin in response to perceived body defect in body dysmorphic disorder).

Question 4

Noting that both trichotillomania and excoriation disorder are of the same spectrum, how would you manage the condition of both sisters?

Answer

Psychotherapy: behavioural therapy, habit reversal therapy (HRT)
Pharmacological options: selective serotonin reuptake inhibitors (SSRIs), glutamatergic agents, antipsychotic medications, naltrexone

Explanation

Behavioural therapy is considered the mainstay therapy in patients who are motivated to cooperate with therapy demands [4]. Pharmacological options should be considered for patients who are unable to cooperate with behavioural therapy or have a strong preference for medications over psychotherapy.

HRT has an emphasis on behavioural change which differs from standard cognitive behavioural therapy (CBT), yet is seen to have additional benefits of taping on techniques from acceptance and commitment therapy (ACT), dialectical behavioural therapy (DBT) and CBT.

Currently, there is no first-line pharmacological management. The medications suggested above have shown clinical improvement in patients as demonstrated in multiple case reports and studies.

 **Exam Essentials**

- Behavioural therapy is considered the first-line treatment in patients who are motivated to cooperate with therapy demands

Diving Deep ...

Amongst patients with trichotillomania, there are different subtypes based on the demonstrated clinical behaviour. These subtypes have slightly different treatments as well as prognoses and associated co-morbidities. The subtypes are focused and automatic pulling. Focused pulling refers to hair-pulling behaviour that the patient is aware of and is often a response to negative feelings or events. Automatic pulling refers to hair pulling outside of the patient's awareness.

Multiple studies [5, 6] have suggested that the nature of automatic hair-pulling behaviour makes these subtypes of patients less amenable to HRT compared to their counterparts with the focused pulling subtype. Therefore, it has been suggested that an increased component of awareness training for the automatic subtype of patients be included in therapy. However, in the clinical setting, many patients exhibit both focused and automatic subtype behaviour and can progressively develop alternate subtype hair-pulling behaviours. Focused pulling was shown to be associated with a comparatively lower quality of life, and increased anxiety and depression.

References

1. World Health Organization. *International classification of diseases*, 11th edition (ICD-11). Geneva: World Health Organization; 2024. Available from: https://icd.who.int/en

2. Grant JE, Redden SA, Medeiros GC, Odlaug BL, Curley EE, Tavares H, et al. Trichotillomania and its clinical relationship to depression and anxiety. *Int J Psychiatry Clin Pract*. 2017 Nov;21(4):302–6.

3. American Psychiatric Association. *Diagnostic and statistical manual of mental disorders*, 5th edition, text revision (DSM-5-TR). Washington, DC: American Psychiatric Association Publishing; 2022. Available from: www.psychiatry.org/psychiatrists/practice/dsm

4. Boland RJ, Verduin ML, Ruiz P, Shah A, Sadock BJ, editors. *Kaplan & Sadock's synopsis of psychiatry*, 12th edition. Philadelphia: Wolters Kluwer; 2022.

5. Grant JE, Chamberlain SR. Trichotillomania and skin-picking disorder: an update. *Focus (Am Psychiatr Publ)*. 2021 Oct;19(4):405–12.

6. Grant JE, Chamberlain SR. Automatic and focused hair pulling in trichotillomania: valid and useful subtypes? *Psychiatry Res*. 2021 Dec;306:114269.

Case 14: Hoarding Disorder

What a mess

Fiona, a 58-year-old lady, has been hospitalised for recurrent falls. The medical social worker and occupational therapist made a home visit and found her living conditions to be excessively cluttered. There was minimal space even to constitute a walkway and, concerningly, newspapers were found inside her oven. Suggestions were made to clear up the home environment to reduce fall hazards. However, on follow-up visits by the allied health professionals, the house remained in a similar state. When help was offered to clear up the house, Fiona expressed strong objection and reluctance to throw away the objects, stating they had sentimental value. Fiona refused to meet the team again, and a referral was made to the psychiatric department.

- **Question 1: What is the diagnosis?**

- **Question 2: What are the risk factors associated with hoarding disorder?**

- **Question 3: What are the possible alternative causes of hoarding?**

- **Question 4: What are the common psychiatric co-morbidities of hoarding?**

- **Question 5: How would you manage hoarding disorder?**

Answers to Case 14

Question 1
What is the diagnosis?

Answer
Hoarding disorder

Explanation

> ### Diagnosis of hoarding disorder [1]
>
> 1. Accumulation of possessions that results in living spaces becoming cluttered to the point that their use or safety is compromised is required for diagnosis. Note: if living areas are uncluttered, this is only due to the intervention of third parties (e.g., family members, cleaners, authorities). Accumulation occurs due to both:
>
>   • Repetitive urges or behaviours related to amassing items, which may be passive (e.g., accumulation of incoming flyers or mail) or active (e.g., excessive acquisition of free, purchased or stolen items)
>
>   • Difficulty discarding possessions due to a perceived need to save items, and distress associated with discarding them

In hoarding disorder, the difficulty of discarding is more persistent than merely the result of transient life circumstances leading to excessive clutter. The main reasons for the persistence of difficulty in discarding include perceived utility, aesthetic value or strong sentimental attachment. The intentional saving of possessions is a distinguishing feature from a passive accumulation of items or absence of distress when items are removed. Clutter refers to unrelated or marginally related objects piled together in a disorganised fashion in spaces designed for other purposes. The cluttering of 'active' living areas of the home, which hinders the intended use of these areas, is distinguished from the more peripheral areas, such as garages, attics or basements.

 **Exam Essentials**

• Hoarding disorder is likely to be egosyntonic as compared to OCD, which is often egodystonic

• Explore the risk of falls, fires from storing flammable items and harm to others (i.e., those involved in decluttering)

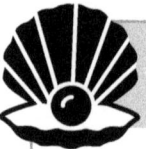

Clinical Pearls

- Diogenes syndrome is a form of hoarding in older people, which is associated with extreme self-neglect and domestic squalor
- Hoarding disorder is not diagnosed if the act of hoarding occurs as a direct consequence of a neurodegenerative disorder (e.g., dementia)

Question 2
What are the risk factors associated with hoarding disorder?

Answer
Risk factors can be split into modifiable and non-modifiable:

- Modifiable: low household income

- Non-modifiable: increased age, male, positive family history for hoarding

Explanation
Household income is inversely related to the development of hoarding disorders [2, 3]. Hoarding is known to be three times more common in the elderly population [3]. Hoarding behaviour is familial; more than 50% of individuals who hoard report having a relative who also hoards. Twin studies indicate that approximately 50% of the variability in hoarding behaviour is attributable to additive genetic factors and the rest to non-shared environmental factors [2, 3].

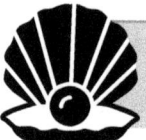

Clinical Pearls

- Hoarding disorder often starts in early adolescence and persists throughout a lifetime, **worsening in severity with age**

Question 3
What are the possible alternative causes of hoarding?

Answer
Organic causes: dementia, brain injuries, cerebrovascular accidents, Prader–Willi syndrome
Psychiatric causes: obsessive–compulsive disorder, major depressive disorder, schizophrenia, autism

Explanation

Hoarding disorder is diagnosed only when alternative organic and psychiatric causes have been ruled out. Organic causes could impair an individual's judgement, ability to sort or physical ability to clear out the clutter. Hoarding has been found in patients with brain injuries and dementia [4, 5]. Psychiatric causes can cause a lack of motivation or psychotic states, which leave patients unable to clear out the clutter.

Exam Essentials

- Hoarding disorder is diagnosed only when alternative organic and psychiatric causes have been ruled out

Question 4

What are the common psychiatric co-morbidities of hoarding?

Answer

The following are common psychiatric co-morbitides of hoarding [6–10]:

- Generalised anxiety disorder (31–37%)
- Major depressive disorder (26–31%)
- Panic disorder (17%)
- Obsessive–compulsive disorder (15–20%)
- Social anxiety disorder (14%)
- Post-traumatic stress disorder (14%)

Explanation

Patients typically present with their psychiatric co-morbidities rather than for hoarding disorder as their main complaint [11].

Question 5

How would you manage hoarding disorder?

Answer

Multidisciplinary management and engaging community resources including specialised cognitive behavioural therapy (CBT) as well as pharmacological options [12–14]:

- CBT: Similar to that used to treat OCD (exposure and response prevention therapy)
- Pharmacological options include selective serotonin reuptake inhibitors (SSRIs), venlafaxine, naltrexone, augmentation with quetiapine

135

- Referrals to allied health including the occupational therapist, medical social worker and community resources

Explanation

Specific CBT elements for hoarding disorder include restriction on the acquisition, sorting and discarding practises and cognitive restructuring to challenge thoughts and beliefs about attachment to items. Psychotherapy is seen to outdo pharmacological therapy in such patients. However, it is common for patients to have poor insight, and be poorly motivated towards treatment.

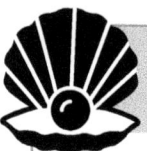

Clinical Pearls

- Management of patients with hoarding disorder is usually difficult due to the patient's limited insight into hoarding as a problem

- Only 18% of patients with hoarding disorder responded to medication and CBT [15]

Diving Deep ...

The Clutter Image Rating Scale (CIRS) [16] developed by the International OCD Foundation works by asking patients to compare photos on the CIRS to that of their own homes. There are nine images in increasing order of clutter, which allows physicians to gauge the impact of hoarding on the patient. Other common assessment instruments include the Hoarding Rating Scale [17, 18], which consists of five Likert-type ratings ranging from 0 (none) to 8 (extreme) and is available in an interview and self-report version.

Various studies have suggested that hoarding runs in the family, with twin studies consistently suggesting that this familiality is largely attributable to genetic factors.

Most hoarders do not perceive their act of hoarding to be a problem as they often view it as part of their identity. The accumulation of items tends to be gradual. Hoarding becomes pathological due to the lack of organisation and often is part of an avoidant behaviour towards making decisions about organising possessions. Although it seems to be a benign accumulation of possessions, hoarding poses a risk to both the individuals as well as to those living with them. The items could attract pest infestations, or even eventually lead to death – as they are a fire hazard or cause death by crushing.

References

1. World Health Organization. *International classification of diseases*, 11th edition (ICD-11). Geneva: World Health Organization; 2024. Available from: https://icd.who.int/en

2. American Psychiatric Association. *Diagnostic and statistical manual of mental disorders*, 5th edition, text revision (DSM-5-TR). Washington, DC: American Psychiatric Association Publishing; 2022. Available from: www.psychiatry.org/psychiatrists/practice/dsm

3. Iervolino AC, Perroud N, Fullana MA, Guipponi M, Cherkas L, Collier DA, et al. Prevalence and heritability of compulsive hoarding: a twin study. *Am J Psychiatry*. 2009 Oct;166(10):1156–61.

4. Anderson SW, Damasio H, Damasio AR. A neural basis for collecting behaviour in humans. *Brain*. 2005 Jan;128(Pt 1):201–12.

5. Ayers CR, Najmi S, Mayes TL, Dozier ME. Hoarding disorder in older adulthood. *Am J Geriatr Psychiatry*. 2015 Apr;23(4):416–22.

6. Pertusa A, Frost RO, Fullana MA, Samuels J, Steketee G, Tolin D, et al. Refining the diagnostic boundaries of compulsive hoarding: a critical review. *Clin Psychol Rev*. 2010 Jun;30(4):371–86.

7. Nordsletten AE, Reichenberg A, Hatch SL, Fernández de la Cruz L, Pertusa A, Hotopf M, et al. Epidemiology of hoarding disorder. *Br J Psychiatry*. 2013 Dec;203(6):445–52.

8. Frost RO, Steketee G, Tolin DF. Comorbidity in hoarding disorder. *Depress Anxiety*. 2011 Oct 3;28(10):876–84.

9. Fullana MA, Vilagut G, Rojas-Farreras S, Mataix-Cols D, de Graaf R, Demyttenaere K, et al. Obsessive–compulsive symptom dimensions in the general population: results from an epidemiological study in six European countries. *J Affect Disord*. 2010 Aug;124(3):291–9.

10. Mataix-Cols D, Billotti D, Fernández de la Cruz L, Nordsletten AE. The London field trial for hoarding disorder. *Psychol Med*. 2013 Apr;43(4):837–47.

11. Tolin DF, Meunier SA, Frost RO, Steketee G. Hoarding among patients seeking treatment for anxiety disorders. *J Anxiety Disord*. 2011 Jan;25(1):43–8.

12. Piacentino D, Pasquini M, Cappelletti S, Chetoni C, Sani G, Kotzalidis GD. Pharmacotherapy for hoarding disorder: how did the picture change since its excision from OCD? *Curr Neuropharmacol*. 2019;17(8):808–15.

13. Boland RJ, Verduin ML, Ruiz P, Shah A, Sadock BJ, editors. *Kaplan & Sadock's synopsis of psychiatry*, 12th edition. Philadelphia: Wolters Kluwer; 2022.

14. Harrison PJ, Cowen P, Burns T, Fazel M. *Shorter Oxford textbook of psychiatry*, 7th edition. Oxford: Oxford University Press; 2018.

15. Black DW, Monahan P, Gable J, Blum N, Clancy G, Baker P. Hoarding and treatment response in 38 nondepressed subjects with obsessive–compulsive disorder. *J Clin Psychiatry*. 1998;59:420–5.

16. Frost RO, Steketee G, Tolin DF, Renaud S. Development and validation of the Clutter Image Rating. *J Psychopathol Behav Assess*. 2008 Sep;30(3):193–203.

17. Tolin DF, Fitch KE, Frost RO, Steketee G. Hoarding Rating Scale–Self-Report. Available from: https://doi.org/10.1037/t35976-000

18. Tolin DF, Frost RO, Steketee G. A brief interview for assessing compulsive hoarding: the Hoarding Rating Scale-Interview. *Psychiatry Res*. 2010 Jun 30;178(1):147–52.

Case 15: Anorexia Nervosa

A phantom reflection

Jessica is a 14-year-old girl brought to your clinic after an episode of fainting in school. This is the second time Jessica has fainted in school after ballet class. On both occasions, she felt lethargic and weak midway through the lesson. Before fainting, she was well and had no chest pain, shortness of breath or palpitations. Earlier today, she consumed only an apple for breakfast and skipped lunch afterwards. Jessica admits to deliberately restricting her dietary intake to one meal daily for six months. Her diet consists mainly of fruits or salads. She reports a loss of weight from 45 kg to 32 kg. She worries about gaining weight despite a body mass index (BMI) of 15.2 and feels 'fat'. She has a BMI goal of less than 14.0. She denies hearing any voices telling her to lose weight and denies deliberately inducing vomiting or using laxatives to lose weight. There is no binge eating behaviour.

- **Question 1: What is Jessica's diagnosis?**

- **Question 2: What are the physical examination findings that may occur in a patient with anorexia nervosa?**

On examination, you noted the following:

- Temperature 35.5 °C

- Lying blood pressure 98/60 mmHg. Standing blood pressure 77/51 mmHg

- Heart rate 50 beats per minute

Clinical examination:

- Thin (BMI 15.2) and emaciated

- Mucous membranes and tongue dry

- Lanugo body hair present

- Heart, lungs and abdominal examinations were unremarkable

- No physical injuries from her syncopal event

- **Question 3: Would you admit Jessica as an inpatient? Please justify your answer.**

You admit Jessica to the ward and perform point-of-care and biochemical tests.

- **Question 4: What abnormalities in the medical investigations would you expect to find?**

The inpatient team commenced Jessica on a new feeding regime. On day three of her new feeding regimen, she complained of swelling in her hands and feet. Her vitals showed a resting heart rate of 80 beats per minute and her blood pressure was noted to be 130/80 mmHg. Electrolyte abnormalities such as hypophosphataemia, hypokalaemia and hypomagnesaemia were noted in her latest biochemistry results.

- **Question 5: What is Jessica most likely suffering from, as a complication of her new feeding regime?**

Jessica was placed under closer monitoring. Aggressive corrections of her hypophosphataemia, hypokalaemia and hypomagnesaemia were carried out with supplementations. She underwent nutritional rehabilitation during her inpatient stay.

- **Question 6: What is the next step of management of anorexia nervosa after Jessica is medically stable?**

Answers to Case 15

Question 1
What is Jessica's diagnosis?

Answer
Anorexia nervosa – restricting type

Explanation

Diagnosis of anorexia nervosa [1]

1. Significantly low body weight for the individual's height, age, developmental stage or weight history is required for diagnosis. A commonly used threshold is a BMI of less than 18.5 kg/m² in adults and a BMI for age under the 5th percentile in children and adolescents. Rapid weight loss (e.g., more than 20% of total body weight within six months) may replace the essential feature of low body weight, as long as other diagnostic requirements are met. Children and adolescents may exhibit failure to gain weight as expected based on the individual developmental trajectory rather than weight loss

2. Low body weight is not better accounted for by another medical condition or the unavailability of food

3. The presentation is characterised by a persistent pattern of restrictive eating or other behaviours aimed at establishing or maintaining abnormally low body weight, typically associated with extreme fear of weight gain. Behaviours may be aimed at reducing energy intake by fasting, choosing low-calorie food, excessively slow eating of small amounts of food, and hiding or spitting out food, as well as by purging behaviours such as self-induced vomiting and use of laxatives, diuretics or enemas, or omission of insulin doses in individuals with diabetes. Behaviours may also be aimed at increasing energy expenditure through excessive exercise, motor hyperactivity, deliberate exposure to cold and use of medication that increases energy expenditure (e.g., stimulants, weight-loss medication, herbal products for reducing weight, thyroid hormones)

4. Excessive preoccupation with body weight or shape is apparent. Low body weight is overvalued and central to the person's self-evaluation, or the person's body weight or shape is inaccurately perceived to be normal or even excessive. Preoccupation with weight or shape, when not explicitly reported, may be manifested in behaviours such as repeatedly checking body weight using scales; repeatedly checking body shape using tape measures or reflection in mirrors; constantly monitoring the calorie content of food or searching for information on how to lose weight; or exhibiting extreme avoidant behaviours, such as refusal to have mirrors at home, avoidance of tight-fitting clothes, or refusal to know one's weight or to purchase clothing with specified sizing

In addition, she fulfils the restricting pattern of anorexia nervosa as she has not engaged in recurrent episodes of binge eating or purging behaviour in the past three months, and the weight loss is accomplished primarily through dieting, fasting and/or excessive exercise.

The binge-eating/purging type of anorexia nervosa describes an individual who has engaged in recurrent episodes of binge eating or purging behaviour.

Rates of eating disorders are much higher in ballet or modelling schools (7%). Incidence is 10 times higher in females than males [2].

Exam Essentials

- Ask specifically for types of compensatory behaviours:
  - Restricting (e.g., excessive exercising, fasting)
  - Purging (e.g., self-induced vomiting, misuse of laxatives, diuretics)

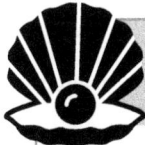

Clinical Pearls

- Severity markers based on BMI kg/m^2:
  - Mild: > 17
  - Moderate: 16–16.9
  - Severe: 15–15.9
  - Extreme: < 15

- The SCOFF screening questions [3] act as a preliminary screening instrument if there is suspicion of an eating disorder

- Rating scales such as the self-rated Eating Attitudes Test (EAT-26) [4] may be used to measure symptoms and concerns characteristic of eating disorders

Question 2

What are the physical examination findings that may occur in a patient with anorexia nervosa?

Answer

System	Physical signs
Nervous	Impaired concentration Slowed cognitive performance Peripheral neuropathy

System	Physical signs
Dermatology	Dry skin Brittle hair Hair loss Lanugo body hair Pallor Hypercarotenaemia (yellow skin and sclera) Hypothermia
Cardiovascular	Bradycardia Low blood pressure, postural hypotension
Musculoskeletal	Myopathy Loss of muscle mass
Reproductive	Atrophy of breasts
Gastrointestinal	Swollen and tender abdomen (intestinal dilatation due to reduced motility and constipation)

Explanation

The categorisation of physical examination findings of anorexia nervosa can be done from a head-down approach or via a systems approach.

Exam Essentials

- **Russell's sign** refers to calloused skin over the interphalangeal joints from repeated self-induced vomiting via finger

- Other signs of repeated self-induced vomiting include erosion of tooth enamel, dental caries and parotid gland enlargement

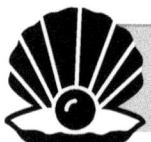

Clinical Pearls

- The most common cardiac complication is bradycardia (< 60 beats per minute)

Question 3
Would you admit Jessica as an inpatient? Please justify your answer.

Answer
Yes, Jessica should be admitted. She presented with syncope, a marker of the severity of her condition. This is further supported by the presence of orthostatic hypotension and bradycardia suggesting medical instability.

Explanation
The indications for inpatient care include [2, 5]:

- Weight: body mass index < 15 kg/m^2 or ideal body weight < 70%

- Behavioural concerns: difficult disordered eating habits, which are challenging to manage as an outpatient

- Medical compromise:
  - Pulse < 40 beats per minute
  - Blood pressure < 80/60 mmHg
  - Orthostatic increase in pulse (> 20 beats per minute) or decrease in systolic blood pressure (> 20 mmHg)
  - Cardiac dysrhythmia (e.g., QTc > 499 msec), or any rhythm other than normal sinus rhythm or sinus bradycardia
  - Cardiovascular, hepatic or renal compromise requiring medical stabilisation
  - Marked dehydration
  - Serious medical complications of malnutrition (e.g., electrolyte imbalance, hypo-glycaemia or syncope)

- Psychiatric co-morbidity/risks: severe co-morbid psychiatric conditions and any suicidal thought, intent or plan

- Treatment-related: failure of outpatient treatment or lack of resources for outpatient weight restoration

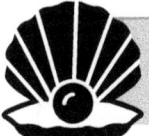

Clinical Pearls

- Anorexia nervosa has **one of the highest mortality rates** among mental illnesses (10–15%) [2, 6]

Question 4
What abnormalities in the medical investigations would you expect to find?

Answer

Investigation	Abnormalities
Full blood count	Anaemia Thrombocytopenia Leucopenia
Electrolyte panel	Raised urea and creatinine Hyponatraemia Hypokalaemia Hypophosphataemia Hypomagnesaemia Hypocalcaemia
Thyroid function tests	Low T3, T4
Liver panel	Transaminitis
Glucose level	Hypoglycaemia
ECG	Sinus bradycardia, prolonged QTc

Explanation

Investigation	Abnormalities
Full blood count	Cytopenias and bone marrow changes are reversible with nutritional rehabilitation
Electrolyte panel	Due to poor oral intake, electrolytes are depleted. Patients may be dehydrated and demonstrate a reduced glomerular filtration rate
Thyroid function tests	A 'euthyroid-sick' pattern of thyroid function tests is commonly seen due to chronic undernutrition
Liver panel	Weight loss and fasting can elevate liver function tests (aspartate aminotransferase and alanine aminotransferase)
Glucose level	Prolonged starvation and low glycogen stores
ECG	The cause of bradycardia appears to be increased parasympathetic (vagal) activity with unchanged sympathetic tone. Anorexia nervosa can cause QT interval prolongation, which predisposes patients to life-threatening ventricular arrhythmias such as torsade de pointes

Question 5
What is Jessica most likely suffering from, as a complication of her new feeding regime?

Answer
Refeeding syndrome

Explanation
Refeeding syndrome is a potentially fatal condition that occurs when patients whose food intake has been severely restricted are given nutrition via oral, enteral or parenteral routes. The sudden reversal of prolonged starvation by the reintroduction of food leads to rapid shifts of electrolytes back into cells from which they had, during starvation, been leached out. Refeeding syndrome usually occurs within 72 hours of refeeding, with a range of two to five days [7].

Features include:

- Hypophosphataemia

- Hypokalaemia

- Seizures

- Congestive heart failure

- Peripheral oedema

- Respiratory insufficiency

- Rhabdomyolysis

- Haemolysis

In Jessica's case, her heart rate of 80 beats per minute should raise alarm bells. We expect to see bradycardia and therefore a seemingly 'normal' heart rate may instead suggest cardiac compromise (relative tachycardia). During the early stages of refeeding, a resting heart rate > 70 beats per minute may suggest heart failure and refeeding syndrome.

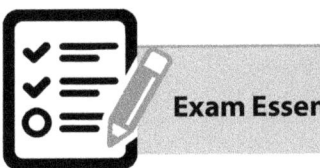

Exam Essentials

- **Hypophosphataemia** is the hallmark manifestation of **refeeding syndrome**
- Refeeding syndrome is potentially fatal and early recognition is essential

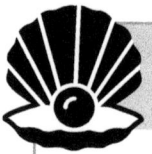

Clinical Pearls

- Regular blood monitoring (potassium, phosphate, magnesium) and ECG monitoring for refeeding syndrome should be done when patients with chronic starvation begin weight restoration treatment, in the first one to two weeks

- Intravenous replacement of phosphate should be initiated if the hypophosphataemia is severe. Replace other electrolytes and vitamin B

- The risk of developing refeeding syndrome is directly related to the amount of weight loss during the current episode and the rapidity of the weight restoration process

Question 6

What is the next step of management of anorexia nervosa after Jessica is medically stable?

Answer

Dietary counselling

Psychological: anorexia nervosa-focused family therapy for children and young people

Pharmacological: medications should not be used as the sole treatment

Explanation

The cornerstone treatment of anorexia nervosa consists of nutritional rehabilitation and psychotherapy. A target weight gain of 0.5–1 kg per week should be set [8, 9], and focus should be placed on multidisciplinary team members such as nurses, dieticians, physicians and family members if deemed appropriate to assist Jessica in her inpatient treatment.

For adults with anorexia nervosa, consider one of:

- Individual eating-disorder-focused cognitive behavioural therapy

- Maudsley Anorexia Nervosa Treatment for Adults (MANTRA)

- Specialist supportive clinical management

For children and young people, consider:

- Anorexia nervosa-focused family therapy for children and young people, delivered as single-family therapy or a combination of single and multi-family therapy

- Family-based treatment, also known as the Maudsley Model, can also be used

Psychotropics, in the setting of anorexia nervosa, are used mainly in the treatment of co-morbid psychiatric illnesses [5, 10, 11].

Exam Essentials

- Poor prognostic factors for anorexia nervosa:
  - Male sex
  - Late age of onset
  - Chronic illness
  - Excessive weight loss
  - Bulimic features (vomiting/purging)
  - Poor parental relationships
  - Poor childhood social adjustment

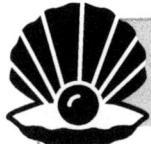

Clinical Pearls

- Treatment of anorexia nervosa requires a multidisciplinary approach and patients will benefit from a community-based, age-appropriate eating disorder service for further assessment or treatment
- **Bupropion, an antidepressant, should be avoided** because it is associated with a higher incidence of seizures in patients with eating disorders, particularly patients who binge-eat and purge. Bupropion can also potentially reduce appetite

Diving Deep …

Avoidant/restrictive food intake disorder (ARFID) is a differential to anorexia nervosa. While restriction in food intake is seen in both conditions, the underlying motivations are different. Patients with anorexia nervosa have body image distortions and a fear of weight gain, while patients with ARFID avoid or restrict food intake due to a lack of interest in food, the sensory characteristics of food or a conditioned negative response associated with food intake following an aversive experience (e.g., choking).

Cardiac complications may increase the incidence of sudden death in anorexia nervosa, especially in patients who weigh less than 80% of their ideal body weight [12]. The weakened heart muscle and hypotension generally improve with weight gain, and heart size normalises with clinical recovery over weeks to months. Total cholesterol levels may be elevated in as many as 50% of patients due to a high level of cardioprotective high-density lipoprotein (HDL) and insignificant elevations in low-density lipoprotein (LDL) [13]. Statin therapy is not needed. The presumptive cause of elevated HDL is excessive exercise and weight loss.

Hypophosphataemia occurs in refeeding syndrome due to a response to carbohydrates, in which the rise in glucose causes a release of insulin, triggering cellular uptake of phosphate (and potassium and magnesium) and a decrease in serum phosphorus levels. Insulin also causes cells to produce a variety of depleted molecules that require phosphate (e.g., adenosine triphosphate and 2,3-diphosphoglycerate), further depleting the body's phosphate stores. Hypophosphataemia causes tissue hypoxia, myocardial dysfunction, respiratory failure due to an inability of the diaphragm to contract, haemolysis, rhabdomyolysis and seizures.

Amenorrhoea is a known complication of anorexia nervosa and may precede weight loss in up to 20% of women with the condition [14]. However, patients with anorexia nervosa may still become pregnant despite being in an amenorrhoeic state [15]. Reproductive function is restored in approximately 80–90% of women following treatment of anorexia nervosa [16].

References

1. World Health Organization. *International classification of diseases*, 11th edition (ICD-11). Geneva: World Health Organization; 2024. Available from: https://icd.who.int/en

2. Semple D, Smyth R. *Oxford handbook of psychiatry*, 4th edition. Oxford: Oxford University Press; 2019.

3. Morgan JF, Reid F, Lacey JH. The SCOFF questionnaire: a new screening tool for eating disorders. *West J Med*. 2000 Mar;172(3):164–5.

4. Garner DM, Olmsted MP, Bohr Y, Garfinkel PE. Eating Attitude Test-26. American Psychological Association; 2013. Available from: http://doi.apa.org/getdoi.cfm?doi=10.1037/t07770-000

5. American Psychiatric Association. *Treatment of patients with eating disorders*, 3rd edition. American Psychiatric Association; 2006.

6. Arcelus J, Mitchell AJ, Wales J, Nielsen S. Mortality rates in patients with anorexia nervosa and other eating disorders. A meta-analysis of 36 studies. *Arch Gen Psychiatry*. 2011 Jul;68(7):724–31.

7. Ponzo V, Pellegrini M, Cioffi I, Scaglione L, Bo S. The refeeding syndrome: a neglected but potentially serious condition for inpatients. A narrative review. *Intern Emerg Med.* 2021 Jan;16(1):49–60.

8. American Dietetic Association. Position of the American Dietetic Association: nutrition intervention in the treatment of anorexia nervosa, bulimia nervosa, and other eating disorders. *J Am Diet Assoc.* 2006 Dec;106(12):2073–82.

9. Golden NH, Meyer W. Nutritional rehabilitation of anorexia nervosa. Goals and dangers. *Int J Adolesc Med Health.* 2004;16(2):131–44.

10. Claudino AM, Hay P, Lima MS, Bacaltchuk J, Schmidt U, Treasure J. Antidepressants for anorexia nervosa. *Cochrane Database Syst Rev.* 2006 Jan 25;2005(1):CD004365.

11. National Institute for Health and Care Excellence (NICE). Eating disorders: recognition and treatment. NICE guideline [NG69]. NICE; 2017. Available from: www.nice.org.uk/guidance/ng69

12. Goldberg SJ, Comerci GD, Feldman L. Cardiac output and regional myocardial contraction in anorexia nervosa. *J Adolesc Health Care.* 1988 Jan;9(1):15–21.

13. Mehler PS, Lezotte D, Eckel R. Lipid levels in anorexia nervosa. *Int J Eat Disord.* 1998 Sep;24(2):217–21.

14. Katz MG, Vollenhoven B. The reproductive endocrine consequences of anorexia nervosa. *BJOG.* 2000 Jun;107(6):707–13.

15. Bulik CM, Hoffman ER, Von Holle A, Torgersen L, Stoltenberg C, Reichborn-Kjennerud T. Unplanned pregnancy in women with anorexia nervosa. *Obstet Gynecol.* 2010 Nov;116(5):1136–40.

16. Chaer R, Nakouzi N, Itani L, Tannir H, Kreidieh D, El Masri D, et al. Fertility and reproduction after recovery from anorexia nervosa: a systematic review and meta-analysis of long-term follow-up studies. *Diseases.* 2020 Dec 16;8(4):46.

Case 16: Bulimia Nervosa

The cycles of excess and regret

Diane is a 22-year-old student who was brought to the clinic by her concerned sister who noted a change in Diane's eating habits over the past year. Diane has been eating large quantities of snacks (e.g., three bags of chips in one sitting) before visiting the bathroom for a long duration after each meal. Diane perceived her weight to be higher than desired and had been self-inducing vomiting after meals. The vomiting makes her feel less guilty after having eaten large quantities of food. She became anxious and was afraid to eat in front of others. She did not want others to see her 'lose control' while eating and would often eat alone to avoid others. On examination, Diane's body mass index (BMI) is 23, and her physical examination revealed thickened calluses over her right knuckles but no other abnormalities.

- **Question 1: What is the most likely diagnosis?**

Diane's sister enquired if the diagnosis could be binge-eating disorder.

- **Question 2: Does Diane fulfil the diagnostic criteria for binge-eating disorder?**

- **Question 3: What are some complications of self-induced vomiting?**

- **Question 4: What are some co-morbidities seen in bulimia nervosa?**

Answers to Case 16

Question 1
What is the most likely diagnosis?

Answer
Bulimia nervosa

Explanation
Bulimia nervosa is characterised by indulgence in binge eating, and inappropriate compensatory behaviours to prevent weight gain. Binge eating and compensatory behaviours both occur at least once a week for three months. Self-induced vomiting is a common inappropriate compensatory method. Individuals who purge may also use laxatives, diuretics or enemas as compensatory behaviours, and many of these products can cause serious medical consequences, which should be screened during your encounter with Diane.

Diagnosis of bullimia nervosa [1]

1. Frequent, recurrent episodes of binge eating (e.g., once a week or more over a period of at least 1 month) are required for diagnosis. Binge eating is defined as a discrete period of time (e.g., two hours) during which the individual experiences a loss of control over their eating behaviour, and eats notably more or differently than usual. Loss of control over eating may be described by the individual as feeling like they cannot stop or limit the amount or type of food eaten; having difficulty stopping eating once they have started; or giving up even trying to control their eating because they know they will end up overeating

2. The presentation is characterised by repeated inappropriate compensatory behaviours to prevent weight gain (e.g., once a week or more over a period of at least one month). The most common compensatory behaviour is self-induced vomiting, which typically occurs within an hour of binge eating. Other inappropriate compensatory behaviours include fasting or using diuretics to induce weight loss, using laxatives or enemas to reduce the absorption of food, omission of insulin doses in individuals with diabetes and strenuous exercise to greatly increase energy expenditure

3. Excessive preoccupation with body weight or shape is apparent. Preoccupation with weight or shape, when not explicitly reported, may be manifested in behaviours such as repeatedly checking body weight using scales; repeatedly checking body shape using tape measures or reflection in mirrors; constantly monitoring the calorie content of food or searching for information on how to lose weight; or exhibiting extreme avoidant behaviours, such as refusal to have mirrors at home, avoidance of tight-fitting clothes or refusal to know one's weight or to purchase clothing with specified sizing

4. There is marked distress about the pattern of binge eating and inappropriate compensatory behaviour, or significant impairment in personal, family, social, educational, occupational or other important areas of functioning. During the early phases of the disorder, symptoms may be concealed and functioning maintained through significant additional effort

5. The symptoms do not meet the diagnostic requirements for anorexia nervosa

The severity of bulimia nervosa is dependent on the frequency of inappropriate compensatory behaviours [2].

Severity of bulimia nervosa as defined by the DSM-5-TR [2]	Number of inappropriate compensatory behaviours per week
Mild	1–3
Moderate	4–7
Severe	8–13
Extreme	≥ 14

Exam Essentials

- An important distinction from anorexia nervosa is that a **diagnosis of anorexia nervosa requires low body weight (BMI < 18)**, whereas this is not a diagnostic criterion for bulimia nervosa. Patients with anorexia nervosa tend to have amenorrhoea while bulimia nervosa patients tend to have normal menses

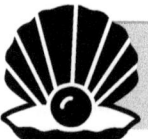

Clinical Pearls

- Both bulimia nervosa and anorexia nervosa patients have body image issues
- Bulimia nervosa patients tend to have fewer medical complications as compared to anorexia nervosa

Question 2
Does Diane fulfil the diagnostic criteria for binge-eating disorder?

Answer
No

Explanation

Diagnosis of binge-eating disorder [1]

1. Frequent, recurrent episodes of binge eating (e.g., once a week or more over a period of three months) are required for diagnosis. Binge eating is defined as a discrete period of time (e.g., two hours) during which the individual experiences a loss of control over their eating behaviour and eats notably more or differently than usual. Loss of control over eating may be described by the individual as feeling like they cannot stop or limit the amount or type of food eaten; having difficulty stopping eating once they have started; or giving up even trying to control their eating because they know they will end up overeating

2. The binge-eating episodes are not regularly accompanied by inappropriate compensatory behaviours aimed at preventing weight gain

The severity of binge-eating disorder is dependent on the frequency of episodes of binge eating [2].

Severity of binge-eating disorder as defined by the DSM-5-TR [2]	Number of binge-eating episodes per week
Mild	1–3
Moderate	4–7
Severe	8–13
Extreme	≥ 14

Binge-eating disorder is characterised primarily by episodes of recurrent binge-eating without compensatory purging behaviours. You may also notice that patients with bulimia nervosa typically restrict their diet between binge-eating episodes to influence their body shape. In contrast, those with binge-eating disorder do not limit their intake in between events.

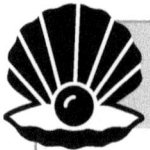

Clinical Pearls

- Patients with binge-eating disorder often suffer from obesity as a co-morbidity, and usually seek treatment for weight reduction

Question 3
What are some complications of self-induced vomiting?

Answer
Common complications [3] include dental enamel erosion, salivary gland hypertrophy, gastro-oesophageal reflux disease and laryngopharyngeal reflex. More serious complications such as Mallory–Weiss syndrome, electrolyte derangement and cardiac arrhythmias should be screened.

Explanation
Dental enamel erosion is a result of gastric acid washing over teeth. Patients often brush their teeth immediately after purging, which can accelerate dental erosion. The clinician should instruct patients who persist in vomiting to rinse their mouths with water or fluoride rather than brush their teeth within 30 minutes of each purging episode.

Salivary gland hypertrophy (sialadenosis) is a common physical sign, which can be detected via physical examination as a swelling around the parotids.

Gastro-oesophageal reflux disease can increase the risk of Barrett's oesophagus (development of abnormal columnar mucosa, which may increase the risk of oesophageal cancer) [4]. Laryngopharyngeal reflux may result in chronic cough.

Mallory–Weiss syndrome can occur due to forceful contraction of the stomach when a patient vomits and may develop into a serious complication known as Boerhaave syndrome (oesophageal rupture).

Cardiac arrhythmia can be caused by hypokalaemia from vomiting leading to QTc prolongation, or the abuse of medications such as ipecac to assist with purging. Ipecac can also cause congestive heart failure and death in severe cases.

Exam Essentials

- Amylase levels are frequently elevated in patients with bulimia nervosa. This may be due to the binge-eating episodes, as well as the purging behaviour

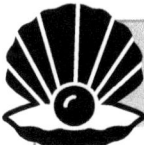

Clinical Pearls

- Complications of laxative, diuretic and enema use should be screened (e.g., chronic abuse of stimulant laxatives such as senna or bisacodyl can result in cathartic colon syndrome)

Question 4
What are some co-morbidities seen in bulimia nervosa?

Answer
Common co-morbid conditions include [2, 5, 6]:

- Unipolar depression: 76%
- Alcohol use disorder: 61%
- Borderline personality disorder: 48%
- Nicotine use disorder: 43%
- Post-traumatic stress disorder: 32%
- Generalised anxiety disorder: 26%

Explanation
Amongst substance use disorders, stimulant use often begins in an attempt to control appetite and weight.

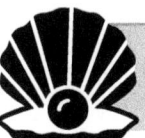

Clinical Pearls

- Patients who abuse stimulants such as cocaine and amphetamine experience weight loss through increased metabolism

Question 5
How would you manage bulimia nervosa?

Answer
Psychotherapy is the first-line treatment, with cognitive behavioural therapy (CBT) having the strongest evidence.

155

Fluoxetine is the only United States Food and Drug Administration (FDA)-approved agent for the treatment of bulimia nervosa.

Explanation

Combination treatment with pharmacotherapy plus psychotherapy is more efficacious than either treatment alone.

Enhanced CBT (CBT-E) is a manualised outpatient therapy which is helpful for eating disorders and is usually given to those who are medically stable and not underweight. Interpersonal psychotherapy is as effective but generally takes longer to achieve results than CBT. Patients who complete psychotherapy have an 80% overall reduction in symptoms [7].

Fluoxetine is the first-line pharmacological agent for bulimia nervosa and is generally well tolerated by patients. Antidepressants have shown efficacy in reducing the frequency of symptoms by 50% [7].

Exam Essentials

- The prognosis for bulimia nervosa is generally good unless there is:
  - Significant low self-esteem
  - A severe personality disorder

Diving Deep ...

Other diagnoses which may present with hyperphagia include Prader–Willi syndrome (a genetic disorder that can present with hyperphagia and obesity, associated with mental disability and hypogonadism, angry outbursts and oppositional behaviour), and Klein–Levin syndrome (a disorder that primarily affects adolescent males and also causes increased appetite, hypersomnia and behavioural disturbances). Compensatory purging behaviour is typically absent in both syndromes.

Other specified feeding or eating disorder (OSFED) is a formal diagnostic category including heterogeneous nosological entities, such as atypical anorexia nervosa, purging disorder, subthreshold bulimia nervosa, subthreshold binge-eating disorder and night eating syndrome.

References

1. World Health Organization. *International classification of diseases*, 11th edition (ICD-11). Geneva: World Health Organization; 2024. Available from: https://icd.who.int/en

2. American Psychiatric Association. *Diagnostic and statistical manual of mental disorders*, 5th edition, text revision (DSM-5-TR). Washington, DC: American Psychiatric Association Publishing; 2022. Available from: www.psychiatry.org/psychiatrists/practice/dsm

3. Forney KJ, Buchman-Schmitt JM, Keel PK, Frank GKW. The medical complications associated with purging. *Int J Eat Disord*. 2016 Mar;49(3):249–59.

4. Dessureault S, Coppola D, Weitzner M, Powers P, Karl RC. Barrett's esophagus and squamous cell carcinoma in a patient with psychogenic vomiting. *Int J Gastrointest Cancer*. 2002;32(1):57–61.

5. Udo T, Grilo CM. Psychiatric and medical correlates of DSM-5 eating disorders in a nationally representative sample of adults in the United States. *Int J Eat Disord*. 2019 Jan;52(1):42–50.

6. Nobles CJ, Thomas JJ, Valentine SE, Gerber MW, Vaewsorn AS, Marques L. Association of premenstrual syndrome and premenstrual dysphoric disorder with bulimia nervosa and binge-eating disorder in a nationally representative epidemiological sample. *Int J Eat Disord*. 2016 Jul;49(7):641–50.

7. Harrison PJ, Cowen P, Burns T, Fazel M. *Shorter Oxford textbook of psychiatry*, 7th edition. Oxford: Oxford University Press; 2018.

Case 17: Pica and Rumination Disorder

You shouldn't eat that!

Tommy is a 5-year-old boy who was brought to the clinic by his mother for concerns over his eating habits. Tommy was observed to be eating hair and paper for over one month, despite warnings from his mother to stop. This has resulted in him suffering constipation. Tommy does not have any other significant medical conditions.

- **Question 1: What is the diagnosis?**

- **Question 2: What co-morbidities are common in patients with pica?**

- **Question 3: How does pica differ from rumination disorder?**

- **Question 4: What are the risk factors for rumination disorder?**

Answers to Case 17

Question 1
What is the diagnosis?

Answer
Pica

Explanation

Diagnosis of pica [1]

1. Regular consumption of non-nutritive substances, such as non-food objects and materials (e.g., clay, soil, chalk, plaster, plastic, metal and paper) or raw food ingredients (e.g., large quantities of salt or corn flour), is required for diagnosis

2. The ingestion of non-nutritive substances is persistent or severe enough to require clinical attention. That is, the behaviour causes damage or significant risk to health or impairment in functioning due to the frequency, amount or nature of the substances or objects ingested

3. Based on age and level of intellectual functioning, the individual would be expected to distinguish between edible and non-edible substances. In typical development, this occurs at approximately two years of age

4. The symptoms or behaviours are not a manifestation of another medical condition (e.g., nutritional deficiency)

Pica is not usually diagnosed where the ingestion of non-food items is part of a culturally sanctioned practice. A minimum age of two years is suggested for a pica diagnosis to exclude developmentally normal mouthing of objects by infants that results in ingestion.

Differential diagnoses include anorexia nervosa, avoidant/restrictive food intake disorder, factitious disorder and non-suicidal self-injury.

Treatment involves decreasing exposure to the craved substance, such as reducing access or providing an appropriate substitute with a similar texture. Nutritional supplementation, such as iron, zinc and other nutrients, should be carried out if deficiencies are identified. Behavioural treatment and mild aversion therapy might be effective in patients with mental disabilities [2]. In mild aversion therapy, pica behaviour is associated with negative consequences while the child receives positive reinforcement for eating normal foods. Differential reinforcement works by teaching the patient to focus on other behaviours and activities and avoiding pica behaviour.

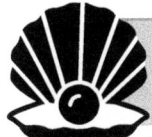

Clinical Pearls

- Pica can lead to severe medical sequelae, including poisoning and obstructions or perforations in the gastrointestinal tract. In some instances, it is associated with appetite loss and reduced intake, weight loss and, in extreme cases, can be fatal.

Question 2
What co-morbidities are common in patients with pica?

Answer

Common co-morbidities include [3]:

- Intellectual developmental disorder

- Autism spectrum disorder

- Avoidant/restrictive food intake disorder

- Obsessive–compulsive disorder

- Schizophrenia

Explanation

Pica is most common in children with intellectual developmental disorder or autism spectrum disorder, but may also occur in maltreated or neglected young children.

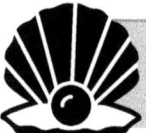

Clinical Pearls

- **Iron studies** should be considered in patients with pica as iron deficiency anaemia has been implicated [4, 5]. Treatment with iron supplementation has been shown to lead to the resolution of symptoms in some cases.

Question 3

How does pica differ from rumination disorder?

Answer

Rumination disorder is characterised by the repeated regurgitation of food that has been swallowed. The regurgitate is then re-chewed (rumination) and swallowed again or spat out. This is in contrast to pica where non-nutritive substances are eaten in large amounts.

Explanation

Diagnosis of rumination disorder [1]

1. The intentional and repeated bringing up of previously swallowed food back to the mouth (regurgitation), which may be re-chewed and re-swallowed (rumination), or may be deliberately spat out (but not as in vomiting), is required for diagnosis

2. The regurgitation behaviour is frequent (at least several times per week) and sustained over a period of at least several weeks

3. The diagnosis should only be assigned to individuals who have reached a developmental age of at least two years

4. The regurgitation behaviour is not a manifestation of another medical condition that directly causes regurgitation (e.g., oesophageal strictures or neuromuscular disorders affecting oesophageal functioning) or causes nausea or vomiting (e.g., pyloric stenosis)

The regurgitation of food occurs without undue effort and is not associated with nausea. Repeated regurgitation can be associated with significant medical problems, such as malnutrition, low weight, dental problems, bad breath and oesophagitis. Rumination disorder occurs in children and adults, in those with intellectual disability as well normally developing individuals. It can be associated with reduced intake and weight loss. Common co-morbidities include generalised anxiety disorder, autism spectrum disorder and intellectual developmental disorder.

Exam Essentials

- Remember to rule out eating disorders

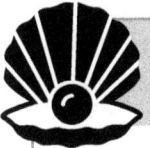

Clinical Pearls

- Remember to rule out organic gastrointestinal causes (e.g., vomiting and gastroesophageal reflux)

Question 4
What are the risk factors for rumination disorder?

Answer
Emotional neglect (in infants) [6]

Emotional stress [6]

Presence of mental health diagnoses such as obsessive–compulsive disorder, anxiety, depression, adjustment disorder, post-traumatic stress disorder and attention deficit hyperactivity disorder [7–9]

Developmental delay

Fibromyalgia [10]

Explanation

The etiology of rumination disorder is likely multifactorial; however, the exact causes are poorly understood [11].

Diving Deep ...

Types of ingested items are variable, including but not limited to earth (geophagy), raw starches (amylophagy), ice (pagophagia), charcoal, ash, paper, chalk, cloth, baby powder, coffee grounds and eggshells. Geophagy is a practice common across sub-Saharan Africa [12] where it is culturally sanctioned to deliberately eat clay or soil. It is prevalent among pregnant women across Sub-Saharan African countries, such as Kenya, Ghana, Rwanda, Nigeria, Tanzania and South Africa. It is the local belief that the consumption of soil may be used to treat morning sickness, nausea and vomiting.

Regurgitation of food in rumination disorder may have a soothing function, playing a role in anxiety management or emotion regulation. It is often a secretive disorder and can be associated with significant impairment to social development and functioning. Common pitfalls include a failure to ask questions related to the possible presence of rumination disorder, which can hinder the identification and diagnosis.

References

1. World Health Organization. *International classification of diseases*, 11th edition (ICD-11). Geneva: World Health Organization; 2024. Available from: https://icd.who.int/en

2. Matson JL, Hattier MA, Belva B, Matson ML. Pica in persons with developmental disabilities: approaches to treatment. *Res Dev Disabil*. 2013 Sep;34(9):2564–71.

3. American Psychiatric Association. *Diagnostic and statistical manual of mental disorders*, 5th edition, text revision (DSM-5-TR). Washington, DC: American Psychiatric Association Publishing; 2022. Available from: www.psychiatry.org/psychiatrists/practice/dsm

4. Roy A, Fuentes-Afflick E, Fernald LCH, Young SL. Pica is prevalent and strongly associated with iron deficiency among Hispanic pregnant women living in the United States. *Appetite*. 2018 Jan 1;120:163–70.

5. Sadeghzadeh M, Khoshnevisasl P, Sadeghzadeh S. The relation between pica and iron deficiency in children in Zanjan, Islamic Republic of Iran: a case–control study. *East Mediterr Health J*. 2017 Aug 20;23(6):404–7.

6. Fleisher DR. Functional vomiting disorders in infancy: innocent vomiting, nervous vomiting, and infant rumination syndrome. *J Pediatr*. 1994 Dec;125(6 Pt 2):S84–94.

7. Barba E, Burri E, Accarino A, Malagelada C, Rodriguez-Urrutia A, Soldevilla A, et al. Biofeedback-guided control of abdominothoracic muscular activity reduces regurgitation episodes in patients with rumination. *Clin Gastroenterol Hepatol*. 2015 Jan;13(1):100–106.e1.

8. Levine DF, Wingate DL, Pfeffer JM, Butcher P. Habitual rumination: a benign disorder. *Br Med J (Clin Res Ed)*. 1983 Jul 23;287(6387):255–6.

9. Halland M, Parthasarathy G, Bharucha AE, Katzka DA. Diaphragmatic breathing for rumination syndrome: efficacy and mechanisms of action. *Neurogastroenterol Motil.* 2016 Mar;28(3):384–91.

10. Almansa C, Rey E, Sánchez RG, Sánchez AA, Díaz-Rubio M. Prevalence of functional gastrointestinal disorders in patients with fibromyalgia and the role of psychologic distress. *Clin Gastroenterol Hepatol.* 2009 Apr;7(4):438–45.

11. Kusnik A VS. *Rumination disorder. StatPearls.* Treasure Island, FL: StatPearls Publishing; 2023. Available from: www.ncbi.nlm.nih.gov/books/NBK576404

12. Nyanza EC, Joseph M, Premji SS, Thomas DS, Mannion C. Geophagy practices and the content of chemical elements in the soil eaten by pregnant women in artisanal and small scale gold mining communities in Tanzania. *BMC Pregnancy Childbirth.* 2014 Apr 15;14:144.

Case 18: Acute Stress Disorder, Post-Traumatic Stress Disorder and Adjustment Disorder

When will my nightmares stop?

The ward nurse has called you to assess Kiandra, a 23-year-old lady currently recovering in the burns intensive care unit (ICU). Kiandra has been tearful, irritable and withdrawn since admission. The nurses also noted that Kiandra appeared hypersensitive to the beeping sounds from the ICU equipment and would get startled easily. She has been unable to sleep well and experiences nightmares and screams in her sleep. She refused to discuss her injury and did not allow her family or neighbours to visit. She was irritable and had trouble concentrating when spoken to. You reviewed the electronic notes and discovered that Kiandra was a victim of a hate crime near her neighbourhood and was set on fire by two perpetrators five days ago. Kiandra says her memory of the events is 'fuzzy' but that she would have frequent flashbacks.

- **Question 1: What is the most likely diagnosis?**

- **Question 2: What are some differential diagnoses you will consider?**

- **Question 3: What are some risk factors for developing acute stress reaction and PTSD?**

- **Question 4: How would you manage Kiandra's acute stress reaction?**

The DSM-5-TR [1] characterises a similar disorder termed 'acute stress disorder', which is similar to acute stress reaction with slight differences in time course. Acute stress disorder requires symptoms to be present for at least three days up to one month while acute stress reaction describes symptoms that appear within hours to days following the stressful event.

- **Question 5: How many patients with acute stress disorder (DSM-5-TR diagnostic entity) develop PTSD in future?**

- **Question 6: Should Kiandra continue to have symptoms for more than a month after the event and fulfil the criteria for PTSD, how would you treat her condition?**

- **Question 7: What are the negative sequelae of untreated PTSD?**

You have started Kiandra on sertraline. Three months later, she continued to report nightmares every night.

- **Question 8: What medication can you consider prescribing for the treatment of nightmares in patients with PTSD?**

You are called to assess Kiandra's cousin, Eunice, a 12-year-old girl who was admitted to the ward after she was found unconscious with an empty bottle of paracetamol next to her. Eunice was quiet and appeared to be zoning out during the clinical interview. For the past one month, her mother noticed that Eunice had been having more nightmares and was tearful at times. She had poor sleep, poor appetite and was withdrawn from her family and friends. After rapport was built, she reveals to you that one month ago her stepfather had raped her and threatened to kill her if she told anyone else about the incident.

- **Question 9: What are the principles of safeguarding a patient who has experienced childhood sexual abuse?**

- **Question 10: What psychiatric disorders are commonly associated with childhood sexual abuse?**

Answers to Case 18

Question 1
What is the most likely diagnosis?

Answer
Acute stress reaction

Explanation
Acute stress reaction is diagnosed in patients after they have experienced a major traumatic event. The duration of symptoms should be between three days and a month.

Diagnosis of acute stress reaction [2]

1. Exposure to an event or situation (either short- or long-lasting) of an extremely threatening or horrific nature is required for diagnosis. Such events include, but are not limited to, directly experiencing natural or human-made disasters, combat, serious accidents, torture, sexual violence, terrorism; assault, acute life-threatening illness (e.g., a heart attack); witnessing the threatened or actual injury or death of others in a sudden, unexpected or violent manner; and learning about the sudden, unexpected or violent death of a loved one

2. There is a response to the stressor that is considered to be normal, given the severity of the stressor. The response to the stressor may include transient emotional, somatic, cognitive or behavioural symptoms, such as being in a daze, confusion, sadness, anxiety, anger, despair, overactivity, inactivity, social withdrawal, amnesia, depersonalisation, derealisation or stupor. Autonomic signs of anxiety (e.g., tachycardia, sweating, flushing) are common, and may be the presenting feature

3. Symptoms typically appear within hours to days following the stressful event, and usually begin to subside within a few days after the event or following removal from the threatening situation, when this is possible. In cases where the stressor is ongoing or removal is not possible, symptoms may persist, but are usually greatly reduced within approximately one month as the person adapts to the changed situation

---

The development of post-traumatic stress disorder (PTSD) is usually within six months after the traumatic event; however, approximately 25% experience a delayed onset after six months or more [3]. PTSD is the incorrect answer as Kiandra did not experience these symptoms for more than a month.

The term 'acute stress reaction' is based on the ICD-10 classification with an equivalent diagnosis in the DSM classification termed 'acute stress disorder'. It should be noted that in ICD-11, the diagnosis of acute stress reaction is no longer regarded as a diagnostic entity but a 'factor influencing health status' as such reactions are considered to be normal brief periods of emotional distress that people experience in response to traumatic experiences and are expected to be resolved within a short period of time.

Exam Essentials

- Symptoms of acute stress reaction last < one month, while those of PTSD last ≥ one month

- Symptoms of trauma-related disorder – **HEARD**

    ○ **H**yperarousal
    ○ **E**motional numbing
    ○ **A**voidance
    ○ **R**ecurrent intrusions
    ○ **D**issociation

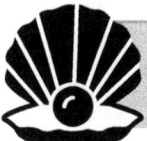

Clinical Pearls

- In patients who present with cognitive impairment, always ascertain if there is a head injury and whether investigations have been done

- Always ask if the patient is seeking any compensation or is involved in legal proceedings. This may perpetuate the symptoms, known as **'compensation neurosis'**

- Often, closure is needed before symptoms may improve

Question 2
What are some differential diagnoses you will consider?

Answer
PTSD, depression, adjustment disorder

Explanation

Diagnosis of PTSD [2]

1. Exposure to an event or situation (either short- or long-lasting) of an extremely threatening or horrific nature is required for diagnosis. Such events include, but are not limited to, directly experiencing natural or human-made disasters, combat, serious accidents, torture, sexual violence, terrorism, assault or acute life-threatening illness (e.g., a heart attack); witnessing the threatened or actual injury or death of others in a sudden, unexpected or violent manner; and learning about the sudden, unexpected or violent death of a loved one

2. Following the traumatic event or situation, the development of a characteristic syndrome lasting for at least several weeks consists of all three of the following core elements:

   A. The traumatic event is re-experienced in the present: it is not just remembered but is experienced as occurring again in the here and now. This typically occurs in the form of vivid intrusive memories or images; flashbacks, which can vary from mild (there is a transient sense of the event occurring again in the present) to severe (there is a complete loss of awareness of present surroundings); or repetitive dreams or nightmares that are thematically related to the traumatic event. Re-experiencing is typically accompanied by strong or overwhelming emotions, such as fear or horror, and strong physical sensations. Re-experiencing in the present can also involve feelings of being overwhelmed or immersed in the same intense emotions that were experienced during the traumatic event, without a prominent cognitive aspect, and may occur in response to reminders of the event. Reflecting on or ruminating about the event and remembering the feelings experienced at that time are not sufficient to meet the re-experiencing requirement

   B. Reminders likely to produce re-experiencing of the traumatic event are deliberately avoided. Deliberate avoidance may take the form either of active internal avoidance of thoughts and memories related to the event, or external avoidance of people, conversations, activities or situations reminiscent of the event. In extreme cases, the person may change their environment (e.g., move to a different city or change jobs) to avoid reminders.

   C. There are persistent perceptions of heightened current threat – for example, as indicated by hypervigilance or an enhanced startle reaction to stimuli such as unexpected noises. Hypervigilant people constantly guard themselves against danger, and feel themselves or others close to them to be under immediate threat either in specific situations or more generally. They may adopt new behaviours designed to ensure safety (e.g., not sitting with their back to the door, repeatedly checking in vehicles' rear-view mirrors)

PTSD should always be considered when a patient is diagnosed with acute stress reaction, as the symptoms may progress and remain for more than a month, requiring more intensive treatment. Depression should also be considered as a differential and a co-morbid condition as she was noted to be tearful. Adjustment disorder is also a possible diagnosis, but the event is traumatic and would fit the diagnosis of acute stress reaction better.

Refer to the Diving Deep section for more information on adjustment disorder.

Exam Essentials

- Traumatic events include exposure to actual or threatened
  ◦ Death
  ◦ Serious injury
  ◦ Sexual violation
- Always screen for substance misuse as a co-morbid condition in PTSD

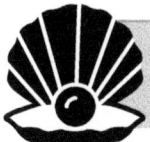

Clinical Pearls

- PTSD includes a dissociative subtype, whereas, in acute stress disorder, depersonalisation and derealisation are included as symptoms under the dissociative heading
- Rating scales such as the Clinician-Administered PTSD Scale (CAPS-5) [4], and the self-administered PTSD Checklist for DSM-5 (PCL-5) [5], may help with diagnosis

Question 3
What are some risk factors for developing acute stress reaction and PTSD?

Answer
Female sex, previous history of psychiatric disorder, previous trauma, increased severity of the traumatic incident, prolonged duration before help is received or lack of social support.

Explanation

PTSD is two to three times more common in females than in males [6]. It is also found that intentional human-inflicted acts such as rape are a risk factor.

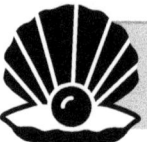

Clinical Pearls

- Common co-morbidities such as depression, anxiety disorders, personality disorders and substance use disorders should be screened: up to 80% of patients with PTSD have another mental disorder [7]

Question 4

How would you manage Kiandra's acute stress reaction?

Answer

One should consider mainly psychological management, including supportive counselling or cognitive behavioural therapy (CBT).

Explanation

You will want to choose a psychological treatment instead of pharmacological treatment in those with acute stress reaction. Psychological debriefing has been found to have no benefit in preventing PTSD [8]. Instead, more extensive, multiple-session cognitive-behavioural interventions appear effective.

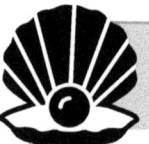

Clinical Pearls

- Acute stress reaction may or may not predict the development of PTSD

Question 5

How many patients with acute stress disorder (DSM-5-TR diagnostic entity) develop PTSD in future?

Answer

Between 40% and 80% of cases

Explanation

Studies showed 40–80% of those with acute stress disorder develop PTSD, while 40–70% of those with PTSD did not meet the criteria for acute stress disorder in the acute phase

[1, 9–12]. Hence, the absence of acute stress disorder does not exclude the possibility of PTSD in future.

Question 6
Should Kiandra continue to have symptoms for more than a month after the event and fulfil the criteria for PTSD, how would you treat her condition?

Answer
Consider pharmacological methods such as a selective serotonin reuptaker inhibitor (SSRI), and psychological methods such as trauma-focused CBT.

Explanation
SSRIs and CBT are first-line treatments in many guidelines. The American Psychiatric Association (APA) recommends sertraline or paroxetine, which are also United States Food and Drug Administration (FDA) approved. The United Kingdom's National Institute for Health and Care Excellence (NICE) guideline also endorses the use of sertraline or paroxetine as first-line treatment options.

Exam Essentials

- **Do not offer benzodiazepines as first-line treatment, as this**
  - Increases the risk of addiction
  - May affect the memory of events

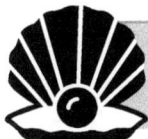

Clinical Pearls

- For patients who have difficulty talking about the trauma, eye movement desensitisation and reprocessing (EMDR) therapy may be considered instead of trauma-focused CBT

Question 7
What are the negative sequelae of untreated PTSD?

Answer
There can be dysfunction in occupation, education and interpersonal relationships. PTSD is related to higher mortality such as cardiovascular disease and diabetes. PTSD patients are also at higher risk of suicide.

171

Explanation

They are more likely to experience occupational problems, have poorer social support and have more disability. PTSD may also be associated with higher mortality in certain circumstances. Symptoms of depression in women with PTSD are associated with a nearly four times greater risk of death (e.g., cardiovascular, diabetes, suicide) compared with women with no PTSD or depression [13]. PTSD may increase the risk of attempted suicide.

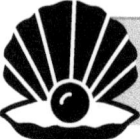

Clinical Pearls

- Complex PTSD may occur in certain patients and includes not only the symptoms of PTSD but also disturbances in three key domains:
  - Emotion regulation
  - Self-identity
  - Relational capacities
- Refer to the Diving Deep section for more information

Question 8

What medication can you consider prescribing for the treatment of nightmares in patients with PTSD?

Answer

Prazosin

Explanation

Prazosin, an alpha-1 receptor antagonist, may help with symptoms such as nightmares and hypervigilance.

Question 9

What are the principles of safeguarding a patient who has experienced childhood sexual abuse?

Answer

While local policies may differ slightly, the following principles are generally true:

1. Suspicion or recognition of child abuse lead to referral to child protection social services

2. Establish the need for immediate protection

3. Initiate investigations

   - Interviewing the child
   - Medical examination of the child

- ◦ Initial assessment of the family
- ◦ Interagency discussion

4. Hold an initial child protection case conference and come up with a protection plan and a more comprehensive assessment

5. Implementation of plans and review

6. Possible criminal prosecution

7. Therapy and closure

Explanation

The principal consideration throughout each step of management is the safety of the child. When sexual abuse is first disclosed, the physician should explain to the child that confidentiality has to be broken in their best interest to ensure their safety. Care should be taken to avoid contamination of information and the physician should seek advice and discuss the case with the lead consultant who deals with child abuse issues.

The social work department and the police both hold the main responsibility for investigations of child abuse and the physician should avoid delay in informing social services. If there is an immediate threat to the child's safety the police should be informed concurrently. Another healthcare worker should sit with the child while the physician makes a referral to the duty social worker in the local social service team. The child should not be left alone until social services come to assess the child and determine placement. A mental state examination by the psychiatrist will assist social services in determining the best placement for the child (e.g., hospitalisation etc.).

Next, inform whoever has the parental responsibility over the child. The parents need to be informed that social services have been contacted and that depending on their assessment the child may be placed in alternative accommodation. Consideration should be given whether the patient's siblings may be at risk as well. Aim to resolve interpersonal conflicts surrounding the child and ensure optimal development for the child following cessation of abuse.

Exam Essentials

- • Involve child protection social services early
- • Care should be taken to **avoid contamination of information** and the physician should seek advice and discuss the case with the lead consultant who deals with child abuse issues

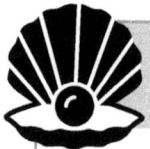

Clinical Pearls

- One in 20 children may experience childhood sexual abuse [14]

Question 10
What psychiatric disorders are commonly associated with childhood sexual abuse?

Answer
Adjustment disorder, PTSD, dissociative disorders, depression, anxiety, deliberate self-harm, suicidality, substance misuse, borderline personality disorder, eating disorders and paraphilias.

Explanation
The National Comorbidity Survey [15] conducted in the United States indicated a relationship between childhood sexual abuse and the subsequent onset of psychiatric disorders. The study revealed that 78% of women and 82% of men who reported childhood sexual abuse met diagnostic criteria for at least one lifetime psychiatric disorder versus 49% and 51%, respectively, among those who did not report childhood sexual abuse.

Diagnosis of adjustment disorder [2]

1. A maladaptive reaction to an identifiable psychosocial stressor or multiple stressors (e.g., single stressful event, ongoing psychosocial difficulty or a combination of stressful life situations) that usually emerges within a month of the stressor is required for diagnosis. Examples include divorce or loss of a relationship, loss of a job, diagnosis of an illness, recent onset of a disability and conflicts at home or work

2. The reaction to the stressor is characterised by preoccupation with the stressor or its consequences, including excessive worry, recurrent and distressing thoughts about the stressor or constant rumination about its implications

3. The symptoms are not better accounted for by another mental disorder (e.g., a mood disorder, another disorder specifically associated with stress)

4. Once the stressor and its consequences have ended, the symptoms resolve within six months

5. Failure to adapt to the stressor results in significant impairment in personal, family, social, educational, occupational or other important areas of functioning. If functioning is maintained, it is only through significant additional effort

Diving Deep ...

The lifetime prevalence of PTSD ranges from 6.1% to 9.2% in national samples of the general adult population in the United States and Canada with a female-to-male ratio of 2:1 [1, 12, 16–18]. The risk of developing PTSD after a traumatic event is 8–13% for men, 20–30% for women.

The underlying aetiology for acute stress disorder and PTSD includes psychological (dissociation, 'working through'), biological (dysregulation of neurotransmitters such as catecholamines, serotonin, gamma-aminobutyric acid (GABA), opioids and glucocorticoids) and genetic (higher concordance rates in monozygotic than dizygotic twins) factors. Remodelling underlying schemas requires holding trauma experiences in 'active' memory until the process of working through (the repeated examination and integration of unconscious psychological issues with the therapist to resolve internal conflict and gain insight) is complete. Dissociation is a mechanism which allows one to avoid overwhelming emotion. Neurophysiological changes lead to permanent neuronal changes as a result of the effects of chronic stress or persistent re-experiencing of the stressful event.

In PTSD, neuroimaging may show reduced hippocampal volume. Dysfunction of the amygdala, hippocampus, septum and prefrontal cortex may lead to enhanced fear response. High arousal appears to be mediated by the anterior cingulate, medial prefrontal cortex and thalamus. Dissociation appears to be mediated by the parietal, occipital and temporal cortexes. There are similarities between PTSD symptoms and opioid withdrawal, leading to speculation that opioid function is disturbed in PTSD.

In ICD-11 diagnostic criteria, patients with complex PTSD fulfil the diagnosis of PTSD, with severe and pervasive problems in affect regulation, persistent beliefs about oneself as diminished and worthless, accompanied by deep and pervasive feelings of shame and guilt related to the traumatic event, and persistent difficulty in sustaining a relationship and in feeling close to others.

References

1. American Psychiatric Association. *Diagnostic and statistical manual of mental disorders*, 5th edition, text revision (DSM-5-TR). Washington, DC: American Psychiatric Association Publishing; 2022. Available from: www.psychiatry.org/psychiatrists/practice/dsm

2. World Health Organization. *International classification of diseases*, 11th edition (ICD-11). Geneva: World Health Organization; 2024. Available from: https://icd.who.int/en

3. Smid GE, Mooren TTM, van der Mast RC, Gersons BPR, Kleber RJ. Delayed posttraumatic stress disorder: systematic review, meta-analysis, and meta-regression analysis of prospective studies. *J Clin Psychiatry*. 2009 Nov;70(11):1572–82.

4. Weathers FW, Bovin MJ, Lee DJ, Sloan DM, Schnurr PP, Kaloupek DG, et al. The Clinician-Administered PTSD Scale for DSM-5 (CAPS-5): development and initial psychometric evaluation in military veterans. *Psychol Assess*. 2018 Mar;30(3):383–95.

5. Blevins CA, Weathers FW, Davis MT, Witte TK, Domino JL. The Posttraumatic Stress Disorder Checklist for DSM-5 (PCL-5): development and initial psychometric evaluation. *J Trauma Stress*. 2015 Dec;28(6):489–98.

6. Olff M. Sex and gender differences in post-traumatic stress disorder: an update. *Eur J Psychotraumatol*. 2017 Sep 29;8(Suppl 4):1351204.

7. Brady KT. Posttraumatic stress disorder and comorbidity: recognizing the many faces of PTSD. *J Clin Psychiatry*. 1997;58(Suppl 9):12–5.

8. Rose SC, Bisson J, Churchill R, Wessely S. Psychological debriefing for preventing post traumatic stress disorder (PTSD). *Cochrane Database Syst Rev*. 2002 Apr;2002(2):CD000560.

9. Harvey AG, Bryant RA. The relationship between acute stress disorder and posttraumatic stress disorder: a prospective evaluation of motor vehicle accident survivors. *J Consult Clin Psychol*. 1998 Jun;66(3):507–12.

10. Brewin CR, Andrews B, Rose S, Kirk M. Acute stress disorder and posttraumatic stress disorder in victims of violent crime. *Am J Psychiatry*. 1999 Mar;156(3):360–6.

11. Bryant RA. Acute stress disorder as a predictor of posttraumatic stress disorder: a systematic review. *J Clin Psychiatry*. 2011 Feb;72(2):233–9.

12. Semple D, Smyth R. *Oxford handbook of psychiatry*, 4th edition. Oxford: Oxford University Press; 2019.

13. Roberts AL, Kubzansky LD, Chibnik LB, Rimm EB, Koenen KC. Association of posttraumatic stress and depressive symptoms with mortality in women. *JAMA Netw Open*. 2020 Dec 1;3(12):e2027935.

14. Gifford J. Is it child sexual abuse? A general paediatrician's guide. *Paediatr Child Health*. 2023 Jan;33(1):1–5.

15. Kessler RC, Berglund P, Demler O, Jin R, Merikangas KR, Walters EE. Lifetime prevalence and age-of-onset distributions of DSM-IV disorders in the National Comorbidity Survey Replication. *Arch Gen Psychiatry*. 2005 Jun;62(6):593–602.

16. Goldstein RB, Smith SM, Chou SP, Saha TD, Jung J, Zhang H, et al. The epidemiology of DSM-5 posttraumatic stress disorder in the United States: results from the National Epidemiologic Survey on Alcohol and Related Conditions-III. *Soc Psychiatry Psychiatr Epidemiol*. 2016 Aug;51(8):1137–48.

17. Van Ameringen M, Mancini C, Patterson B, Boyle MH. Post-traumatic stress disorder in Canada. *CNS Neurosci Ther*. 2008;14(3):171–81.

18. Koenen KC, Ratanatharathorn A, Ng L, McLaughlin KA, Bromet EJ, Stein DJ, et al. Posttraumatic stress disorder in the World Mental Health Surveys. *Psychol Med*. 2017 Oct;47(13):2260–74.

Case 19: Illness Anxiety Disorder and Somatic Symptom Disorder

I have a brain tumour

Jose is a 31-year-old male who reports mild subjective intermittent numbness over his hands for the past three weeks. He is preoccupied with worries such as 'Do I have cancer? Do I have an autoimmune disease? Am I going to die?'. These thoughts have gotten worse recently and have been affecting his sleep for the past three weeks. He has seen various neurologists, and multiple brain imaging scans have proven to be normal. He spends many hours on the internet reading up on his symptoms, hoping to arrive at a diagnosis. Despite reassurances from multiple physicians and family members, his anxiety cannot be allayed. Over the past three years, he has seen multiple specialists over fears of having acquired diseases such as HIV, bladder cancer, neurofibromatosis-1, etc.

- **Question 1: What is the most likely diagnosis? Which differential diagnoses would you consider?**

- **Question 2: What is the key defining difference between hypochondriasis and bodily distress disorder?**

- **Question 3: How would you differentiate bodily distress disorder from factitious disorder and malingering?**

- **Question 4: How would you manage Jose's hypochondriasis?**

Answers to Case 19

Question 1
What is the most likely diagnosis? Which differential diagnoses would you consider?

Answer
Hypochondriasis (health anxiety disorder)

Differential diagnoses include: bodily distress disorder and generalised anxiety disorder.

Explanation
Jose is preoccupied with acquiring a serious illness. He frequently worries that his numbness may be due to cancer or an autoimmune condition, and his somatic complaint is mild in intensity. He is easily alarmed by his health status as evidenced by previous episodes of frequent and excessive health examinations over mild symptoms within three years. This extends to excessive checking on the internet about his symptoms. Though his episode of numbness is only for three weeks, it is important to note that the similar pattern of behaviour over three years for different conditions fulfils the time criterion of at least six months.

Diagnosis of hypochondriasis (health anxiety disorder) [1]

1. Persistent preoccupation or fear about the possibility of having one or more serious, progressive or life-threatening illnesses is required for diagnosis

   The preoccupation is accompanied by either:

   • Repetitive and excessive health-related behaviours, such as repeatedly checking the body for evidence of illness, spending inordinate amounts of time searching for information about the feared illness or repeatedly seeking reassurance (e.g., arranging multiple medical consultations); or

   • Maladaptive avoidance behaviour related to health (e.g., avoiding medical appointments)

As for the differential diagnoses:

Condition	Defining feature(s)
Bodily distress disorder	Jose does have a somatic symptom – numbness – which is the cause of his worry. Additionally, this causes him to have persistent thoughts about the seriousness of his numbness, high levels of anxiety and, to a certain degree, excessive time and energy devoted to seeking the cause of his numbness. However, his numbness has only been around for a few weeks, and he was previously well without any symptoms

Condition	Defining feature(s)
Generalised anxiety disorder	Jose does complain of anxiety that bothers him throughout the day, which affects his sleep and causes him some irritability. However, there is no free-floating anxiety reported. Additionally, he does not suffer from other physical symptoms of generalised anxiety disorder

Exam Essentials

- **Always rule out medical causes before labelling bodily distress disorder**: it has implications for future medical care

- For hypochondriasis and bodily distress disorder, always ask for the patient's illness perception, degree of health consciousness and personal/family history of physical illness

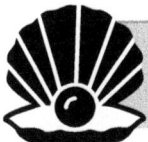

Clinical Pearls

- The two specifiers for hypochondriasis include [2]:
  - Care-seeking
  - Care avoidant

- For patients with suggestive features of bodily distress disorder, do a thorough exploration of symptoms in the domains of sensory, neurological, gastrointestinal, genitourinary, etc. and refer to appropriate specialists if necessary

Question 2
What is the key defining difference between hypochondriasis and bodily distress disorder?

Answer

	Hypochondriasis	Bodily distress disorder
Presence of symptoms	Most often absent	Present
Patient's main concern	Having a serious illness	Having severe symptom(s)

Diagnosis of bodily distress disorder [1]

1. The presence of bodily symptoms that are distressing to the individual is required for diagnosis. Typically, this involves multiple bodily symptoms that may vary over time. Occasionally, the focus is limited to a single symptom: usually pain or fatigue

2. Excessive attention is directed towards the symptoms, which may manifest in:

   • Persistent preoccupation with the severity of the symptoms or their negative consequences in individuals who have an established medical condition that may be causing or contributing to the symptoms, and a degree of attention related to the symptoms that is clearly excessive in relation to the nature and severity of the medical condition

   • Repeated contacts with healthcare providers related to the bodily symptoms that are substantially in excess of what would be considered medically necessary

3. Excessive attention to the bodily symptoms persists, despite appropriate clinical examination and investigations or appropriate reassurance from healthcare providers.

4. Bodily symptoms are persistent; that is, some symptoms are present (although not necessarily the same symptoms) on most days during a period of at least several months (e.g., three months or more)

Question 3
How would you differentiate bodily distress disorder from factitious disorder and malingering?

Answer
Patients with bodily distress disorder experience actual symptom(s) involuntarily as compared to those with a factitious disorder, whose symptoms are reproduced/staged deliberately and intentionally.

Explanation

Patients with bodily distress disorder may evoke negative emotions in clinicians as they repeatedly seek medical attention. Hence, clinicians may start to wonder if such patients have factitious disorder. However, it is prudent to note that patients with bodily distress disorder are suffering from symptoms which are very real to them, while those who have factitious disorder usually have complete resolution of symptoms once their gain is achieved.

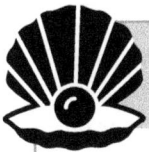

Clinical Pearls

- Patients with bodily distress disorder may have medical conditions that cause physical symptoms, but the experienced symptoms may be exaggerated and **out of proportion to the condition**

Question 4

How would you manage Jose's hypochondriasis?

Answer

Biological: selective serotonin reuptake inhibitors, serotonin–noradrenaline reuptake inhibitors

Psychological: cognitive behavioural therapy (CBT)

Social: frequent follow-ups with a consistent primary care physician and/or psychiatrist, group therapies

Explanation

CBT is considered a first-line treatment for hypochondriasis [3]. CBT involves treating dysfunctional maladaptive cognitive beliefs by behavioural modification, addressing habits of excessive body checking for signs of illness and education on normal somatic sensations and variations. Antidepressants can be considered as second-line treatment and are effective for hypochondriasis. A maintenance treatment course of six months to a year is recommended and should be used together with psychotherapy.

The primary physician and psychiatrist, ideally the same treating clinicians, need to maintain frequent regular follow-ups with the patient, to reduce visits to the various healthcare systems.

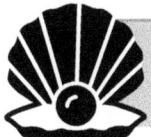

Clinical Pearls

- Once organic causes have been ruled out, the aim is to avoid overutilisation of the medical system, unnecessary investigations and referrals

181

Diving Deep ...

The estimated prevalence rate of hypochondriasis in the general population is set at 0.1% [1], while that of bodily distress disorder is estimated to be 5–7% of the general population, with a higher female representation of 10:1 (female to male). In the primary care population, 17% of patients have been found to suffer from bodily distress disorder. Despite the pre-existing pool of bodily distress disorder patients within the primary care population, these patients are often missed by primary care physicians. Hence this might lead to underdiagnosis of bodily distress disorder that translates into higher healthcare utilisation, higher morbidity and lower health-related quality of life. In countries with overloaded primary healthcare, this leads to added stress on the practitioners as well as increasing healthcare costs as a whole.

References

1. World Health Organization. *International classification of diseases*, 11th edition (ICD-11). Geneva: World Health Organization; 2024. Available from: https://icd.who.int/en

2. American Psychiatric Association. *Diagnostic and statistical manual of mental disorders*, 5th edition, text revision (DSM-5-TR). Washington, DC: American Psychiatric Association Publishing; 2022. Available from: www.psychiatry.org/psychiatrists/practice/dsm

3. Boland RJ, Verduin ML, Ruiz P, Shah A, Sadock BJ, editors. *Kaplan & Sadock's synopsis of psychiatry*, 12th edition. Philadelphia: Wolters Kluwer; 2022.

Case 20: Conversion Disorder and Factitious Disorder

You don't believe me?

You are currently working in the neurology team when you clerked Sofia, a 55-year-old lady, who was admitted for left-sided dense hemiplegia. However, the brain imaging was unremarkable, and her neurological exam revealed findings which were inconsistent and not reproducible. Sofia's lack of distress over the dense hemiplegia and apparent lack of interest in treatment options struck the team as peculiar. Your consultant has ruled out the possibility of an organic medical condition and wants you to speak to the psychiatry team to seek their advice.

- **Question 1: In the absence of an organic cause, what is the most likely diagnosis?**

- **Question 2: What are the differential diagnoses?**

'Sofia's lack of distress over the dense hemiplegia and apparent lack of interest in treatment options struck the team as peculiar.'

- **Question 3: What is this phenomenon in the case description known as?**

- **Question 4: How would you manage a patient with conversion disorder?**

Sofia subsequently reveals that she has had longstanding unhappiness with her husband, who refuses to do their housework, and her son, who is often not at home. She states that since her admission, her husband has taken on some responsibilities in buying groceries, and her son is now coming home earlier to prepare the home environment for her discharge. You hence diagnosed her with conversion disorder with a psychological stressor.

- **Question 5: What is her prognosis and please give evidence supporting your answer.**

Answers to Case 20

Question 1
In the absence of an organic cause, what is the most likely diagnosis?

Answer
Dissociative neurological symptom disorder (also known in the DSM-5-TR as functional neurological symptom disorder/conversion disorder)

Explanation
Sofia displays one or more symptoms of altered voluntary motor or sensory function leading to functional impairment, with clinical findings showing no evidence of any recognised neurological or medical conditions, which is consistent with conversion disorder.

Diagnosis of dissociative neurological symptom disorder (conversion disorder) [1]

1. Involuntary disruption or discontinuity in the normal integration of motor, sensory or cognitive functions, lasting at least several hours, is required for diagnosis

2. Clinical findings are not consistent with a recognised disease of the nervous system (e.g., a stroke) or another medical condition (e.g., a head injury)

3. The symptoms do not occur exclusively during episodes of trance disorder, possession trance disorder, dissociative identity disorder or partial dissociative identity disorder

4. The symptoms are not due to the effects of a substance or medication on the central nervous system (including withdrawal effects), do not occur exclusively during hypnagogic or hypnopompic states and are not due to a sleep–wake disorder (e.g., sleep-related rhythmic movement disorder, recurrent isolated sleep paralysis)

Exam Essentials

- Conversion disorder usually presents as a loss in function, while somatic disorder is a gain in symptom – both occur along the spectrum of disorders with underlying emotional difficulties that may be difficult to express

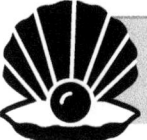

Clinical Pearls

- Always ensure that all medical causes/investigations are complete before considering a psychiatric cause

Question 2
What are the differential diagnoses?

Answer
Factitious disorder (previously known as Munchausen syndrome)
Malingering

Explanation

Diagnosis of factitious disorder [1]

Factitious disorder imposed on self:

1. The presentation is characterised by feigning, falsifying or intentionally inducing medical, psychological or behavioural signs and symptoms or injury associated with identified deception. If a pre-existing disorder or disease is present, the individual intentionally aggravates existing symptoms or falsifies or induces additional symptoms

2. The individual seeks treatment or otherwise presents themselves as ill, injured or impaired based on the feigned, falsified or self-induced signs, symptoms or injuries

3. The deceptive behaviour is not solely motivated by obvious external rewards or incentives (e.g., obtaining disability payments or evading criminal prosecution)

Factitious disorder imposed on another (previously factitious disorder by proxy)*:

1. The presentation is characterised by feigning, falsifying or intentionally inducing medical, psychological or behavioural signs and symptoms or injury in another person – most commonly a child dependant – associated with identified deception. If a pre-existing disorder or disease is present in the other person, the individual intentionally exaggerates or aggravates existing symptoms, or falsifies or induces additional symptoms

2. The individual seeks treatment for the other person or otherwise presents them as ill, injured or impaired based on the feigned, falsified or induced signs, symptoms or injuries

3. The deceptive behaviour is not solely motivated by obvious external rewards or incentives (e.g., obtaining disability payments or avoiding criminal prosecution for child or elder abuse)

*The perpetrator, not the victim, receives this diagnosis.

Factitious disorder is seen in patients with the intentional production of symptoms to assume a sick role as a primary gain. We will need more history, such as corroborative accounts from family members, current and old medical records and longitudinal observations to diagnose this in Sofia.

Apart from factitious disorder, malingering is a possibility but should always be the last differential diagnosis. This diagnosis should only be made after careful exploration with sufficient evidence. Patients with factitious disorder deliberately create symptoms for primary gain, while those with malingering deliberately create symptoms consciously for secondary gain.

Exam Essentials

- **Primary gain** is an internal motivation to obtain the sick role and be cared for. For example, an individual who feels guilty about not being able to perform a task may experience diminished guilt if there is a medical condition which justifies this inability

- **Secondary gain** is an external motivation to obtain something desired (such as food and shelter), or avoiding responsibility (such as missing a court date)

Question 3
What is this phenomenon in the case description known as?

Answer
La belle indifference

Explanation
La belle indifference is a paradoxical absence of psychological distress despite having a serious medical illness or symptoms related to a health condition. The mere presence of la belle indifference does not confirm the diagnosis of conversion disorder; however, la belle indifference is most commonly seen in patients with conversion disorder.

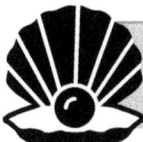

Clinical Pearls

- **Hoover's sign** [2] is a common clinical sign elicited to differentiate between the organic and functional weakness of pyramidal origin
- Patients with conversion disorder may have inconsistent fluctuating symptoms that change over time

Question 4
How would you manage a patient with conversion disorder?

Answer
Management includes psychoeducation, cognitive behavioural therapy (CBT) and physiotherapy.

Explanation
The most common form of treatment is to suggest that the conversion symptoms will gradually improve, by starting with reassuring news that the investigations are unremarkable and that recovery is certain. Specific suggestions with gradual rehabilitation goals are also key to successful treatment. Confrontation is seldom helpful as patients can be sensitive to the idea that an authoritative person has dismissed their suffering.

Behavioural interventions such as CBT (which may include self-help therapy explaining the changes in the nervous system as influenced by psychological and behavioural factors), physiotherapy (as first-line treatment as well as secondary prevention of weakness or true deficits due to initial functional symptoms) and reassurance are crucial, particularly for less verbal patients.

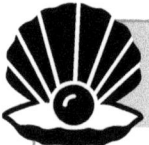

Clinical Pearls

- Getting patients to understand the concept of **mind–body connection** helps direct treatment

Question 5
What is her prognosis and please give evidence supporting your answer.

Answer
The prognosis is good in view of an acute presentation, recognition of potential stressors and early diagnosis.

Explanation
For acute conversion symptoms, especially those with a clear precipitant, the prognosis is good, with 70–90% attaining complete resolution at subsequent follow-up [3]. A positive patient–doctor relationship and early diagnosis of the condition also promote a good prognosis. Those with multiple, longer-lasting and well-established symptoms have poorer outcomes, and up to 20–25% of patients develop recurrent conversion symptoms one year after discharge [4].

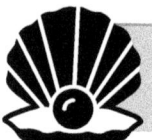

Clinical Pearls

- Often, there is a trauma, adverse life event or stressor preceding the symptoms of conversion disorder. However, the absence of a stressor does not exclude the diagnosis

Diving Deep …

Conversion disorder is two to three times more common in women than men for most symptom presentations [5]. Patients of lower socioeconomic class and with less education have higher incidences of conversion disorder. Age of onset is variable across most of the life span with different manifestations of the illness.

Factitious disorder, also known as Munchausen syndrome, may be imposed on self, or imposed by another/proxy. Some classical presentations include polymicrobial blood cultures in those who self-inject foreign liquid into the body, or low C-peptide levels in those who self-inject insulin to create hypoglycaemic episodes. Patients with factitious disorder are usually well known to the healthcare system due to multiple visits to physicians or hospitalisations. Pseudologia fantastica (production of intricate and colourful stories or fantasies) is a form of pathological lying which is seen in those with factitious disorder. Risk factors for factitious disorder include female gender, a history of abuse, being unmarried and having borderline personality disorder [6].

Malingering is not a psychiatric disorder but a behaviour that patients may display. Malingering involves the conscious feigning, induction or exacerbation of physical or psychological symptoms for conscious gain. Involvement in the legal system is a risk factor for malingering, particularly among patients who are referred for examination by an attorney. Those with poor coping skills and utilisation of immature defence mechanisms are also at risk of malingering. The presence of a secondary gain is not absolute evidence of malingering – one must be careful not to miss the diagnosis of a true medical condition in this population!

	Behaviour	Type of incentive
Bodily distress disorder	Involuntary production of symptoms, or exaggerated psychological behaviours towards existing symptoms	May be psychological or due to underlying health concerns
Conversion disorder	Involuntary loss of function	Psychological/ unconscious
Factitious disorder	Voluntary production of symptoms	Primary gain/ unconscious
Malingering	Voluntary production of symptoms	Secondary gain/ conscious

References

1. World Health Organization. *International classification of diseases*, 11th edition (ICD-11). Geneva: World Health Organization; 2024. Available from: https://icd.who.int/en

2. Mehndiratta MM, Kumar M, Nayak R, Garg H, Pandey S. Hoover's sign: clinical relevance in neurology. *J Postgrad Med*. 2014;60(3):297–9.

3. Semple D, Smyth R. *Oxford handbook of psychiatry*, 4th edition. Oxford: Oxford University Press; 2019.

4. Feinstein A. Conversion disorder: advances in our understanding. *CMAJ.* 2011 May 17;183(8):915–20.

5. American Psychiatric Association. *Diagnostic and statistical manual of mental disorders,* 5th edition, text revision (DSM-5-TR). Washington, DC: American Psychiatric Association Publishing; 2022. Available from: www.psychiatry.org/psychiatrists/practice/dsm

6. Jaghab K, Skodnek KB, Padder TA. Munchausen's syndrome and other factitious disorders in children: case series and literature review. *Psychiatry (Edgmont).* 2006 Mar;3(3):46–55.

Case 21: Delirium and Neurocognitive Disorders

Why is my memory failing?

Mary is a 72-year-old lady brought to the clinic by her daughter for gradually increasing 'forgetfulness' over the past five years. She has been misplacing her personal belongings more frequently and once forgot to turn off the kitchen stove after cooking. While still able to carry out activities of daily living (ADLs) independently (e.g., toileting and showering), she has increasing difficulty performing some more complex instrumental activities and requires assistance. For example, she now needs to write down a list before grocery shopping and refers to her cookbook more when preparing meals for her family. Mary admits that her memory is 'fuzzy' and sometimes feels frustrated but chalks it up to 'getting old'.

- **Question 1: What is the most likely diagnosis?**

- **Question 2: Other than Alzheimer's disease, what are the three most common causes of dementia?**

- **Question 3: What are the risk factors for Alzheimer's disease?**

- **Question 4: What other standardised instruments can be used in the evaluation of a patient presenting with possible cognitive impairment?**

- **Question 5: What investigations would you perform for Mary?**

The investigations for Mary came back unremarkable and she was diagnosed with mild neurocognitive disorder due to Alzheimer's disease. Mary and her daughter are keen on non-pharmacological methods of management.

- **Question 6: What strategies would you offer in the management of her condition?**

Two years later, Mary returns for a follow-up appointment. Her daughter reports that her mother's memory loss has progressed and the repeat Mini-Mental State Examination (MMSE) scores reveal a decline from 22/30 to 18/30. With a further decline in functioning, both Mary and her daughter are now keen on a trial of pharmacological treatment.

- **Question 7: What medications would you offer her in the treatment of her mild to moderate Alzheimer's disease?**

Before starting on donepezil, Mary and her daughter would like to know the potential adverse effects of the medication.

- **Question 8: What are the side effects of donepezil?**

Mary was started on donepezil with subsequent stabilisation in cognitive symptoms. Four years later, Mary is brought to your clinic by her daughter for 'worsening confusion'. In the preceding three days, Mary had developed a cough and fever, since then she has become increasingly disoriented. She is often unable to tell the time or recognise her location. Occasionally she mistakes her daughter for someone else and becomes agitated. Conversations are challenging as Mary appears distractible and replies inappropriately. Mary's confusion fluctuates throughout the day and her sleep has been affected (reduced). On examination, she was found to be tachypnoeic, febrile with crepitations and reduced air entry auscultated over her left anterior chest.

- **Question 9: What is the likely cause of her current altered mental status?**

- **Question 10: Following an inpatient admission, how would you manage Mary's delirium?**

Mary's delirium was managed, and she was eventually discharged. During a follow-up appointment five years later, Mary's daughter expressed concerns that Mary's symptoms were worsening. Mary was found to be wandering and lost outside of her home on multiple occasions. Her family now discourages her from leaving home without a companion. In recent months, she has been increasingly agitated and suspicious of the family's domestic helper. Mary claims the helper has been stealing her belongings, although, on investigations by her daughter, these items were found to be misplaced instead of stolen. When alone, Mary reports voices talking to her about her helper's ill intentions. These episodes of agitation worsen in the evenings. Last week, Mary had threatened to slap the domestic helper unless she returned the 'stolen items'. An interval MMSE test showed a further decline in scores from 18/30 to 13/30.

- **Question 11: What is Mary's revised diagnosis?**

Similarly to the non-pharmacological approach to treating delirium, you investigate and treat the various exacerbating factors of Mary's BPSD. Her daughter was educated on the diagnosis and taught strategies involving distraction, redirection and the provision of structured routines to calm Mary. You reviewed her medications and suggested other environmental supportive measures as well.

- **Question 12: What are the pharmacological measures which can be used to manage Mary's moderate to severe Alzheimer's disease and the presence of BPSD?**

Answers to Case 21

Question 1
What is the most likely diagnosis?

Answer
Mild neurocognitive disorder due to Alzheimer's disease

Explanation

Diagnosis of mild neurocognitive disorder [1]

1. The presence of mild impairment in one or more cognitive domains (e.g., attention, executive function, language, memory, perceptual–motor abilities, social cognition) relative to expectations for age and general pre-morbid level of neurocognitive functioning is required for diagnosis

2. Impairment represents a decline from the individual's previous level of functioning

3. Neurocognitive impairment is not severe enough to interfere significantly with an individual's ability to perform activities related to personal, family, social,

educational and/or occupational functioning or other important functional areas

4. Evidence of mild neurocognitive impairment is based on:

- Information obtained from the individual, an informant or clinical observation

- Objective evidence of impairment as demonstrated by standardised neuropsychological/cognitive testing or, in its absence, another quantified clinical assessment

5. Neurocognitive impairment is not attributable to normal ageing

6. Neurocognitive impairment may be attributable to an underlying acquired disease of the nervous system, a trauma, an infection or other disease process affecting the brain, use of specific substances or medications, nutritional deficiency or exposure to toxins, or the aetiology may be undetermined

7. The symptoms are not better explained by another neurocognitive disorder, substance intoxication or substance withdrawal or another mental disorder (e.g., attention deficit hyperactivity disorder or other neurodevelopmental disorder, schizophrenia or another primary psychotic disorder, mood disorder, post-traumatic stress disorder or dissociative disorder)

From the DSM-5 onwards, 'major neurocognitive disorder' has been used as the preferred term over 'dementia'; however, ICD-11 still uses the term 'dementia'.

Diagnosis of dementia [1]*

1. Marked impairment in two or more cognitive domains relative to the level expected given the individual's age and general pre-morbid level of neurocognitive functioning, which represents a decline from the individual's previous level of functioning, is required for diagnosis

2. Memory impairment is present in most forms of dementia, but neurocognitive impairment is not restricted to memory and may be present in other cognitive domains. The six cognitive domains are: complex attention, executive function, learning and memory, language, social cognition and perceptual–motor functioning

3. Evidence of neurocognitive impairment is based on:

- Information obtained from the individual, an informant or clinical observation

- Substantial impairment in neurocognitive performance as demonstrated by standardised neuropsychological/cognitive testing or, in its absence, another quantified clinical assessment

4. Behavioural changes (e.g., changes in personality, disinhibition, agitation, irritability) may also be present and, in some forms of dementia, may be the presenting symptom

*Specify the underlying subtype (e.g., Alzheimer's disease, frontotemporal degeneration, Lewy body disease, etc.)

Features	Mild dementia	Major dementia
Cognitive function	Mild decline	Significant decline
Cognitive performance*	Modest impairment	Substantial impairment
Capacity for independence in everyday activities**	No interference, or managed with greater compensatory strategies	Interference present

*   Standardised neuropsychological testing or quantified clinical assessment.

**   That is, complex instrumental ADLs.

When measuring cognitive ability, it is important to consider the following:

- Evidence of significant cognitive decline from a previous level of performance in one or more cognitive domains

- The decline does not occur exclusively in the context of delirium

- Cognitive deficits are not better explained by another mental disorder

Dementia is a syndrome characterised by progressive, usually irreversible, global cognitive deficits. Alzheimer's disease is the most common form of dementia [2, 3]. The onset of Alzheimer's disease tends to occur after 60 years old. The cardinal symptoms include memory impairment which has a distinctive pattern of insidious and slow onset with episodic memory (memory of events occurring at a particular time and place) affected first. Executive function and judgement are also affected in the early stages of Alzheimer's disease and can be reflected as disorganisation and inability to multitask.

In patients with a history or symptoms suggestive of depression, pseudodementia should be considered as a differential diagnosis. Features which may indicate pseudodementia include:

- Patient is poorly motivated when attempting the cognitive assessment. May repeat 'I don't know'

- Memory loss is patchy (short-term memory loss and long-term memory loss) and inconsistent

- Attention is predominantly affected
- Low mood occurs before cognitive problems and is more prominent clinically
- Cognition improves with mood improvement

Exam Essentials

- Cognitive domains – **SPELL-C**
    - **S**ocial cognition
    - **P**erceptual motor function
    - **E**xecutive function
    - **L**anguage
    - **L**earning
    - **C**omplex attention

- There may be patients who complain of subjective memory issues, but the cognitive assessment is normal and there is no functional impairment. This is termed '**subjective cognitive impairment**'. It is worthwhile to follow them up to monitor any progressive decline in cognition and rule out other mental illnesses (i.e., depression or anxiety)

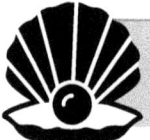

Clinical Pearls

- As patients may lack insight into their cognitive decline, a corroborative history is important

- If the patient presents with an acute onset of cognitive decline, rule out delirium and organic causes

- Assess risks associated with cognitive decline:
    - Exploitation/Abuse (physical, emotional, financial)
    - Driving
    - Flooding, fire
    - Falls
    - Inappropriate medication intake
    - Wandering/getting lost

Question 2

Other than Alzheimer's disease, what are the other three most common causes of dementia?

Answer

Vascular neurocognitive disorder

Neurocognitive disorder due to multiple aetiologies (Alzheimer's disease + vascular dementia)

Neurocognitive disorder with Lewy body dementia (LBD)

Explanation

Causes of dementia [3] can be divided into irreversible and reversible causes.

Irreversible causes	Reversible causes
Alzheimer's disease (62%) Vascular dementia (15%) Dementia due to multiple aetiologies (Alzheimer's disease + vascular dementia) (10%) Lewy body dementia (4%) Frontotemporal dementia (2%) Other causes (3%) (e.g., progressive supranuclear palsy, corticobasal degeneration, multiple system atrophy, Creutzfeldt–Jakob disease, Parkinson's disease dementia, Huntington's disease)	Subdural haematoma Normal pressure hydrocephalus Intracranial lesions Metabolic disorder (e.g., vitamin B12 deficiency) Hypothyroidism

Vascular dementia is caused by cerebrovascular disease or impaired cerebral blood flow and cognitive decline typically follows a clinically diagnosed stroke or brain imaging findings of a vascular brain injury. Neuroimaging allows for the diagnosis of strokes and silent manifestations of cerebrovascular disease that impair cognition. It tends to have a stepwise pattern of cognitive decline.

The pathological hallmark of Lewy body dementia is the presence of eosinophilic intra-cytoplasmic inclusions called Lewy bodies that contain aggregated alpha-synuclein. Lewy body dementia is characterised by visual hallucinations, parkinsonism, cognitive fluctuations, dysautonomia, sleep disorders (REM sleep behavioural disorder, etc.) and neuroleptic sensitivity.

Frontotemporal dementia is defined by the degeneration of frontal and/or temporal lobes with prominent changes in social behaviour and personality or aphasia. It is one of the more common causes of early-onset neurocognitive disorders, with an average age of symptom onset in the 60s. Clinical features of the behavioural-variant type include disinhibition, apathy, hyperorality, preference for sweet food, speech problems and perseverative, stereotyped or compulsive ritualistic behaviours. Other subtypes include semantic and progressive non-fluent aphasia types.

Exam Essentials

- Vascular dementia often presents as a stepwise deterioration, whereas Alzheimer's disease presents with an insidious and gradual decline in cognition

- In Lewy body dementia, cognitive and motor symptoms occur within a year, while in dementia due to Parkinson's disease, the parkinsonism symptoms precede the cognitive symptoms by more than one year

- Disinhibition is commonly seen in those with frontal lobe symptoms

- Remember to rule out mania and substance use

- Behavioural issues in frontotemporal dementia may include disinhibition or apathy (two extreme ends)

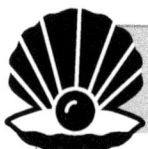

Clinical Pearls

- Bedside cognitive tests such as the Frontal Assessment Battery (FAB) may be used to screen for frontal lobe dysfunction

- Always ask for a family history of dementia or neurodegenerative diseases in patients with early-onset symptoms

- Some patients with frontotemporal dementia may have motor symptoms too – with motor neuron disease

Question 3
What are the risk factors for Alzheimer's disease?

Answer

Risk factors for Alzheimer's disease		
Genetic	**Acquired**	**Environmental**
Family history of dementia Presence of apolipoprotein E epsilon 4 (APOE4) allele Rare dominantly inherited mutations in genes, affecting brain amyloid (e.g., amyloid precursor protein, presenilin 1, and presenilin 2)	Hypertension Dyslipidaemia Cerebrovascular disease Peripheral atherosclerosis Type 2 diabetes and obesity Brain trauma Medications (e.g., benzodiazepines, anticholinergics, antihistamines, opioids)	Second-hand smoke Air pollution Occupational or environmental exposure to pesticides
Possible protective factors for Alzheimer's disease		
APOE2 allele Higher level of physical activity Oestrogen (e.g., hormone replacement therapy) Non-steroidal anti-inflammatory drugs (NSAIDs) Vitamin E Higher level of pre-morbid education		

Explanation

The most clearly established risk factors for Alzheimer's disease include increasing age, family history of dementia, autosomal dominant genes that impact amyloid in the brain and the APOE4 allele.

Question 4

What other standardised instruments can be used in the evaluation of a patient presenting with possible cognitive impairment?

199

Exam Essentials

- The presence of the APOE4 allele increases the risk of developing Alzheimer's disease, while the APOE2 allele decreases the risk of developing the disease [4, 5]

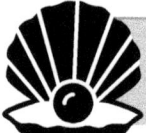

Clinical Pearls

- Physically active individuals have a lower incidence and prevalence of cognitive decline, including Alzheimer's disease [6]

Answer

Bedside screening instruments:

- Abbreviated Mental Test (AMT) [7]

- Clock drawing [8]

Scales with moderate assessment times:

- MMSE [9]

- Montreal Cognitive Assessment (MoCA) [10]

Scales with longer assessment times:

- Addenbrooke's Cognitive Examination – Revised (ACE-R) [11]

Explanation

The AMT is a 10-item questionnaire testing orientation, memory and concentration. It is a useful bedside test for rapid screening for cognitive impairment – indicated by a score of 7 or less out of 10. Note that some of the questions involved are contextualised to the country the patient is based in (e.g., current president/prime minister).

In clock drawing, the patient is asked to draw a large clock face with the time shown at ten past five. It is a useful bedside screening technique to test for executive functioning, which is sensitive to organisation and planning as well as constructional ability (visuo-spatial–constructional domain).

The MMSE takes approximately 10 minutes to administer and is one of the most commonly used and studied standardised instruments with a variety of uses in the psychiatric context. It is based almost entirely on verbal assessment of memory and attention. Different cut-off scores are used based on the patient's education level [12–14]. The limitations of the MMSE include a low sensitivity.

The MoCA is similarly well studied and scored on a 30-point scale. A score of ≤ 26/30 may suggest cognitive impairment. The MoCA is more difficult and appears to be more sensitive in detecting mild cognitive decline compared to the MMSE. The MoCA also contains components to assess the frontal lobe.

The ACE-R is a detailed, 100-item, clinician-administered bedside test of cognitive function. It covers five areas of function: attention and orientation, memory, verbal fluency, language and visuospatial awareness. It has a sensitivity of 94% and a specificity of 89% for dementia with a cut-off score of 88/100 [11].

Question 5
What investigations would you perform for Mary?

Exam Essentials

- Components of the bedside FAB include:

  ○ Similarities
  ○ Lexical fluency
  ○ Motor series ('Luria's test')
  ○ Conflicting instructions and alternating sequence/Go–No-Go
  ○ Judgement question
  ○ Prehension behaviour (grasp reflex)
  ○ Cognitive estimates

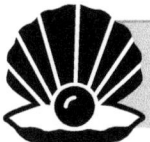

Clinical Pearls

- Always check the **baseline education level of the patient**. MMSE and MoCA scores may be normal in high-functioning patients. You may consider formal neuropsychological assessment for such individuals

- The MoCA is freely available online (with various languages and versions which one can alternate). This helps to prevent practice effect

Answer

Category	Investigations
Point-of-care test	ECG Capillary blood glucose
Biochemistry	Full blood count Liver function test Renal panel and electrolytes* Vitamin B12/D and folate levels* C-reactive protein, blood cultures Thyroid function test* HIV/syphilis screening*
Imaging	CT or MRI brain imaging Lumbar puncture* Electroencephalogram*

* If clinically indicated.

Explanation

Biochemical investigations are useful in patients with a presentation that is possibly acute or subacute in whom delirium is a differential. They are also useful in investigating for a reversible cause of cognitive impairment, and to guide further treatment of the cause.

The American Academy of Neurology [15] recommends structural neuroimaging with either a non-contrast CT or MRI brain in the routine initial evaluation of all patients with dementia. MRI is preferred over CT brain imaging because it is more sensitive for a broad range of potential pathologies while avoiding exposure to ionising radiation. A CT brain scan is used when contraindications to MRI exist (e.g., pacemaker in situ). MRI brain should also be considered for patients with earlier-onset and/or ambiguous symptoms.

Structural MRI findings in Alzheimer's disease include both generalised and focal atrophy, as well as white matter lesions. In general, these findings are non-specific. The most characteristic focal finding in Alzheimer's disease is reduced hippocampal volume or medial temporal lobe atrophy.

Other MRI findings to look out for include:

- Focal versus generalised atrophy

- Hyperintensities

- White matter changes

- Microbleeds

- Extent of vascular burden

- Mass lesions

Question 6
What strategies would you offer in the management of her condition?

Answer
Non-pharmacological methods:

- Cognitive rehabilitation programmes

- Occupational therapy with a specific programme designed for patients with dementia

- Adequate nutrition

- Risk factor control

- Avoiding adverse drug effects (e.g., polypharmacy, benzodiazepines)

- Formal exercise programmes

- Support for caregivers

- Actively addressing safety issues

- End-of-life care

Explanation
Cognitive rehabilitation aims to help patients in the early stages of a neurocognitive disorder to maintain memory and higher cognitive function and to devise strategies to compensate for declining function [16]. Occupational therapy with a specific programme designed for patients with a neurocognitive disorder has been shown to improve motor and process skills and ADLs [17]. Inadequate nutrition in Alzheimer's disease is associated with increased morbidity and mortality [18]. Identification and treatment of risk factors for stroke and cardiovascular disease may help in slowing the progression of cognitive decline. Formal exercise programmes carry the benefits of improved physical functioning and improved ability of people with dementia to perform ADLs, slowing the progression of functional decline in patients with Alzheimer's disease [19–21]. However, they do not appear to improve cognitive functioning in adults with dementia. Counselling and participation in support groups can be beneficial as caregivers are at risk of burnout and significant stress. Assess the patient's fitness to drive, fall risk, wandering risk and risk of injuries while cooking. Community services should be activated for patients who live alone and may be at risk of self-neglect. Patients should consider discussing their end-of-life plans including lasting power of attorney, will and advanced care plans, before mental capacity is lost.

Question 7

What medications would you offer her in the treatment of her mild to moderate Alzheimer's disease?

Answer

Acetylcholinesterase inhibitors (ACheIs; e.g., donepezil, rivastigmine, galantamine)

Explanation

Patients with Alzheimer's disease have reduced cerebral content of choline acetyltransferase and impaired cortical cholinergic function. ACheIs increase cholinergic transmission at the synaptic cleft and provide modest symptomatic benefit in some patients with dementia. ACheIs provide a small improvement in cognition, neuropsychiatric symptoms and ADLs. ACheIs are typically used as monotherapies in the treatment of mild or major dementia (MMSE, 10–26) as recommended by the NICE guidelines [22].

Vitamin E (alpha-tocopherol) and selegiline (a monoamine oxidase inhibitor) have antioxidant properties but showed mixed results from randomised trials [23, 24]. There are no dietary supplements that have convincingly been shown to have symptomatic or preventive benefits in patients with mild cognitive impairment due to Alzheimer's disease.

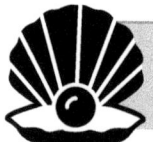 **Clinical Pearls**

- Ginkgo biloba supplement may be considered but is not shown to be effective in reducing the incidence of Alzheimer's disease or all-cause dementia and did not slow cognitive decline in individuals with either normal cognition or mild cognitive impairment at baseline [25, 26]

- Be aware of bleeding risks when prescribing Ginkgo supplements

Question 8

What are the side effects of donepezil?

Answer

Common class side effects of ACheIs:

- Nausea and diarrhoea

- Anorexia and weight loss

- Bradycardia and hypotension

- Sleep disturbances: insomnia, vivid dreams

- Headaches

Donepezil-specific side effects:

- Avoid in patients with asthma

- Avoid in patients with peptic ulcer disease (gastrointestinal bleeding)

Explanation

Adverse effects of ACheIs are related to excessive cholinergic effects:

Acetylcholinesterase inhibitors			
	Donepezil	**Galantamine**	**Rivastigmine**
Indications	Alzheimer's disease, Vascular dementia	Alzheimer's disease	Alzheimer's disease, LBD
Enzymes inhibited*	AchE	AchE	AchE and BchE
Route of administration	Oral	Oral	Oral and transdermal patch
Contraindications	Asthma Peptic ulcer disease (risk of gastrointestinal bleed)	End-stage kidney disease Severe hepatic impairment	-
Bradycardia or known cardiac conduction system disease			

* AchE = acetylcholinesterase, BchE = butyrylcholinesterase.

Always moderate expectations of patients and family members about the effects of anti-dementia medications: 30–50% of patients show no observable benefit from ACheIs [27, 28]. Ultimately, progression of dementia is irreversible.

Exam Essentials

- ACheIs are contraindicated in patients with baseline bradycardia or known cardiac conduction system disease

- ACheIs are indicated for mild–moderate severity of dementia, while memantine is indicated for moderate–severe cases

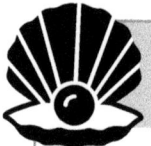

Clinical Pearls

- Rivastigmine is available as a transdermal patch, which may be a preferred choice for those who are non-compliant with oral medications – monitor for skin allergic reaction

- A combination of AChels with memantine may be considered for patients with more severe symptoms

- Patients with Parkinson's disease dementia/Lewy body dementia may benefit from rivastigmine, improving behaviour and psychotic symptoms

- Those with vascular aetiology may also benefit from rivastigmine

Question 9
What is the likely cause of her current altered mental status?

Answer
Delirium due to pneumonia

Explanation
Mary displays features of delirium: acute onset and fluctuating course of inattention and disorganised thinking. The underlying infective process (pneumonia) is the likely precipitant.

The CAM is a simple bedside screening tool for delirium. A background of cognitive impairment predisposes patients to delirium.

Diagnosis of delirium using the Confusion Assessment Method (CAM) [29]

1. Acute onset and fluctuating course

2. Inattention

3. Disorganised thinking

4. Altered level of consciousness

The diagnosis of delirium requires the presence of features 1 and 2 plus either 3 OR 4

Exam Essentials

- Three types of delirium:
  - Hyperactive
  - Hypoactive
  - Mixed delirium
- Sometimes, hypoactive delirium may be mistaken for depression, especially if patients present with poor oral intake, amotivation or lethargy

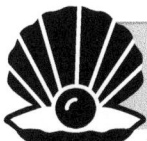

Clinical Pearls

- Delirium is diagnosed in 10–20% of medical and surgical inpatients [30]. Patients with a neurocognitive disorder are at higher risk of developing delirium
- Delirium can be of acute or sub-acute onset

Question 10
Following an inpatient admission, how would you manage Mary's delirium?

Answer
Identify and treat precipitating causes and exacerbating factors
Provide environmental and supportive measures
Management of behavioural problems

Explanation
The cornerstone of delirium management is directed towards treating or correcting the underlying cause of the delirium.

Supportive medical care includes maintaining adequate hydration and nutrition, enhancing mobility and range of motion, treating pain and discomfort, preventing skin breakdown, attention to incontinence and minimising the risk of aspiration pneumonia.

Environmental measures include educating caregivers, ensuring the environment is safe, optimising environment stimulation (e.g., adequate lighting, reducing unnecessary noise, correcting any sensory impairment), frequent reality orientation techniques (e.g., clocks and calendar) and providing clear communication, preferably by the same staff member/family member. Physical restraints should only be used as a last resort.

Melatonin is a safe medication that can help relieve sleep–wake reversal and improve sleep. Sedative medications should be used judiciously and be limited to the treatment of severely agitated patients in hyperactive delirium. Start with a single agent at a low dose and titrate upwards to clinical effect. While benzodiazepines have a more rapid onset of action, antipsychotics (e.g., haloperidol 0.5 to 1 mg used as needed) are preferred as benzodiazepines may worsen delirium (with the exception of alcohol withdrawal delirium). Quetiapine may also be considered especially for those with neuroleptic sensitivity (e.g., Parkinson's disease, Lewy body dementia). Look out for postural hypotension and the presence of QTc prolongation before commencing on antipsychotics.

Exam Essentials

- Sometimes, after the cause of delirium is removed, the patient's confusion may still not improve. Always check for other causes which might still be perpetuating delirium

- Due to poor cognitive reserves in Mary's case, delirium may take weeks to even months to improve. Sometimes, symptoms may not fully resolve, and it may unfortunately be the new baseline mentation for Mary

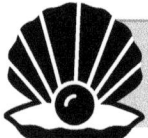

Clinical Pearls

- Always perform medication reconciliation and remove unnecessary prescriptions such as:
  - Painkillers
  - Anticholinergics
  - Antihistamines
  - Benzodiazepines or hypnotics

- Haloperidol or risperidone droplets can allow for even lower doses of 0.2 mg, which limit side effects and allow for easier administration

Question 11
What is Mary's revised diagnosis?

Answer
Dementia (major neurocognitive disorder) with behavioural disturbances (also commonly known as behavioural and psychological symptoms of dementia (BPSD) or neuropsychiatric symptoms of dementia)

Explanation
On a background of progressing dementia, symptoms of wandering, agitation, paranoia and hallucinations are suggestive of behavioural disturbances, commonly known as BPSD.

Symptoms of BPSD include agitation, aggression, delusions, hallucinations, paranoia, wandering, depression, apathy, disinhibition and sleep disturbances. One or more of these symptoms are observed in 60–90% of patients with dementia [31–33]; the prevalence increases with disease severity. Delusions and hallucinations (20–40%) [3] are common in patients with severe Alzheimer's disease.

Factors which support the diagnosis of BPSD include the presence of 'sundowning', where behavioural disturbances peak in the later afternoon or evening. Sundowning occurs in two-thirds of patients with dementia [34].

Exam Essentials

- **Sundowning** refers to the phenomenon where behavioural disturbances peak in the late afternoon or evening. Sundowning may be seen in both delirium and neurocognitive disorders, but patients with the latter usually have a more chronic course, and may not be as disorientated

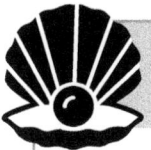

Clinical Pearls

- BPSD causes significant functional impairment and often leads to caregiver stress
- One may use the Zarit Burden Interview to objectively measure the caregiving burden [35]

Question 12
What are the pharmacological measures which can be used to manage Mary's moderate to severe Alzheimer's disease and the presence of BPSD?

Answer
Add on memantine

Judicious use of atypical antipsychotics (e.g., quetiapine, aripiprazole)

Antidepressants such as selective serotonin reuptake inhibitors (SSRIs; e.g., escitalopram) and serotonin antagonists and reuptake inhibitors (e.g., trazodone)

Explanation
Memantine is an N-methyl-D-aspartate receptor antagonist. It can also be used as a single agent among patients who do not tolerate ACheIs. While systematic reviews have concluded that memantine does not significantly improve BPSD symptoms and rarely paradoxically increases agitation and delusions, it can be used in combination with an ACheI in patients with moderate to advanced Alzheimer's disease (MMSE ≤ 18). The combination leads to modest improvements in cognition and global outcomes in patients with advanced disease.

A black box warning exists for antipsychotic use for BPSD [36, 37]: there is a higher risk of mortality and possibly stroke. Nonetheless, atypical antipsychotics are commonly used in the treatment of BPSD. Their benefits include the management of neuropsychiatric symptoms, particularly psychosis, that are severe, debilitating or pose a safety risk.

SSRIs can be useful in the management of agitation and paranoia in patients with Alzheimer's disease, as the symptoms are often driven by a mood disorder that is poorly verbalised. Short-term use of citalopram in non-depressed patients with a neurocognitive disorder may reduce agitation and caregiver distress [38, 39]. Trazodone is used for insomnia in patients with dementia.

Benzodiazepines should be avoided as these drugs have adverse side effects of worsening gait, potential paradoxical agitation and dependence. If required, their use should be limited to brief stressful episodes, such as a change in residence or an anxiety-provoking medical event.

Exam Essentials

- A **black box warning** exists for antipsychotic use for BPSD: there is a higher risk of mortality and possibly stroke

- Memantine may be used for patients with cardiac conduction problems

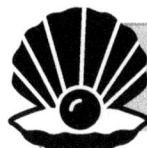

Clinical Pearls

- Memantine has no convincing benefit in mild Alzheimer's disease. While used in moderate to severe Alzheimer's disease, in rare instances it can paradoxically increase agitation and delusional behaviours

- There have been cases of **memantine-induced confusion**. Clinicians may need to stop treatment if the patient becomes more confused

- As memantine is excreted via the kidneys, renal-adjusted doses are needed in those with impaired kidney function

Diving Deep …

The incidence and prevalence of Alzheimer's disease increase exponentially with age, essentially doubling in prevalence every five years after the age of 65 years [40]. Memory impairment is the most common initial symptom of Alzheimer's disease. In patients with the typical form of the illness, deficits in other cognitive domains may appear with or after the development of memory impairment. Executive dysfunction and visuospatial impairment are often present relatively early, while deficits in language and behavioural symptoms often manifest later in the disease course.

Forty per cent of patients have a positive family history of Alzheimer's disease [3]. The American College of Medical Genetics and the National Society of Genetic Counselors do not recommend the use of APOE genotyping to diagnose Alzheimer's disease [41]. APOE is a susceptibility gene, not a determinative gene (i.e., not all patients who are homozygous for the APOE4 allele will develop Alzheimer's disease).

For carriers of the APOE4 allele, the odds of Alzheimer's disease [5, 42, 43] are as follows:

- one allele = 2–3-fold increase

- two alleles = 8–12-fold increase

Pseudodementia is a differential for dementia. Depressed elderly patients with psychomotor retardation may present with pseudodementia (i.e., marked difficulties with concentration and memory). Features suggestive of pseudodementia include a previous history of depression, current depressed mood, poor effort on testing (e.g., 'I don't know', 'it's too difficult') and a clinical response to antidepressant medication.

211

AChels do not slow the progression of dementia. A Cochrane review [44] reporting conversion to dementia gives no strong evidence of a beneficial effect of AChels on the progression to dementia at one, two or three years. The AD2000 study [45] found no significant benefit of donepezil compared with placebo for institutionalisation.

Non-pharmacological management of BPSD includes the use of aromatherapy, music therapy and massages. Light therapy through increased bright-light exposure in the mornings may have benefits independent of melatonin and can lead to improvement in sleep disturbances as well. Physical restraints (both physical and pharmacological) are associated with an increased risk of falls, incontinence and pressure ulcerations.

Haloperidol is a commonly used antipsychotic for delirium. It can be administered orally, intramuscularly or intravenously. The onset of action may be as soon as 5–20 minutes after intravenous administration or longer with the intramuscular or oral route. An immediate response is not expected. Intravenous haloperidol has been associated with clinically significant QT prolongation, requiring additional precautions with its use. High-potency neuroleptics (e.g., haloperidol) should be used with caution in patients with dementia as they are associated with a high incidence of extrapyramidal side effects.

The risk of death with the usage of atypical antipsychotics in patients with dementia is between 1.6 and 1.7 times the risk of death in placebo-treated patients based on the Dementia Antipsychotic Withdrawal Trial study [46]. As such, the American Psychiatric Association recommends that antipsychotic therapy be tapered within four months of initiation in patients who have responded to therapy and who have no prior history of relapse with medication taper.

Most patients with severe dementia will have eating problems in the final stages of their illness. Multiple studies have failed to show evidence for the purported benefits of tube feeding in severe Alzheimer's disease. In the late stage of dementia, the goal of care is primarily focused on comfort and provision of food and drink to the extent that it is enjoyable for the patient [47]. There is no evidence that tube feeding in severe dementia prolongs survival nor has it been shown to improve nutritional status or pressure ulcers [48]. Feeding tubes will not prevent aspiration and these procedures carry antecedent risks such as agitation with greater use of physical and/or chemical restraints and tube-related complications [49].

References

1. World Health Organization. *International classification of diseases*, 11th edition (ICD-11). Geneva: World Health Organization; 2024. Available from: https://icd.who.int/en

2. American Psychiatric Association. *Diagnostic and statistical manual of mental disorders*, 5th edition, text revision (DSM-5-TR). Washington, DC: American Psychiatric

Association Publishing; 2022. Available from: www.psychiatry.org/psychiatrists/practice/dsm

3. Semple D, Smyth R. *Oxford handbook of psychiatry*, 4th edition. Oxford: Oxford University Press; 2019.

4. Castellano JM, Kim J, Stewart FR, Jiang H, DeMattos RB, Patterson BW, et al. Human APOE isoforms differentially regulate brain amyloid-β peptide clearance. *Sci Transl Med.* 2011 Jun 29;3(89):89ra57.

5. Farrer LA, Cupples LA, Haines JL, Hyman B, Kukull WA, Mayeux R, et al. Effects of age, sex, and ethnicity on the association between apolipoprotein E genotype and Alzheimer disease. A meta-analysis. APOE and Alzheimer Disease Meta Analysis Consortium. *JAMA.* 1997 Oct 22;278(16):1349–56.

6. Laurin D, Verreault R, Lindsay J, MacPherson K, Rockwood K. Physical activity and risk of cognitive impairment and dementia in elderly persons. *Arch Neurol.* 2001 Mar 1;58(3). Available from: http://archneur.jamanetwork.com/article.aspx?doi=10.1001/archneur.58.3.498

7. Hodkinson HM. Evaluation of a mental test score for assessment of mental impairment in the elderly. *Age Ageing.* 1972 Nov;1(4):233–8.

8. Hazan E, Frankenburg F, Brenkel M, Shulman K. The test of time: a history of clock drawing. *Int J Geriatr Psychiatry.* 2018 Jan;33(1):e22–30.

9. Folstein MF, Folstein SE, McHugh PR. "Mini-mental state". A practical method for grading the cognitive state of patients for the clinician. *J Psychiatr Res.* 1975 Nov;12(3):189–98.

10. Nasreddine ZS, Phillips NA, Bédirian V, Charbonneau S, Whitehead V, Collin I, et al. The Montreal Cognitive Assessment, MoCA: a brief screening tool for mild cognitive impairment. *J Am Geriatr Soc.* 2005 Apr;53(4):695–9.

11. Mathuranath PS, Nestor PJ, Berrios GE, Rakowicz W, Hodges JR. A brief cognitive test battery to differentiate Alzheimer's disease and frontotemporal dementia. *Neurology.* 2000 Dec 12;55(11):1613–20.

12. Crum RM, Anthony JC, Bassett SS, Folstein MF. Population-based norms for the Mini-Mental State Examination by age and educational level. *JAMA.* 1993 May 12;269(18):2386–91.

13. Tsoi KKF, Chan JYC, Hirai HW, Wong SYS, Kwok TCY. Cognitive tests to detect dementia: a systematic review and meta-analysis. *JAMA Intern Med.* 2015 Sep;175(9):1450–8.

14. Tombaugh TN, McIntyre NJ. The Mini-Mental State Examination: a comprehensive review. *J Am Geriatr Soc.* 1992 Sep;40(9):922–35.

15. Knopman DS, DeKosky ST, Cummings JL, Chui H, Corey-Bloom J, Relkin N, et al. Practice parameter: diagnosis of dementia (an evidence-based review). Report of the Quality Standards Subcommittee of the American Academy of Neurology. *Neurology.* 2001 May 8;56(9):1143–53.

16. Woods B, Aguirre E, Spector AE, Orrell M. Cognitive stimulation to improve cognitive functioning in people with dementia. *Cochrane Database Syst Rev.* 2012 Feb 15;2012(2):CD005562.

17. Graff MJL, Vernooij-Dassen MJM, Thijssen M, Dekker J, Hoefnagels WHL, Rikkert MGMO. Community based occupational therapy for patients with dementia and their care givers: randomised controlled trial. *BMJ.* 2006 Dec 9;333(7580):1196.

213

18. White H. Weight change in Alzheimer's disease. *J Nutr Health Aging*. 1998;2(2):110–2.

19. Forbes D, Forbes SC, Blake CM, Thiessen EJ, Forbes S. Exercise programs for people with dementia. *Cochrane Database Syst Rev*. 2015 Apr 15;2015(4):CD006489.

20. Teri L, Gibbons LE, McCurry SM, Logsdon RG, Buchner DM, Barlow WE, et al. Exercise plus behavioral management in patients with Alzheimer disease: a randomized controlled trial. *JAMA*. 2003 Oct 15;290(15):2015–22.

21. Pitkälä KH, Pöysti MM, Laakkonen ML, Tilvis RS, Savikko N, Kautiainen H, et al. Effects of the Finnish Alzheimer Disease Exercise Trial (FINALEX): a randomized controlled trial. *JAMA Intern Med*. 2013 May 27;173(10):894–901.

22. National Institute for Health and Care Excellence (NICE). Donepezil, galantamine, rivastigmine and memantine for the treatment of Alzheimer's disease. Technology appraisal guidance [TA217]. NICE; 2011. Available from: www.nice.org.uk/guidance/ta217

23. Sano M, Ernesto C, Thomas RG, Klauber MR, Schafer K, Grundman M, et al. A controlled trial of selegiline, alpha-tocopherol, or both as treatment for Alzheimer's disease. The Alzheimer's Disease Cooperative Study. *N Engl J Med*. 1997 Apr 24;336(17):1216–22.

24. Farina N, Llewellyn D, Isaac MGEKN, Tabet N. Vitamin E for Alzheimer's dementia and mild cognitive impairment. *Cochrane Database Syst Rev*. 2017 Jan 27;2017(1):CD002854.

25. Birks J, Grimley Evans J. Ginkgo biloba for cognitive impairment and dementia. *Cochrane Database Syst Rev*. 2009 Jan 21;2009(1):CD003120.

26. DeKosky ST, Williamson JD, Fitzpatrick AL, Kronmal RA, Ives DG, Saxton JA, et al. Ginkgo biloba for prevention of dementia: a randomized controlled trial. *JAMA*. 2008 Nov 19;300(19):2253–62.

27. Cummings JL. Use of cholinesterase inhibitors in clinical practice: evidence-based recommendations. *Am J Geriatr Psychiatry*. 2003;11(2):131–45.

28. Clark CM, Karlawish JHT. Alzheimer disease: current concepts and emerging diagnostic and therapeutic strategies. *Ann Intern Med*. 2003 Mar 4;138(5):400–10.

29. Wei LA, Fearing MA, Sternberg EJ, Inouye SK. The Confusion Assessment Method: a systematic review of current usage. *J Am Geriatr Soc*. 2008 May;56(5):823–30.

30. Burns A. Delirium. *J Neurol, Neurosurg Psychiatry*. 2004 Mar 1;75(3):362–7.

31. Mega MS, Cummings JL, Fiorello T, Gornbein J. The spectrum of behavioral changes in Alzheimer's disease. *Neurology*. 1996 Jan;46(1):130–5.

32. Lyketsos CG, Steinberg M, Tschanz JT, Norton MC, Steffens DC, Breitner JC. Mental and behavioral disturbances in dementia: findings from the Cache County Study on Memory in Aging. *Am J Psychiatry*. 2000 May;157(5):708–14.

33. Lyketsos CG, Lopez O, Jones B, Fitzpatrick AL, Breitner J, DeKosky S. Prevalence of neuropsychiatric symptoms in dementia and mild cognitive impairment: results from the cardiovascular health study. *JAMA*. 2002 Sep 25;288(12):1475–83.

34. Gallagher-Thompson D, Brooks JO, Bliwise D, Leader J, Yesavage JA. The relations among caregiver stress, "sundowning" symptoms, and cognitive decline in Alzheimer's disease. *J Am Geriatr Soc*. 1992 Aug;40(8):807–10.

35. Zarit SH, Reever KE, Back-Peterson J. Relatives of the impaired elderly: correlates of feelings of burden. *Gerontologist* 1980;20:649–55.

36. Atypical antipsychotics in the elderly. *Med Lett Drugs Ther.* 2005 Aug 1;47(1214):61–2.

37. Kuehn BM. FDA warns antipsychotic drugs may be risky for elderly. *JAMA.* 2005 May 25;293(20):2462.

38. Porsteinsson AP, Drye LT, Pollock BG, Devanand DP, Frangakis C, Ismail Z, et al. Effect of citalopram on agitation in Alzheimer disease: the CitAD randomized clinical trial. *JAMA.* 2014 Feb 19;311(7):682–91.

39. Pollock BG, Mulsant BH, Rosen J, Sweet RA, Mazumdar S, Bharucha A, et al. Comparison of citalopram, perphenazine, and placebo for the acute treatment of psychosis and behavioral disturbances in hospitalized, demented patients. *Am J Psychiatry.* 2002 Mar;159(3):460–5.

40. Qiu C, Kivipelto M, von Strauss E. Epidemiology of Alzheimer's disease: occurrence, determinants, and strategies toward intervention. *Dialogues Clin Neurosci.* 2009;11(2):111–28.

41. Goldman JS, Hahn SE, Catania JW, LaRusse-Eckert S, Butson MB, Rumbaugh M, et al. Genetic counseling and testing for Alzheimer disease: joint practice guidelines of the American College of Medical Genetics and the National Society of Genetic Counselors. *Genet Med.* 2011 Jun;13(6):597–605.

42. Slooter AJC, Cruts M, Hofman A, Koudstaal PJ, van der Kuip D, de Ridder M a. J, et al. The impact of APOE on myocardial infarction, stroke, and dementia: the Rotterdam Study. *Neurology.* 2004 Apr 13;62(7):1196–8.

43. Myers RH, Schaefer EJ, Wilson PW, D'Agostino R, Ordovas JM, Espino A, et al. Apolipoprotein E epsilon4 association with dementia in a population-based study: the Framingham study. *Neurology.* 1996 Mar;46(3):673–7.

44. Birks J. Cholinesterase inhibitors for Alzheimer's disease. *Cochrane Database Syst Rev.* 2006 Jan 25;2006(1):CD005593.

45. Courtney C, Farrell D, Gray R, Hills R, Lynch L, Sellwood E, et al. Long-term donepezil treatment in 565 patients with Alzheimer's disease (AD2000): randomised double-blind trial. *Lancet.* 2004 Jun 26;363(9427):2105–15.

46. Ballard C, Hanney ML, Theodoulou M, Douglas S, McShane R, Kossakowski K, et al. The dementia antipsychotic withdrawal trial (DART-AD): long-term follow-up of a randomised placebo-controlled trial. *Lancet Neurol.* 2009 Feb;8(2):151–7.

47. American Geriatrics Society Ethics Committee and Clinical Practice and Models of Care Committee. American Geriatrics Society feeding tubes in advanced dementia position statement. *J Am Geriatr Soc.* 2014 Aug;62(8):1590–3.

48. Finucane TE. Malnutrition, tube feeding and pressure sores: data are incomplete. *J Am Geriatr Soc.* 1995 Apr;43(4):447–51.

49. Finucane TE, Bynum JP. Use of tube feeding to prevent aspiration pneumonia. *Lancet.* 1996 Nov 23;348(9039):1421–4.

Case 22: Mental Capacity Assessment

Can he decide on his own matters?

The general medicine team has referred to the psychiatry consultation team for an opinion on Bill's mental capacity. He is a 79-year-old gentleman with a known history of dementia (major neurocognitive disorder) due to Alzheimer's disease. He was admitted a week ago for treatment of pyelonephritis and had been displaying behavioural issues in the ward, such as fluctuating consciousness, intermittent agitation and reporting that he could see his dead wife in the ward. These symptoms were not present when he was at home. His son has expressed that Bill's memory issues have worsened over the past two years. His son is keen to apply for a nursing home placement for Bill as he is unable to provide care for him at home.

- **Question 1: What is the most likely disease of the mind that he is suffering from at present?**

The medical social worker has reviewed Bill's case and assessed that he is suitable for a nursing home application. The general medicine team is requesting a mental capacity assessment as Bill oscillates between agreeing and disagreeing with his nursing home application.

- **Question 2: How would you advise the general medicine team about the request for a mental capacity assessment?**

Three days later, the general medicine medical officer phoned the psychiatry consultation team to enquire about Bill's mental capacity to decide on consenting to a percutaneous nephrostomy (PCN) tube insertion. The urologist is worried about complications of sepsis and opined that such a procedure is necessary for treatment. Bill's mental state did not improve, and he is still intermittently confused, giving irrelevant answers to questions.

- **Question 3: How would you advise the medical officer about the new request for a mental capacity assessment?**

- **Question 4: When assessing Bill's mental capacity to consent to a PCN tube insertion, what are the principles and general approaches you would use during your assessment?**

Answers to Case 22

Question 1
What is the most likely disease of the mind that he is suffering from at present?

Answer
Delirium superimposed on dementia due to Alzheimer's disease

Explanation
Bill has an acute and recent change in behaviour and mental state in the ward, which should prompt the treating doctors to diagnose him with delirium on top of his previously diagnosed dementia. (Refer to Case 21 for more information.)

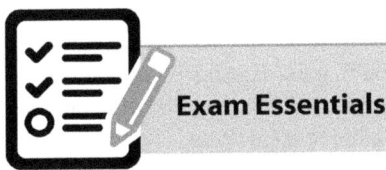

Exam Essentials

- Multiple diseases of the mind such as delirium and dementia can co-exist in a patient

Question 2
How would you advise the general medicine team about the request for a mental capacity assessment?

Answer
As delirium will take time to settle, the mental capacity assessment may need to be postponed until Bill's delirium resolves, as the decision for placement is not medically urgent and can be discussed at a later time as the delirium improves.

Explanation
The request for a mental capacity assessment for a placement decision may be postponed and is not urgent or time-sensitive. Assessors of mental capacity should advocate for the assessment to be made when all possible reversible disease(s) of the mind are treated – in Bill's case, to allow for the delirium to resolve. Even if the assessment is made at this juncture, assessors must caveat that his capacity may fluctuate, and a reassessment will be required at a later time.

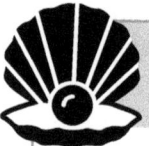

Clinical Pearls

- The timing of the assessment is dependent on the type of decision to be made (i.e., whether the decision is urgent or time-sensitive)

Question 3

How would you advise the medical officer about the new request for a mental capacity assessment?

Answer

The medical officer should be advised to proceed with the mental capacity assessment given that the procedure is time-sensitive and deemed to be necessary at present.

Explanation

As the procedure is time-sensitive and deemed to be necessary, there will be a need to assess his mental capacity at this cross-sectional juncture. There may not be enough time to allow for his delirium to completely resolve as the procedure will address the underlying cause of his delirium. Again, assessors must caveat that his capacity will fluctuate, and that this assessment is decision- and time-specific for the PCN tube insertion, and not for other procedures or matters such as his nursing home application.

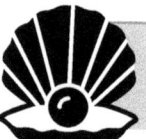

Clinical Pearls

- Types of capacity assessment include:

    ◦ Procedures
    ◦ Treatment
    ◦ Placement
    ◦ At own risk discharge
    ◦ Personal affairs
    ◦ Finances
    ◦ Testamentary (will-making)
    ◦ Lasting power of attorney

Question 4

When assessing Bill's mental capacity to consent to a PCN tube insertion, what are the principles and general approaches you would use during your assessment?

Answer

With reference to the England and Wales Mental Capacity Act (2005) [1], there are five broad guiding principles:

1. Identify the question
   - The question of capacity is assessed in relation to the particular decision required of the patient and the nature of this decision should be established prior to the interview

2. Consider whether the patient has capacity to make the decision
   - If the person can **understand** and **retain** the information relevant to the decision, **weigh** the information as part of the process of making the decision, and **communicate** his or her decision

3. Evaluate the presence of an impairment of, or a disturbance in the functioning of, the mind or brain and determine whether it is influencing the patient's decision

4. Gather additional information
   - What views did the patient previously hold when greater capacity existed (e.g., is there an advance directive? Was his opinion on the matter conveyed to family members before?)
   - What views do the patient's relatives or carers hold? Is there a relative with surrogate decision-making powers? (e.g., lasting power of attorney, court-appointed deputy in England and Wales or guardian in Scotland)

5. Report and document opinion

Explanation

The principles for the purposes of the Mental Capacity Act are as follows:

- **A person must be assumed to have capacity** unless it is established that the person lacks capacity

- A person is not to be treated as unable to make a decision unless **all practicable steps to help the person to do so have been taken** without success

- A person is **not to be treated as unable to make a decision merely because the person makes an unwise decision**

- An act done, or a decision made, under this Act for or on behalf of a person who lacks capacity must be done, or made, in the person's **best interests**

- Before the act is done, or the decision is made, regard must be made to whether the purpose for which it is needed can be as effectively achieved in a way that is **less restrictive** of the person's rights and freedom of action

Do note that, for the first step of the assessment, it does not matter if the impairment or disturbance is permanent or temporary and that a lack of capacity cannot be established merely by reference to age, condition or behaviour which may lead others to have unjustified assumptions.

Exam Essentials

- If the patient declines the procedure, ask if they are aware of any alternative treatments

- Do not assume that the patient lacks mental capacity simply because the individual has cognitive impairment or psychosis. Assessment is still needed to ascertain how their symptoms affect the decision-making

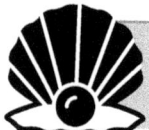

Clinical Pearls

- The four components of a mental capacity assessment include

  ○ Understand
  ○ Retain
  ○ Weigh
  ○ Communicate

- If the patient lacks mental capacity, it is important to ascertain if the incapacity is **temporary or permanent**. If the incapacity is temporary, the patient needs to be reassessed when their condition improves

- Clear documentation is imperative for capacity assessment as this is medicolegal

Diving Deep ...

For one to suspect that an individual has lost his or her capacity, the individual should be established to be suffering from a disease of the mind, which is not limited to delirium, brain tumours, dementia or other mental illnesses. Hence, investigations and bedside assessments such as the Mini-Mental State Examination or Montreal Cognitive Assessment that help to determine the presence of such disease(s) are important and should be performed before a mental capacity assessment is attempted.

The lasting power of attorney is a power of attorney under which the donor confers on the donee(s) authority to make decisions about all or any of the donor's **health**

and welfare and **property and financial affairs** when the donor no longer has the capacity to make such decisions.

Testamentary capacity involves the ability to make complex decisions regarding one's property and affairs through a will. Assessment of testamentary capacity is guided by the Banks v Goodfellow test [2], which requires the following four criteria to be fulfilled:

1. Understand the nature of the will and its effect

2. Understand the extent of the property of which they are disposing under the will

3. Understand the persons for whom they would usually be expected to provide

4. The donor is free from any delusion of the mind or mental disorders that would affect their dispositions to those people

References

1. Parliament of the United Kingdom. Mental Capacity Act 2005, c. 9. Available from: www.legislation.gov.uk/ukpga/2005/9/contents/enacted

2. Banks v Goodfellow (1870) LR 5 QB 549.

Case 23: Attention Deficit Hyperactivity Disorder

The dance of distraction

Josh, a 7-year-old boy, was brought in by his mother Rose to your clinic. She mentions that she has been receiving multiple calls from the school that Josh 'is unable to sit still' and is constantly squirming in his seat, intruding into other people's activities and doesn't finish his schoolwork on time. Josh finds it difficult to make friends – his classmates find him a 'show off' when he blurts out answers in class – and is frequently reprimanded for being too talkative. Rose also acknowledges that he is restless at home, has poor concentration when doing his homework and is unable and reluctant to complete the tasks she has assigned him. Rose also has to purchase multiple stationery items as Josh always loses them. Josh has been doing poorly academically and has failed to complete his examination papers on time, on multiple occasions. As a result, Rose decided to leave her job to spend more time tutoring Josh.

- **Question 1: What is the most likely diagnosis? Which differential diagnoses would you consider?**

- **Question 2: How would you further evaluate Josh to confirm the diagnosis of ADHD?**

- **Question 3: How would you differentiate inattention from learning difficulties?**

- **Question 4: How would you manage Josh's ADHD?**

You started Josh on methylphenidate (Ritalin), but his parents are worried about the side effects of the medication.

- **Question 5: What are the common side effects of methylphenidate?**

After three months of using methylphenidate, Josh started to develop tics.

- **Question 6: What is the difference between a tic and a stereotypy?**

- **Question 7: What is your next course of action in response to Josh getting methylphenidate-related tics?**

Answers to Case 23

Question 1
What is the most likely diagnosis? Which differential diagnoses would you consider?

Answer
Attention deficit hyperactivity disorder (ADHD) – predominantly inattentive presentation

Differentials include oppositional defiance disorder (ODD)

Explanation

Diagnosis of ADHD [1]

A persistent pattern (e.g., over at least six months) of inattention symptoms and/or a combination of hyperactivity and impulsivity symptoms that is outside the limits of normal variation expected for age and level of intellectual development is required for diagnosis. Symptoms vary according to chronological age and disorder severity.

Inattention

- Several symptoms of inattention that are persistent and sufficiently severe that they have a direct negative impact on academic, occupational or social functioning are among the essential components. Symptoms are typically from the following clusters:
  - Having difficulty sustaining attention on tasks that do not provide a high level of stimulation or reward or require sustained mental effort
  - Lacking attention to detail
  - Making careless mistakes in school or work assignments
  - Not completing tasks
  - Being easily distracted by extraneous stimuli or thoughts not related to the task at hand
  - Often seeming not to listen when spoken to directly

- ∘ Frequently appearing to be daydreaming or to have their mind elsewhere
- ∘ Losing things
- ∘ Being forgetful in daily activities
- ∘ Having difficulty remembering to complete upcoming daily tasks or activities
- ∘ Having difficulty planning, managing and organising schoolwork, tasks and other activities

Note: inattention may not be evident when the individual is engaged in activities that provide intense stimulation and frequent rewards.

Hyperactivity–impulsivity

- Several symptoms of hyperactivity–impulsivity that are persistent and sufficiently severe that they have a direct negative impact on academic, occupational or social functioning are among the essential components. These tend to be most evident in structured situations that require behavioural self-control. Symptoms are typically from the following clusters:

  - ∘ Showing excessive motor activity
  - ∘ Leaving their seat when expected to sit still
  - ∘ Often running about
  - ∘ Having difficulty sitting still without fidgeting (younger children)
  - ∘ Displaying feelings of physical restlessness and a sense of discomfort with being quiet or sitting still (adolescents and adults)
  - ∘ Having difficulty engaging in activities quietly
  - ∘ Talking too much
  - ∘ Blurting out answers in school or comments at work
  - ∘ Having difficulty waiting their turn in conversation, games or activities; interrupting or intruding on others' conversations or games
  - ∘ Having a tendency to act in response to immediate stimuli without deliberation or consideration of risks and consequences (e.g., engaging in behaviours with potential for physical injury; impulsive decisions; reckless driving)

- Several symptoms were present before age 12 years

- Symptoms are evident across multiple situations or settings

Condition	Defining feature(s)
ADHD	Josh has been suffering from both inattention and hyperactivity–impulsivity symptoms for years. These symptoms must persist in two or more settings (both in school and at home for Josh's case). This has affected Josh's interpersonal functioning as well as academic functioning

Condition	Defining feature(s)
ODD	Although Josh is unable to comply with requests from authoritative figures or rules, it does not seem to be an active defiance or refusal to comply. He does not have the angry/irritable, argumentative/defiant behaviour or vindictiveness that is seen in ODD

Exam Essentials

- Symptoms of inattention – **SOLID**
    - **S**tarts tasks without finishing
    - **O**rganisation poor
    - **L**oses things necessary for tasks
    - **I**nstructions not followed
    - **D**istraction by external stimuli
- Symptoms of hyperactivity and impulsiveness – **WORST FAIL**
    - **W**aiting for turns causes frustration
    - **O**n the move
    - **R**estless and jittery
    - **S**quirms in seat
    - **T**alks excessively
    - **F**idgets with limbs
    - **A**nswers blurted
    - **I**nterrupting others' conversations
    - **L**oud noises when playing

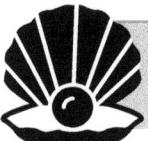

Clinical Pearls

- ADHD has three specifiers
    - Combined presentation
    - Predominantly inattentive
    - Predominantly hyperactive or impulsive
- Always assess for learning difficulties in a hyperactive and/or inattentive child with poor grades as they can be co-morbid in ADHD

Question 2
How would you further evaluate Josh to confirm the diagnosis of ADHD?

Answer
The diagnosing clinician can rely on the following to help confirm the diagnosis:

- Observations by teachers, parents or school counsellors

- ADHD questionnaires

- Computerised performance test (CPT)

- Intellectual quotient (IQ) testing

Explanation
ADHD is often diagnosed clinically and does not have laboratory or radiological tests. The evaluation of the patient is usually done with different rating scales with multiple informants (i.e., teachers and parents). The CPT may also be used as an objective measure of the patient's inattention and impulsivity during the test.

A recent test called the Qbtest [2] has been found to quicken diagnostic decision-making, and consultation time to diagnosis was reduced by 15%. This particular test uses infrared cameras to detect motor activity during the test, and to provide objective measures of attention, impulsivity and activity (the three domains of ADHD).

If clinically indicated, IQ testing may be done to exclude an intellectual disability that is a common masquerade of ADHD.

Clinical Pearls

- Different scales may be used for children and adults to measure the morbidity of ADHD.
  - Children: Conners Rating Scales–Revised (CRS-R) [3] and Vanderbilt ADHD diagnostic parent/teacher rating scales [4]
  - Adults: Adult ADHD Self-Report Scale (ASRS) [5]

Question 3
How would you differentiate inattention from learning difficulties?

Answer
Learning difficulties often present with consistently poor performance whilst inattention presents with fluctuating performance (the patient is able to do well, but not consistently as a result of lapses in attention).

Explanation

The abovementioned is often used as a clinical guide. Research has suggested that ADHD and IQ deficiencies are often related. This association becomes more prominent with age, as patients with ADHD might struggle more in mainstream educational systems as compared to their non-ADHD peers due to inattention, hyperactivity and impulsivity symptoms.

Question 4

How would you manage Josh's ADHD?

Answer

Biological: stimulants (i.e., methylphenidate)

Psychological: behavioural therapy

Social: psychoeducation for family and patient

Explanation

The mainstay of treatment is pharmacological with stimulant options being more effective than non-stimulant options. Stimulants are effective in 70% of patients [6, 7]. Examples of stimulants include methylphenidate, dexamfetamine and lisdexamfetamine. Methylphenidate is typically the first-line medication. Dexamfetamine is less well tolerated than methylphenidate. Lisdexamfetamine is the prodrug which is hydrolysed to dexamfetamine.

Behavioural interventions include modifications in the physical and social environment that are designed to change behaviour using rewards and non-punitive consequences. Behavioural techniques that are used for children with ADHD include positive reinforcement, time out, response cost (withdrawing rewards or privileges when unwanted or problem behaviour occurs) and token economy (a combination of positive reinforcement and response cost).

Psychoeducation is important to help parents understand their child's condition to best support them in their journey to recovery.

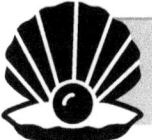 **Clinical Pearls**

- Hyperactivity symptoms tend to improve as the child matures. However, inattention tends to be more persistent in adulthood

Question 5

What are the common side effects of methylphenidate?

Answer

Psychological symptoms: decreased appetite, insomnia, tics, psychosis

Physical symptoms: blood pressure changes, tachycardia, growth stunting

227

Explanation

Side effects were reported in about 51.2% of patients on methylphenidate [8]. The most common side effects are decreased appetite (31.1%) and insomnia (17.9%). Psychostimulants (mainly methylphenidate) have traditionally been associated with the appearance of tics due to the increased dopamine activity caused by stimulants. New-onset psychosis has been noted to occur in approximately 1 in 660 patients who are prescribed methylphenidate [9].

Changes in blood pressure can occur, however not significant enough to be considered hypertension, with systolic blood pressure increases of 3–8 mmHg and diastolic blood pressure increases of 2–14 mmHg [10]. Pulse increases of 3–10 beats per minute may also be found [11]. Growth stunting of approximately 2–4 cm may be noted as well [12].

Exam Essentials

- It is advised to check ECG, weight/height/nutrition before starting methylphenidate

- Extended-release stimulants such as Concerta have a better side-effect profile than immediate release methylphenidate and are recommended for older patients

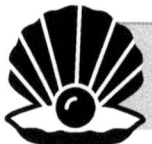

Clinical Pearls

- It is important to counsel parents that despite controversies of potential abuse, there is no evidence that stimulants produce 'euphoric' effects in children when restricted to normal treatment

- Stimulant therapy is associated with reduced risk for subsequent drug and alcohol use disorders [13]

Question 6

What is the difference between a tic and a stereotypy?

Answer

A tic is a sudden, less predictable, non-rhythmic and repetitive motor movement or vocalisation, without any purpose; for example, vocal tics could include grunting, snarling, coprolalia (involuntary utterance of vulgarities) and echolalia. In contrast, a stereotypy is a predictable, rhythmic, repeated, fixed movement that is also seemingly purposeless.

Explanation

	Stereotypy	Tics
Onset	1–4 years	5–7 years
Movement type	Repeated rhythmic movements (i.e., wavelike, jiggling)	Fixed, sudden short aimless movement movements (i.e., blinking, grimacing, jerking)
Suppressibility	By external distraction	Self-directed, concentration dependent
Ego	Egosyntonic	Egodystonic
Response to treatment	None	Neuroepileptics

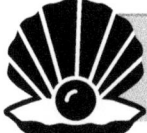

Clinical Pearls

- Always explore co-morbid disorders in ADHD:
  - Learning disorders
  - Depression
  - Anxiety
  - Conduct disorder
  - Tic disorders
  - Obsessive–compulsive disorder
  - Autism spectrum disorder

Question 7
What is your next course of action in response to Josh getting methylphenidate-related tics?

Answer
Medications can be changed to non-stimulants such as atomoxetine, and alpha agonists such as clonidine and guanfacine. Adjunctive alpha agonists can be added to reduce the tics.

229

Explanation

Atomoxetine is a selective noradrenaline reuptake inhibitor with an onset of action of four to six weeks. While less effective than stimulants, it is useful when stimulants are not tolerated or where stimulant diversion is a problem. Side effects include insomnia, mood and appetite changes and, rarely, liver injury. There is also a US Black Box warning of increased risk of suicidal ideation in short-term studies in children or adolescents with ADHD on atomoxetine [14, 15].

Alpha agonists are found to be more effective in younger children than in adults. Guanfacine and clonidine are central alpha-2A-adrenergic receptor agonists with an onset of action of approximately one to five weeks. They are common alternatives to both stimulants and selective noradrenaline reuptake inhibitors. Side effects include constipation, giddiness, dryness of the mouth, sleepiness and headaches.

While studies have suggested decreased fatty acid concentrations in children with ADHD, evidence for the efficacy of fatty acid supplementation in the treatment of core ADHD symptoms is limited [16–18]. The relationship between diet and symptoms of ADHD is controversial and the American Academy of Pediatrics [19], the American Academy of Allergy, Asthma and Immunology [20] and the United Kingdom's National Institute for Health and Care Excellence (NICE) [21] do not recommend the practice of routine elimination diets. However, a short trial of a medically supervised (close follow-up with physician and dietician) elimination diet can be favourable in some children [22–24]. Second-generation antipsychotics may be helpful in patients with autism with symptoms of hyperactivity, but evidence for their use in ADHD alone is limited.

Exam Essentials

- Side effects of atomoxetine include worsening mood and liver dysfunction

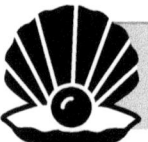

Clinical Pearls

- For patients who cannot tolerate stimulants, bupropion may be considered. This is especially so if the patient has concomitant depression

Diving Deep ...

To fulfil the criteria for a tic disorder, the individual must have experienced tics (either multiple motor tics and/or one vocal tic), and symptom onset should be before the age of 18 and not be due to an underlying substance usage or medical condition.

Tic disorders are subclassified into three main subtypes:

- Tourette's syndrome: both motor and vocal tics for at least one year

- Persistent (chronic) motor or vocal tic disorder: either motor or vocal tics for at least one year

- Provisional tic disorder: motor and/or vocal tics but the duration of symptoms has not met the one-year criterion

Differential diagnoses of tic disorders include transient tic disorder: 25% of children [25]; involving blinks, frowns, grimaces, head flicks, grunts, throat clearing, sniffs from four weeks to one year in duration, with good prognosis.

References

1. World Health Organization. *International classification of diseases*, 11th edition (ICD-11). Geneva: World Health Organization; 2024. Available from: https://icd.who.int/en

2. Hollis C, Hall CL, Guo B, James M, Boadu J, Groom MJ, et al. The impact of a computerised test of attention and activity (QbTest) on diagnostic decision-making in children and young people with suspected attention deficit hyperactivity disorder: single-blind randomised controlled trial. *J Child Psychol Psychiatry*. 2018 Dec;59(12):1298–308.

3. Mueller F, Brozovich R, Johnson CB. Conners' Rating Scales-Revised (CRS-R). *Diagnostique*. 1999 Mar;24(1–4):83–97.

4. Wolraich ML. Psychometric properties of the Vanderbilt ADHD diagnostic parent rating scale in a referred population. *J Pediatr Psychol*. 2003 Dec 1;28(8):559–68.

5. Kessler RC, Adler L, Ames M, Demler O, Faraone S, Hiripi E, et al. The World Health Organization Adult ADHD Self-Report Scale (ASRS): a short screening scale for use in the general population. *Psychol Med*. 2005 Feb;35(2):245–56.

6. Schachter HM, Pham B, King J, Langford S, Moher D. How efficacious and safe is short-acting methylphenidate for the treatment of attention-deficit disorder in children and adolescents? A meta-analysis. *CMAJ*. 2001 Nov 27;165(11):1475–88.

7. Barbaresi WJ, Katusic SK, Colligan RC, Weaver AL, Leibson CL, Jacobsen SJ. Long-term stimulant medication treatment of attention-deficit/hyperactivity disorder: results from a population-based study. *J Dev Behav Pediatr*. 2006 Feb;27(1):1–10.

8. Storebø OJ, Pedersen N, Ramstad E, Kielsholm ML, Nielsen SS, Krogh HB, et al. Methylphenidate for attention deficit hyperactivity disorder (ADHD) in children and adolescents: assessment of adverse events in non-randomised studies. *Cochrane Database Syst Rev*. 2018 May 9;5(5):CD012069.

9. Moran LV, Ongur D, Hsu J, Castro VM, Perlis RH, Schneeweiss S. Psychosis with methylphenidate or amphetamine in patients with ADHD. *N Engl J Med*. 2019 Mar 21;380(12):1128–38.

10. Samuels JA, Franco K, Wan F, Sorof JM. Effect of stimulants on 24-h ambulatory blood pressure in children with ADHD: a double-blind, randomized, cross-over trial. *Pediatr Nephrol*. 2006 Jan;21(1):92–5.

11. Fay TB, Alpert MA. Cardiovascular effects of drugs used to treat attention-deficit/ hyperactivity disorder. Part 2: impact on cardiovascular events and recommendations for evaluation and monitoring. *Cardiol Rev*. 2019;27(4):173–8.

12. Greenhill LL, Swanson JM, Hechtman L, Waxmonsky J, Arnold LE, Molina BSG, et al. Trajectories of growth associated with long-term stimulant medication in the multimodal treatment study of attention-deficit/hyperactivity disorder. *J Am Acad Child Adolesc Psychiatry*. 2020 Aug;59(8):978–89.

13. Wilens TE, Faraone SV, Biederman J, Gunawardene S. Does stimulant therapy of attention-deficit/hyperactivity disorder beget later substance abuse? A meta-analytic review of the literature. *Pediatrics*. 2003 Jan;111(1):179–85.

14. Bangs ME, Tauscher-Wisniewski S, Polzer J, Zhang S, Acharya N, Desaiah D, et al. Meta-analysis of suicide-related behavior events in patients treated with atomoxetine. *J Am Acad Child Adolesc Psychiatry*. 2008 Feb;47(2):209–18.

15. Davies M, Coughtrie A, Layton D, Shakir SAS. Use of atomoxetine and suicidal ideation in children and adolescents: results of an observational cohort study within general practice in England. *Eur Psychiatr*. 2017 Jan;39:11–6.

16. Sonuga-Barke EJS, Brandeis D, Cortese S, Daley D, Ferrin M, Holtmann M, et al. Nonpharmacological interventions for ADHD: systematic review and meta-analyses of randomized controlled trials of dietary and psychological treatments. *Am J Psychiatry*. 2013 Mar;170(3):275–89.

17. Bloch MH, Qawasmi A. Omega-3 fatty acid supplementation for the treatment of children with attention-deficit/hyperactivity disorder symptomatology: systematic review and meta-analysis. *J Am Acad Child Adolesc Psychiatry*. 2011 Oct;50(10):991–1000.

18. Barragán E, Breuer D, Döpfner M. Efficacy and safety of omega-3/6 fatty acids, methylphenidate, and a combined treatment in children with ADHD. *J Atten Disord*. 2017 Mar;21(5):433–41.

19. Wolraich ML, Hagan JF, Allan C, Chan E, Davison D, Earls M, et al. Clinical practice guideline for the diagnosis, evaluation, and treatment of attention-deficit/hyperactivity disorder in children and adolescents. *Pediatrics*. 2019 Oct;144(4):e20192528.

20. Sampson HA, Aceves S, Bock SA, James J, Jones S, Lang D, et al. Food allergy: a practice parameter update – 2014. *J Allergy Clin Immunol*. 2014 Nov;134(5):1016–1025.e43.

21. National Institute for Health and Care Excellence (NICE). Attention deficit hyperactivity disorder: diagnosis and management. NICE guideline [NG87]. NICE; 2018. Available from: www.nice.org.uk/guidance/NG87

22. Rojas NL, Chan E. Old and new controversies in the alternative treatment of attention-deficit hyperactivity disorder. *Ment Retard Dev Disabil Res Rev*. 2005;11(2):116–30.

23. Nigg JT, Lewis K, Edinger T, Falk M. Meta-analysis of attention-deficit/hyperactivity disorder or attention-deficit/hyperactivity disorder symptoms, restriction diet, and synthetic food color additives. *J Am Acad Child Adolesc Psychiatry*. 2012 Jan;51(1):86–97.e8.

24. Millichap JG, Yee MM. The diet factor in attention-deficit/hyperactivity disorder. *Pediatrics*. 2012 Feb;129(2):330–7.

25. Jankovic J, Kurlan R. Tourette syndrome: evolving concepts. *Mov Disord*. 2011 May;26(6):1149–56.

Case 24: Autism Spectrum Disorder and Intellectual Developmental Disorder

Why is my child different?

Jacob is a 3-year-old boy brought to your clinic by his mother for concerns about 'slow development'. Jacob was born through normal vaginal delivery with no antenatal complications. He has always been a 'quiet child', and his first spoken words were at one and a half years old. Since then, he has only been able to say five words in total and has not formed two-word phrases. He can follow one-step commands without gestures but often seems disinterested in engaging with others. His parents describe him as a 'good toddler' who does not demand much attention from them. At children's parties, Jacob is often seen playing alone and not interacting with others. He would only play with toy trains that are yellow and gets upset when other children join in. When Jacob is interested in an object, he does not point at it but instead pulls his parents to it. His parents also noted that he has difficulty maintaining eye contact and often does not respond when his name is called. He repeatedly flaps his hands and rocks his body.

- **Question 1: What is Jacob's diagnosis?**

Jacob's parents asked if he had 'Asperger's syndrome' instead.

- **Question 2: What is Asperger's syndrome?**

- **Question 3: What co-morbid conditions and genetic causes are associated with ASD?**

As intellectual developmental disorder/intellectual disability is a common co-morbidity, Jacob was screened for it.

- **Question 4: What clinical features are suggestive of intellectual developmental disorder/intellectual disability?**

The screening test for intellectual disability was unremarkable and Jacob was diagnosed with ASD without accompanying intellectual impairment.

- **Question 5: What are the risk factors for ASD?**

- **Question 6: Having diagnosed Jacob with ASD, what are the non-pharmacological management options available in the management of ASD?**

Jacob undergoes behavioural therapy with subsequent enrolment into a special needs school. In primary school, he was noted to be disruptive in class with significant explosive outbursts of agitation, such as banging his head against the wall and biting others. Non-pharmacological measures were unsuccessful and there are concerns for his safety and that of his caregivers.

- **Question 7: What pharmacological management options are available in the treatment of aggression in ASD?**

Answers to Case 24

Question 1
What is Jacob's diagnosis?

Answer
Autism spectrum disorder (ASD)

Explanation
Jacob displays core features of ASD: (1) impaired social interactions, (2) restricted behaviour and (3) impaired communication.

Features of ASD can be remembered with the mnemonic 'ABC'	
'A' = Asocial	Few or no sustained relationships Persistent aloofness or awkward interactions with peers Unusually egocentric, with little concern for others or awareness of their viewpoint and limited empathy or sensitivity Lack of awareness of social rules and reciprocity

Features of ASD can be remembered with the mnemonic 'ABC'	
'B' = Behaviour restricted and repetitive	Obsessively pursued and unusually circumscribed interests Unusual routines or rituals, change is often upsetting Focus on rules
'C' = Communication impaired	Odd voice, monotonous, perhaps at an unusual volume talking 'at' (rather than 'to') you, with little awareness about their response Language is superficially good, but too formal/stilted/pedantic and with difficulty in catching any meaning other than literal Impassive appearance, with few gestures and abnormal gaze (i.e., limited non-verbal communicative behaviour) Awkward or odd posture and body language

Differentials for social communicative issues in children include ASD, social communication disorder, social anxiety disorder and intellectual developmental disorder.

Diagnosis of ASD [1]

1. Persistent deficits in initiating and sustaining social communication and reciprocal social interactions that are outside the expected range of typical functioning based on the individual's age and level of intellectual development are required for diagnosis. Specific manifestations of these deficits vary according to chronological age, verbal and intellectual ability and disorder severity. Manifestations may include limitations in the following:

    •   Understanding of, interest in, or inappropriate responses to the verbal or non-verbal social communications of others

    •   Integration of spoken language with typical complementary non-verbal cues, such as eye contact, gestures, facial expressions and body language (these non-verbal behaviours may also be reduced in frequency or intensity)

    •   Understanding and use of language in social contexts and ability to initiate and sustain reciprocal social conversations

    •   Ability to imagine and respond to the feelings, emotional states and attitudes of others.

    •   Ability to make and sustain typical peer relationships

2. Persistent restricted, repetitive and inflexible patterns of behaviour, interests or activities that are clearly atypical or excessive for the individual's age and sociocultural context are an essential component. These may include:

   - Lack of adaptability to new experiences and circumstances, with associated distress, that can be evoked by trivial changes to a familiar environment or in response to unanticipated events

   - Inflexible adherence to particular routines: these may be geographical, such as following familiar routes, or may require precise timing such as mealtimes or transport

   - Excessive adherence to rules

   - Excessive and persistent ritualised patterns of behaviour that serve no apparent external purpose

   - Repetitive and stereotyped motor movements such as whole-body movements, atypical gait, unusual hand or finger movements and posturing (these behaviours are particularly common during early childhood)

   - Persistent preoccupation with one or more special interests, parts of objects or specific types of stimuli (including media), or an unusually strong attachment to particular objects (excluding typical comforters)

   - Lifelong excessive and persistent hypersensitivity or hyposensitivity to sensory stimuli or unusual interest in a sensory stimulus, which may include actual or anticipated sounds, light, textures (especially clothing and food), odours and tastes, heat, cold or pain

3. The onset of the disorder occurs during the developmental period – typically in early childhood – but characteristic symptoms may not become fully manifest until later, when social demands exceed limited capacities

4. The symptoms result in significant impairment in personal, family, social, educational, occupational or other important areas of functioning. Some individuals with autism spectrum disorder are able to function adequately in many contexts through exceptional effort, such that their deficits may not be apparent to others. A diagnosis of autism spectrum disorder is still appropriate in such cases

Exam Essentials

- The loss of skills or stasis in development (social/language skills) in the first three years is a red flag for ASD. If there is no speech production by 12–18 months, alarms should be raised

- Children with ASD may be sensitive to touch and noise. They may also be clumsy with balance coordination issues

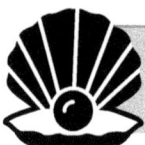

Clinical Pearls

- Delays in language and social interaction alone indicate likely ASD while global developmental delay indicates an alternative pathology instead

- Lack of eye contact may be seen in younger children but may be learned as one gets older

Question 2
What is Asperger's syndrome?

Answer

Asperger's syndrome was a subcategory of ASD described in DSM-4 and ICD-10. Similar to the other subcategories, Asperger's syndrome has been characterised by severe persistent impairment in reciprocal social interactions, repetitive behaviour patterns and restricted interests. It is phenotypically distinct from the other disorders by presenting with normal (or sometimes superior) intellectual quotient (IQ) and normal language development except for social behaviour. There is often mild motor clumsiness as well.

Explanation

A literature search before the publication of DSM-5 concluded that there was insufficient evidence that clinical distinctions between autism and the other subcategories could be made reliably. As a result, the subcategories have been eliminated and replaced with the single diagnosis of 'ASD' [2].

Exam Essentials

- ASD encompasses the spectrum of symptomatology formerly diagnosed as autism, Asperger's syndrome, childhood disintegrative disorder and pervasive developmental disorder

Question 3
What co-morbid conditions and genetic causes are associated with ASD?

Answer
Co-morbid conditions:

- Intellectual developmental disorder/global developmental delay
- Language impairment
- Learning difficulty
- Anxiety disorder
- Attention deficit hyperactivity disorder (ADHD)
- Oppositional defiant disorder and other disruptive behaviour disorders
- Depression
- Schizophrenia
- Tic disorders
- Epilepsy
- Catatonia

Genetic causes:

- Tuberous sclerosis complex
- Fragile X syndrome
- Angelman syndrome
- Rett syndrome
- Cornelia de Lange syndrome

- Cohen syndrome

- Neurofibromatosis type 1

- Down syndrome

- Noonan syndrome

- DiGeorge syndrome

Explanation

Intellectual developmental disorder (20%), anxiety disorder (~50%) and ADHD (30–50%) are common psychiatric co-morbidities [3–8]. Epilepsy occurs in 12.1% of patients with ASD [9].

Clinicians may use specifiers when co-morbid conditions are involved. They can specify whether the patient is:

- With or without disorder of intellectual development

- With or without impairment of functional language

- With or without loss of previously acquired skills

Exam Essentials

- Not all patients with ASD have an intellectual disability

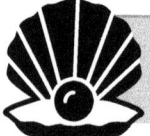

Clinical Pearls

- Patients with ASD can present with transient psychosis. Hence, clinicians need to rule out co-morbid schizophrenia

Question 4

What clinical features are suggestive of intellectual developmental disorder/intellectual disability?

Answer

Language delay
Immature behaviour, play or self-help skills
Learning difficulties
A younger sibling 'overtaking' the child in development

Explanation

Diagnosis of intellectual developmental disorder (intellectual disability) [1]

1. The presence of significant limitations in intellectual functioning across various domains such as perceptual reasoning, working memory, processing speed and verbal comprehension is required for diagnosis. There is often substantial variability in the extent to which any of these domains are affected in an individual. Whenever possible, performance should be measured using appropriately normed, standardised tests of intellectual functioning and found to be approximately two or more standard deviations below the mean (i.e., approximately less than the 2.3rd percentile). In situations where appropriately normed and standardised tests are not available, assessment of intellectual functioning requires greater reliance on clinical judgement based on appropriate evidence and assessment, which may include the use of behavioural indicators of intellectual functioning

2. The presence of significant limitations in adaptive behaviour, which refers to the set of conceptual, social and practical skills that have been learned and are performed by people in their everyday lives, is an essential component. Conceptual skills are those that involve the application of knowledge (e.g., reading, writing, calculating, solving problems and making decisions) and communication; social skills include managing interpersonal interactions and relationships, social responsibility, following rules and obeying laws and avoiding victimisation; and practical skills are involved in areas such as self-care, health and safety, occupational skills, recreation, use of money, mobility and transportation, as well as use of home appliances and technological devices. Expectations of adaptive functioning may change in response to environmental demands that change with age. Whenever possible, performance should be measured with appropriately normed, standardised tests of adaptive behaviour and the total score found to be approximately two or more standard deviations below the mean (i.e., approximately less than the 2.3rd percentile). In situations where appropriately normed and standardised tests are not available, assessment of adaptive behaviour functioning requires greater reliance on clinical judgement based on appropriate assessment, which may include the use of behavioural indicators of adaptive behaviour skills

3. Onset occurs during the developmental period. Among adults with intellectual developmental disorder who come to clinical attention without a previous diagnosis, it is possible to establish developmental onset through the person's history (retrospective diagnosis)

Intellectual disability is usually diagnosed in children over the age of five years. It describes the onset of deficits during the developmental period in areas of intellectual functions and adaptive functioning. Adaptive impairments occur in at least one of three

241

domains: conceptual, social and practical. Impaired intellectual functioning corresponds to an IQ that is two standard deviations or more below the mean (i.e., an IQ score < 70).

The severity of intellectual disability is defined by the DSM-5-TR [2] according to the level of adaptive impairment and the level of support needed. Similarly, the ICD-11 revision codes [1] suggest that IQ scores should not be used in isolation as a diagnostic requirement but rather as a proxy measure of the significant limitations in intellectual functioning. In the DSM-IV, IQ score cut-offs were used to define intellectual disability: mild intellectual disability, IQ level of 50–55 to approximately 70; moderate intellectual disability, IQ level of 35–40 to 50–55; severe intellectual disability, IQ level of 20–25 to 35–40; profound intellectual disability, IQ level below 20–25.

Global developmental delay is reserved for children under the age of five years when the clinical severity level cannot be reliably assessed during early childhood and comprehensive standardised testing cannot be accurately and reliably completed. It is diagnosed in individuals who fail to meet expected developmental milestones in multiple areas of intellectual functioning. Not all children with global developmental delay meet the criteria for intellectual disability as they grow older.

Exam Essentials

- Intellectual disability may be further categorised as syndromic or non-syndromic intellectual disability

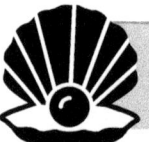

Clinical Pearls

- Patients with intellectual disability are more likely to suffer neglect, discrimination and maltreatment

Question 5
What are the risk factors for ASD?

Answer
Pre-natal:

- Male sex

- Genetic factors (family history of ASD, associated genetic syndromes)

- Advanced parental age

- Pre-natal infections (e.g., rubella)

- Maternal conditions (e.g., diabetes, preeclampsia)

- *In utero* exposure to medications (e.g., sodium valproate)

Antenatal:

- Obstetric complications (e.g., hypoxia, meconium aspiration)

- Preterm birth

- Low birth weight

- Immigrant mothers

Explanation
ASD is three to four times more common in males than females [10]. The cumulative risk of ASD by age 20 years was approximately 3% for cousins, 10% for full siblings [11, 12] and 59% for monozygotic twins [11, 12].

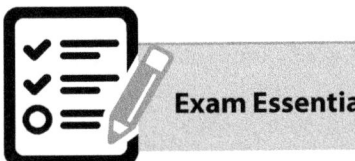

Exam Essentials

- There is no association between mumps, measles and rubella (MMR) vaccinations and the development of ASD [13, 14]

Question 6
Having diagnosed Jacob with ASD, what are the non-pharmacological management options available in the management of ASD?

Answer
Early intervention: behavioural and educational therapy
Family education

Explanation
While there is no cure for ASD, the goals of ASD treatment are to maximise functioning, independence and quality of life. Treatment for ASD must be individualised depending upon the specific strengths, weaknesses and needs of the child and family.

Intervention is more effective when initiated early, improving behaviour, functional skills and communication. Symptoms can decrease over time and in a small minority be minimised to the extent that they no longer cause disability. Parents should be counselled on the diagnosis, and parental support and training in management are essential.

When the child is at a school-going age, enrolling them into a school with a dedicated autism educational program may be more appropriate. Ideally, such programmes would

243

have features such as a high staff-to-student ratio, individualised programming for each child, teachers with special expertise in working with children with autism and a curriculum emphasising attention, imitation, communication, play, social interaction, regulation and self-advocacy, etc.

Question 7

What pharmacological management options are available in the treatment of aggression in ASD?

Answer

Atypical antipsychotic agents (e.g., risperidone or aripiprazole)

Explanation

Psychopharmacological interventions are used to ameliorate behavioural symptoms and psychiatric co-morbidity, rather than core features of ASD.

Risperidone and aripiprazole are the only United States Food and Drug Administration (FDA) approved medications to treat irritability and self-injurious and aggressive behaviours in children (> 5 years old and < 6 years old, respectively) with ASD [15, 16]. Additional symptoms ameliorated include improvements in repetitive behaviours and restricted interests, but these medications have no effects on social function or communication.

Repetitive behaviours and rigidity are core symptoms of ASD and, if thought to be related to anxiety, can be treated with antidepressants (selective serotonin reuptake inhibitors (SSRIs) are the first-line agents). Patients with significant symptoms of obsessive–compulsive disorder and depression may benefit from antidepressants.

Patients with co-morbid ADHD and symptoms of hyperactivity and inattention can be treated with stimulant medications, alpha-2-adrenergic agonists, atomoxetine, atypical antipsychotics and anticonvulsant mood stabilisers.

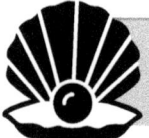

Clinical Pearls

- Children with ASD are prone to adverse effects of medications. Hence, always start low and slow when prescribing medications

Diving Deep ...

Theory of mind is the ability to attribute subjective mental states to oneself and others. Children with ASD have an impairment in this ability and hence experience difficulties in inferring the feelings or emotional state of others around them.

The controversy surrounding the association between MMR vaccinations and ASD first arose in 1998 in a study proposed by the British academic Andrew Wakefield, which suggested a link between the recent injection of MMR vaccine and the onset of symptoms of ASD and enterocolitis. However subsequent studies failed to replicate his findings and, in 2004, 10 of the 13 authors of the study published a statement retracting its interpretation, and the *Lancet* fully retracted the paper in 2010. An investigative reporter found inconsistencies in the study and subsequent investigations determined Wakefield had been guilty of fraud. In addition, Wakefield had a conflict of interest, which was later established.

Due to the increased risk of adverse effects from psychotropics, when antidepressants are used in children with ASD, care should be taken to observe for increased incidence of behavioural activation (impulsivity, silliness, agitation and disinhibition) and other side effects.

Social (pragmatic) communication disorder is a differential for ASD. Social communication disorder is characterised by persistent difficulties in the social use of verbal and non-verbal communication (deficits in using communication for social purposes, inability to change communication to match context or the needs of the listener, difficulties following rules for conversation and storytelling and difficulties understanding what is not explicitly stated). It is distinguished from ASD by the absence of restricted, repetitive patterns of behaviour, interests or activities.

Borderline intellectual functioning is applied when there is both an IQ of about one to two standard deviations below the mean (equalling an IQ between 70 and 85) and functional impairment. This category can be used when an individual's borderline intellectual functioning is the focus of clinical attention or has an impact on the individual's treatment or prognosis.

References

1. World Health Organization. *International classification of diseases*, 11th edition (ICD-11). Geneva: World Health Organization; 2024. Available from: https://icd.who.int/en

2. American Psychiatric Association. *Diagnostic and statistical manual of mental disorders*, 5th edition, text revision (DSM-5-TR). Washington, DC: American Psychiatric Association Publishing; 2022. Available from: www.psychiatry.org/psychiatrists/practice/dsm.

3. Semple D, Smyth R. *Oxford handbook of psychiatry*, 4th edition. Oxford: Oxford University Press; 2019.

4. White SW, Oswald D, Ollendick T, Scahill L. Anxiety in children and adolescents with autism spectrum disorders. *Clin Psychol Rev*. 2009 Apr;29(3):216–29.

5. Kirsch AC, Huebner ARS, Mehta SQ, Howie FR, Weaver AL, Myers SM, et al. Association of comorbid mood and anxiety disorders with autism spectrum disorder. *JAMA Pediatr*. 2020 Jan 1;174(1):63–70.

6. Simonoff E, Pickles A, Charman T, Chandler S, Loucas T, Baird G. Psychiatric disorders in children with autism spectrum disorders: prevalence, comorbidity, and associated factors in a population-derived sample. *J Am Acad Child Adolesc Psychiatry*. 2008 Aug;47(8):921–9.

7. Gargaro BA, Rinehart NJ, Bradshaw JL, Tonge BJ, Sheppard DM. Autism and ADHD: how far have we come in the comorbidity debate? *Neurosci Biobehav Rev*. 2011 Apr;35(5):1081–8.

8. Leitner Y. The co-occurrence of autism and attention deficit hyperactivity disorder in children: what do we know? *Front Hum Neurosci*. 2014;8:268.

9. Lukmanji S, Manji SA, Kadhim S, Sauro KM, Wirrell EC, Kwon CS, et al. The co-occurrence of epilepsy and autism: a systematic review. *Epilepsy Behav*. 2019 Sep;98 (Pt A):238–48.

10. Loomes R, Hull L, Mandy WPL. What is the male-to-female ratio in autism spectrum disorder? A systematic review and meta-analysis. *J Am Acad Child Adolesc Psychiatry*. 2017 Jun;56(6):466–74.

11. Ozonoff S, Young GS, Carter A, Messinger D, Yirmiya N, Zwaigenbaum L, et al. Recurrence risk for autism spectrum disorders: a Baby Siblings Research Consortium study. *Pediatrics*. 2011 Sep;128(3):e488–95.

12. Sandin S, Lichtenstein P, Kuja-Halkola R, Larsson H, Hultman CM, Reichenberg A. The familial risk of autism. *JAMA*. 2014 May 7;311(17):1770–7.

13. Dales L, Hammer SJ, Smith NJ. Time trends in autism and in MMR immunization coverage in California. *JAMA*. 2001 Mar 7;285(9):1183–5.

14. Deer B. How the case against the MMR vaccine was fixed. *BMJ*. 2011 Jan 5;342 (jan05 1):c5347.

15. McDougle CJ, Scahill L, Aman MG, McCracken JT, Tierney E, Davies M, et al. Risperidone for the core symptom domains of autism: results from the study by the autism network of the research units on pediatric psychopharmacology. *Am J Psychiatry*. 2005 Jun;162(6):1142–8.

16. Abilify (aripiprazole). *US Food & Drug Administration (FDA) approved product information*. US National Library of Medicine; 2014. Available from: www.dailymed .nlm.nih.gov

Case 25: Alcohol Use Disorder

Seeing elephants in the ward

John is a 48-year-old male who was brought to the emergency department after he was found unconscious by the roadside with an empty whiskey bottle in his hand. You noted that John had six emergency room visits over the past two years for alcohol intoxication. He was previously given a follow-up appointment with a gastroenterologist for deranged liver function tests but had defaulted on the appointment. There is difficulty in obtaining a history from John, who is agitated and disoriented to time, place and person. His speech is slurred and he answers incomprehensibly. You note the presence of alcohol fetor with nystagmus and an unsteady gait. The rest of the physical examination and vital signs are unremarkable.

- **Question 1: The working diagnosis is acute alcohol intoxication. What initial investigations will you perform?**

A bedside capillary blood glucose (GBG) test showed hypoglycaemia of 3.4 mmol/L. An intravenous cannula is inserted to administer a dextrose-containing drip. As John had presented in a comatose state, 500 mg of parenteral thiamine is also administered to prevent Wernicke's encephalopathy. He is subsequently admitted to a medical ward for further management. John's sister arrives and reports that John drinks six cans of beer a day and has been increasing his alcohol intake over the past 20 years with difficulties in cutting down his alcohol use. You are concerned about alcohol dependence (ICD-11)/alcohol use disorder (DSM-5-TR) [1, 2].

- **Question 2: What other features will you elicit to clinch the diagnosis of alcohol dependence when John is more alert?**

- **Question 3: What are common co-morbid psychiatric disorders of alcohol dependence?**

John reveals that his alcohol intake has slowly increased over the years with intermittent episodes of binge drinking. He finds himself needing to drink a can of beer each morning to steady himself. As a result of his drinking habit, he lost his job and has repeatedly fought with his family members, leaving him estranged. He tried multiple times to cut down on his alcohol use but was unsuccessful, with frequent cravings. With the elicited history, you diagnose him with alcohol dependence. The next morning, John wakes up feeling increasingly irritable, restless and anxious. He complains of a headache which was accompanied by nausea. On examination, he is tachycardic at 110 beats per minute with a blood pressure of 140/100 mmHg. He is tremulous with beads of sweat on his forehead.

- **Question 4: What syndrome is John experiencing?**

While reviewing John, he becomes increasingly agitated and verbally abusive. He becomes disoriented to time, place and person. He reports seeing miniature elephants crawling along the blood pressure machine and little dwarfs running around the ward, which are not seen by others. He is tachycardic and diaphoretic, with coarse tremors seen in both hands.

- **Question 5: What is the most appropriate diagnosis given the constellation of symptoms John is experiencing?**

John subsequently reports a right upper-quadrant abdominal pain with tenderness on physical examination. The liver panel shows transaminitis of two times the normal upper limit. He was diagnosed with mild alcoholic hepatitis.

- **Question 6: How will you manage delirium tremens?**

After his alcohol withdrawals and alcoholic hepatitis have been treated, he is discharged with plans for outpatient detoxification with community support services. He is scheduled for two regular outpatient visits with healthcare staff members over the first week to ensure that he is doing well upon discharge. He also joined Alcoholics Anonymous, a peer support group, to aid in his rehabilitation process. His goal is for complete abstinence as opposed to controlled drinking.

- **Question 7: Keeping in mind his history of alcoholic hepatitis, what pharmacological interventions can be used in the maintenance treatment of his alcohol dependence?**

Answers to Case 25

Question 1

The working diagnosis is acute alcohol intoxication. What initial investigations will you perform?

Answer

For patients with moderate to severe but uncomplicated alcohol intoxication (e.g., not requiring intubation, not initially hypoglycaemic, no trauma), routine biochemical (basic electrolytes, liver function test (LFT)) and point-of-care tests (CBG) may be obtained. Further investigations to rule out other causes of altered mental status are based on clinical suspicion.

Explanation

A suggestive history accompanied by typical clinical signs allows for the diagnosis of acute alcohol intoxication. Laboratory studies are unnecessary in patients with isolated mild alcohol intoxication. In moderate to severe cases, acute alcohol intoxication can induce multiple metabolic derangements, including hypoglycaemia, hyperlactataemia, hypokalaemia, hypomagnesaemia, hypocalcaemia, and hypophosphataemia. Serum alcohol concentration level or breath analysis can be done.

If clinically indicated, further investigations may be ordered to rule out more serious conditions such as head trauma (CT of the brain) or hepatic encephalopathy (LFT and ammonia levels).

Serum and urine toxicology screens are useful in detecting co-ingested substances. However, results take time and will not affect the immediate management of John.

Wernicke's encephalopathy can also present with confusion, ataxia and oculomotor dysfunction, which can be difficult to distinguish from acute alcohol intoxication. Clinicians should watch for the persistence of symptoms even after the acute intoxication phase and empirical treatment can be started in patients with significant chronic alcohol use.

 **Exam Essentials**

- National Institute on Alcohol Abuse and Alcoholism [3] defines binge drinking as ≥ 5 units (males) or ≥ 4 units (females) on a single occasion

- Risky use of alcohol refers to drinking > 21 units (males) or > 14 units (females) in a week

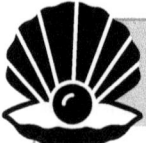

Clinical Pearls

- One unit is equivalent to eight grams of alcohol

- Investigations that ascertain if the patient has been abusing alcohol include increased gamma-glutamyl transferase (GGT) and mean corpuscular volume (MCV)

Question 2

What other features will you elicit to clinch the diagnosis of alcohol dependence when John is more alert?

Answer

Diagnosis of substance dependence [1]

1. A pattern of recurrent episodic or continuous use of a psychoactive substance is required for diagnosis, with evidence of impaired regulation of use of that substance that is manifested in two or more of the following:

   - Impaired control over substance use (i.e., onset, frequency, intensity, duration, termination, context)

   - Increasing precedence of substance use over other aspects of life, including maintenance of health, and daily activities and responsibilities, such that substance use continues or escalates despite the occurrence of harm or negative consequences (e.g., repeated relationship disruption, occupational or scholastic consequences, negative impact on health)

   - Physiological features indicative of neuroadaptation to the substance, including tolerance to the effects of the substance or a need to use increasing amounts of the substance to achieve the same effect; withdrawal symptoms following cessation or reduction in use of that substance; or repeated use of the substance or pharmacologically similar substances to prevent or alleviate withdrawal symptoms

2. The features of dependence are usually evident over a period of at least 12 months, but the diagnosis may be made if use is continuous (daily or almost daily) for at least three months

Course specifiers for alcohol dependence are used to describe the pattern of substance use or remission. A distinction is made between continuous and episodic use.

Exam Essentials

- Thiamine needs to be co-administered with dextrose saline; oral thiamine should be prescribed after stopping intravenous thiamine

- Symptoms of Wernicke's encephalopathy:

    ◦ Confusion
    ◦ Ataxia
    ◦ Ophthalmoplegia

- Diagnosis of Wernicke's encephalopathy is clinical with a high index of suspicion

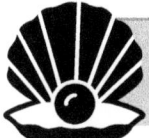

Clinical Pearls

- Patients with alcoholic hepatitis have an aspartate to alanine amino-transferase ratio of greater than 2.0

- Questionnaire to screen for at-risk drinking – **CAGE** [4]

    ◦ Felt like **C**utting down
    ◦ **A**nnoyed by people asking
    ◦ Felt **G**uilty drinking
    ◦ **E**ye-opener drink

- Each question is scored 1 for 'yes' and 0 for 'no'. A total score of 2 or greater is considered clinically significant and should prompt further assessments.

- The cause of Wernicke's encephalopathy and Korsakoff syndrome is vitamin B1 deficiency, which can be seen in:

    ◦ Alcoholism
    ◦ Starvation in anorexia nervosa
    ◦ Dietary deficiency
    ◦ Effects of chemotherapy

Question 3
What are common co-morbid psychiatric disorders of alcohol dependence?

Answer
Depression, bipolar disorder, anxiety, schizophrenia, dementia and antisocial personality disorder are associated with alcohol use disorder.

Explanation
Chronic alcohol use has been associated with alcohol-induced dementia, presenting with decreased intellectual functioning, cognitive abilities and memory. Brain functioning tends to improve with abstinence, but approximately half have permanent deficits in memory and thinking.

Alcohol-induced psychotic disorder occurs in patients with heavy alcohol use or alcohol withdrawal. Experiencing hallucinations in a clear sensorium is a distinct entity experienced during withdrawal and is termed 'alcohol hallucinosis'. Morbid jealousy is a form of delusional disorder and up to 34% of people with alcohol use disorder suffer from morbid jealousy [5].

Alcohol use appears to have a temporary effect of inducing depressive symptoms, with symptoms of sadness resolving within days to weeks of abstinence. Thirty to forty per cent of chronic alcohol users also fulfil the criteria for major depressive disorder in their lifetime. It is estimated that 10–15% of patients with alcohol-related disorders complete suicide [6].

Twenty to fifty per cent of chronic alcohol users suffer from anxiety disorders. Phobias and panic disorder are the two more common co-morbid anxiety disorders [6].

Antisocial personality disorder is the most common personality disorder related to alcohol use.

Question 4
What syndrome is John experiencing?

Answer
Alcohol withdrawal

Explanation
Symptoms of alcohol withdrawal begin after cessation of (or reduction in) alcohol use that has been heavy and prolonged.

Diagnosis of substance withdrawal [1]

1. The presentation is characterised by a clinically significant cluster of symptoms, behaviours and/or physiological features that occurs upon cessation or reduction in the use of a substance in individuals who have developed

dependence on that substance, or have used the substance for a prolonged period or in large amounts. (Note: substance withdrawal can occur when prescribed psychoactive medications (e.g., opioids, anxiolytics, stimulants) have been used in standard therapeutic doses)

2. The specific features of substance withdrawal depend on the pharmacological properties of the specified substance, and are consistent with those recognised as occurring upon cessation or reduction of the particular substance or other members of the same pharmacological group of substances. The symptoms also vary in degree of severity and duration, depending on the substance and the amount and pattern of prior use

3. The symptoms are not better accounted for by another medical condition or another mental disorder

Substance-specific features of alcohol withdrawal

Presenting features of alcohol withdrawal may include autonomic hyperactivity (e.g., tachycardia, hypertension, perspiration), increased hand tremor, nausea, retching or vomiting, insomnia, anxiety, psychomotor agitation, depressed or dysphoric mood, transient visual, tactile or auditory illusions or hallucinations and distractibility. Less commonly, alcohol withdrawal is complicated by seizures.

Symptoms of alcohol withdrawal generally begin within 6–12 hours of the last drink or a sudden reduction in chronic alcohol drinking. Features of mild or moderate withdrawal typically last for 3–7 days after cessation of alcohol use [1].

Factors that increase the risk for the development of alcohol withdrawal include the consumption of more drinks per occasion and the presence of alcohol-related complications. Prophylactic treatment must be considered in any patient with the following features [7]:

• History of dependence

• Previous episodes of withdrawal syndromes

• Consumption of > 10 units of alcohol daily for the previous 10 days

• Currently experiencing withdrawal

Seizures are a complication of alcohol withdrawal and usually present as generalised tonic–clonic convulsions that occur within 6–48 hours after the last alcoholic drink.

Exam Essentials

- Screen early for other substance use through urine drug screen or toxicology screen

- Symptoms of benzodiazepine withdrawal are similar to alcohol, and you may see the following:
  - Increasing agitation
  - Insomnia
  - Restlessness
  - Irritability
  - Risk of seizures

Clinical Pearls

- Patients who have no withdrawal symptoms for more than 24 hours after cessation are unlikely to develop such symptoms

- A score of 4 or more on the Alcohol Use Disorders Identification Test – (Piccinelli) Consumption (AUDIT-PC) [8] predicted the development of alcohol withdrawal symptoms

- Patients may use alcohol to alleviate symptoms of anxiety or depression. Remember to screen for other disorders underlying alcohol dependence

- If alcohol dependence occurs in the presence of other conditions, we need to ascertain the temporal sequence to identify the primary psychiatric disorder

Question 5

What is the most appropriate diagnosis given the constellation of symptoms John is experiencing?

Answer

Delirium tremens

Explanation

Delirium tremens, a medical emergency requiring intensive medical care, is defined by an acute confusional state secondary to alcohol withdrawal. It is associated with global clouding of the sensorium and occasionally with haemodynamic instability. Approximately 5% of patients who undergo alcohol withdrawal also suffer from delirium tremens [7]. Untreated delirium tremens has a mortality of up to 37% [9], but with early identification and appropriate management, this is reduced to approximately 5–10% [7].

The hallucinations experienced by patients with delirium tremens are usually visual. Lilliputian hallucinations, visual hallucinations in which the patient sees miniature people or animals, are commonly experienced in those with delirium tremens. Auditory and tactile hallucinations may also occur.

In contrast to withdrawal delirium, alcoholic hallucinosis is not associated with altered cognition such as disorientation, and vital signs are usually normal.

Exam Essentials

- Delirium tremens typically peaks between **48 and 96 hours after the last drink** and lasts one to five days

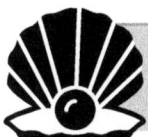

Clinical Pearls

- **Alcoholic hallucinosis occurs** in a clear sensorium, commonly seen in those who decrease their alcohol intake or attempt to abstain completely. In contrast, delirium tremens occurs in a disorientated patient

Question 6
How will you manage delirium tremens?

Answer

Close monitoring	Vitals
	Clinical Institute Withdrawal Assessment Scale for Alcohol – revised (CIWA-Ar) charting [10]
	Fit charting
Pharmacological	Benzodiazepines

Non-pharmacological	Management goals similar to delirious patients Temporary physical restraints as a last resort
Right siting of care	Transfer to high-dependency or intensive care unit if condition worsens

Explanation

Benzodiazepines are the first-line treatment for alcohol withdrawal and delirium tremens. In choosing the type of benzodiazepine, patients with a history of advanced chronic liver disease or acute alcoholic hepatitis (which this patient is suffering from) should be given an agent which is metabolised by conjugation or glucuronidation (e.g., lorazepam), but with more frequent dosing due to its shorter half-life. If no such concerns exist, longer-acting benzodiazepines with active metabolites (e.g., diazepam) are preferred because they result in a smoother clinical course with a lower chance of recurrent withdrawal or seizures.

While antipsychotic medications sedate agitated patients, they may reduce seizure thresholds. Antipsychotic medications with a lower propensity to reduce the seizure threshold include haloperidol and sulpiride. Haloperidol is recommended as it has more evidence supporting its use in delirious patients.

The CIWA-Ar allows for a symptom-triggered approach in treating alcohol withdrawals. CIWA-Ar charting gauges the patient's extent of withdrawal and guides benzodiazepine titration. When the score is elevated (score ≥ 8), additional benzodiazepines can be given to help with withdrawal symptoms. Physical restraints should only be used as a last resort if all other methods of de-escalation fail.

Exam Essentials

- Ascertain when the patient's last drink was as this can be used to estimate the onset of alcohol withdrawal symptoms and delirium tremens

- Check the baseline LFT as it helps decide which benzodiazepine to use (diazepam or lorazepam)

- The absence of transaminitis in the LFT does not exclude liver dysfunction. Do check for liver synthetic function with albumin and coagulation panel (prothrombin time/partial thromboplastin time)

- When the patient becomes delirious, always consider other causes (concurrent infection etc.) if symptoms are not improving with benzodiazepines

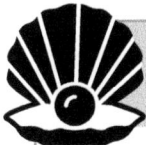

Clinical Pearls

- Benzodiazepines are the drugs of choice for psychomotor agitation from alcohol withdrawal

- Monitoring for respiratory depression and oversedation is essential when prescribing high doses of benzodiazepines. Do not hesitate to consider facilities with higher monitoring such as the high-dependency or intensive care unit

Question 7

Keeping in mind his history of alcoholic hepatitis, what pharmacological interventions can be used in the maintenance treatment of his alcohol dependence?

Answer

Acamprosate

Explanation

Acamprosate modulates glutamate neurotransmission at metabotropic-5 glutamate receptors and is an alternative to naltrexone. It is renally excreted and can be used safely in patients with liver disease. It works by ameliorating some symptoms associated with abstinence and withdrawal, diminishing the desire to return to drinking.

Naltrexone is a first-line therapeutic option for most patients and can be initiated at the point of maximum crisis while patients are still consuming alcohol. Naltrexone is an opioid antagonist, which is involved in modulating the expression of alcohol's reinforcing effects, and hence it should be avoided in individuals using opioids. However, naltrexone has been associated with hepatotoxicity.

Disulfiram should be initiated at least 12 hours after the last alcoholic drink. Disulfiram works by leading to adverse biological effects when alcohol is taken concurrently, and may cause flushing, nausea, palpitations and, more seriously, arrhythmias, hypotension and collapse. A rare complication of disulfiram includes a rapid-onset hepatotoxicity.

Benzodiazepines are used for managing alcohol withdrawals and not for treatment for alcohol dependence.

Antidepressants are used to treat co-morbid psychiatric conditions and not for alcohol dependence alone.

Exam Essentials

- A disulfiram–alcohol reaction occurs when individuals take disulfiram with alcohol, resulting in a severe reaction (hypertension, tachycardia, chest pain, etc.). It can be risky for patients who are ambivalent about quitting and must not be prescribed to patients who may continue drinking

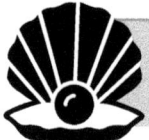

Clinical Pearls

- Naltrexone is a common first-line treatment option, except in patients with liver disease or those prescribed opioids

Diving Deep …

Alcohol affects gamma-aminobutyric acid A (GABA-A) transmission, which results in an anxiolytic effect, but its effects are short-lived and subsequently associated with rebound exacerbation of anxiety and panic attacks when blood levels decline. Alcohol and substance misuse is seen in up to 37% of patients with panic disorder [11].

Risk factors for the development of delirium tremens:

- A history of sustained drinking
- A history of alcohol withdrawal seizures or delirium tremens
- Age > 30 years
- The presence of a concurrent illness
- Significant alcohol withdrawal in the presence of an elevated blood alcohol concentration
- A longer period since the last drink (i.e., patients who present with alcohol withdrawal more than two days after their last drink are more likely to experience delirium tremens than those who present within two days)

Data from the third National Epidemiologic Survey on Alcohol and Related Conditions [12] showed that 14% of adults (age > 18 years) met the criteria for a current alcohol use disorder and 29% had met the criteria for alcohol use disorder in their lifetime.

Wernicke's encephalopathy and Korsakoff syndrome are neurological complications of thiamine (vitamin B1) deficiency. Wernicke's encephalopathy is an acute syndrome characterised by the classic triad:

- Encephalopathy

- Oculomotor dysfunction (nystagmus, lateral rectus palsy and conjugate gaze palsies)

- Gait ataxia

The classic triad is present in approximately one-third of patients [13]. Other symptoms include: being in a stupor or coma, hypotension, hypothermia and peripheral neuropathy. Wernicke's encephalopathy is treated urgently with parenteral administration of thiamine: 500 mg of thiamine is infused over 30 minutes three times daily for two consecutive days and 250 mg once daily for an additional five days, in combination with other B vitamins.

On the other hand, Korsakoff syndrome is a late neuropsychiatric manifestation of Wernicke's encephalopathy. Korsakoff syndrome is characterised by selective anterograde and retrograde amnesia, confabulation, apathy, an intact sensorium and relative preservation of long-term memory and other cognitive skills. The prognosis of Korsakoff syndrome is poor, and patients are usually managed with supervision and social support, either at home or in a chronic care facility.

The transtheoretical model and the stages of change are often employed in the treatment of addiction disorders [14]. The stages of change are (Figure 25.1):

- Pre-contemplation: there is no intention to change behaviour in the foreseeable future

- Contemplation: aware that a problem exists but have not yet committed to taking action

- Preparation: made some reductions in their problem behaviours but have not yet reached effective action

- Action: modify behaviour, experiences and/or environment to overcome their problems

- Maintenance: prevent relapse and consolidate the gains attained during action

- Relapse: the unofficial sixth stage of change is relapse, which is common in the process towards the ultimate goal of termination. Lapsing back to old behavior is typically accompanied by disappointment or feelings of failure

259

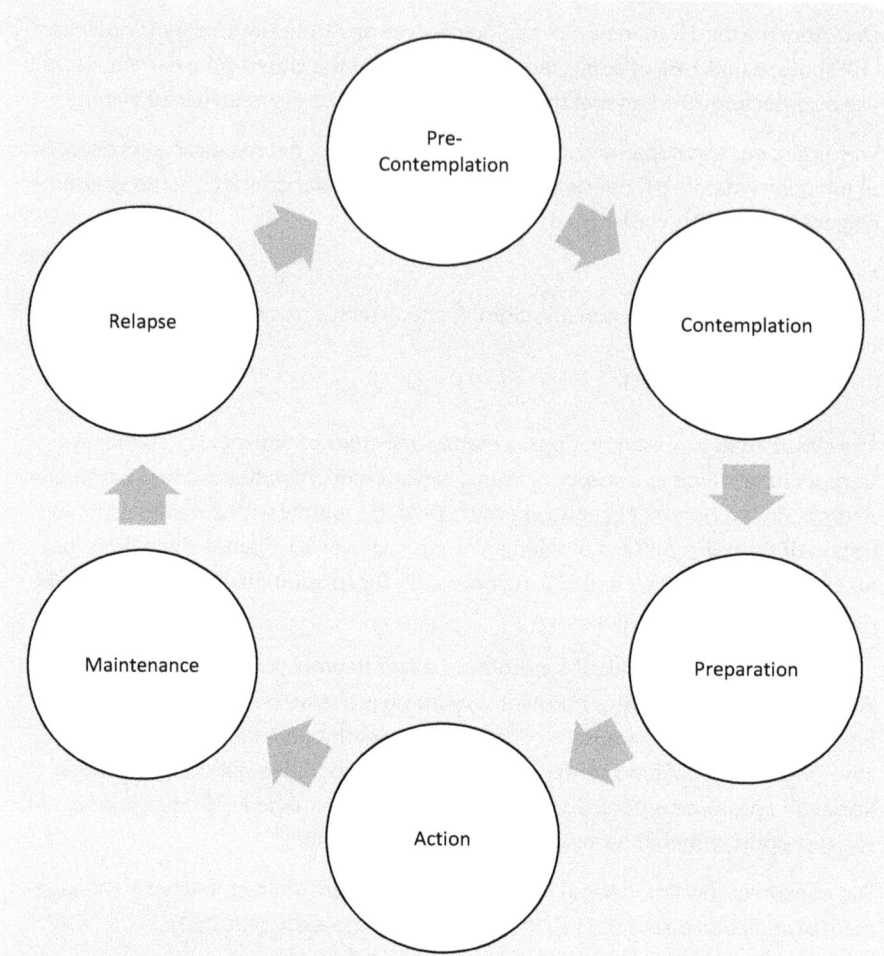

Figure 25.1 The stages of change

Motivational interviewing is effective in the treatment of patients with substance use disorder and has been shown to reduce substance use throughout therapy and up to 12 months later [15]. It elicits behavioural change by helping patients explore their ambivalence towards change. In motivational interviewing, confrontation is avoided; instead, the therapist uses motivational interviewing to build rapport and support the patient in exploring the possibility and value of change about behaviours that are not healthy. A collaborative and autonomy-supporting stance is adopted and the therapist seeks to understand the patient's perspectives on substance use and to help build awareness of the discrepancy between where the patient is at and where they hope to be. Key techniques include engagement, focusing, evoking and planning.

References

1. World Health Organization. *International classification of diseases*, 11th edition (ICD-11). Geneva: World Health Organization; 2024. Available from: https://icd.who.int/en

2. American Psychiatric Association. *Diagnostic and statistical manual of mental disorders*, 5th edition, text revision (DSM-5-TR). Washington, DC: American Psychiatric Association Publishing; 2022. Available from: www.psychiatry.org/psychiatrists/practice/dsm.

3. Willenbring ML, Massey SH, Gardner MB. Helping patients who drink too much: an evidence-based guide for primary care clinicians. *Am Fam Physician*. 2009 Jul 1;80(1):44–50.

4. Ewing JA. Detecting alcoholism. The CAGE questionnaire. *JAMA*. 1984 Oct 12;252(14):1905–7.

5. Michael A, Mirza S, Mirza KA, Babu VS, Vithayathil E. Morbid jealousy in alcoholism. *Br J Psychiatry*. 1995 Nov;167(5):668–72.

6. Boland RJ, Verduin ML, Ruiz P, Shah A, Sadock BJ, editors. *Kaplan & Sadock's synopsis of psychiatry*, 12th edition. Philadelphia: Wolters Kluwer; 2022.

7. Semple D, Smyth R. *Oxford handbook of psychiatry*, 4th edition. Oxford: Oxford University Press; 2019.

8. Saunders JB, Aasland OG, Babor TF, de la Fuente JR, Grant M. Development of the Alcohol Use Disorders Identification Test (AUDIT): WHO Collaborative Project on Early Detection of Persons with Harmful Alcohol Consumption – II. *Addiction*. 1993 Jun;88(6):791–804.

9. Rahman A, Paul M. *Delirium tremens. StatPearls*. Treasure Island, FL: StatPearls Publishing; 2023. Available from:www.ncbi.nlm.nih.gov/books/NBK482134/

10. Sullivan JT, Sykora K, Schneiderman J, Naranjo CA, Sellers EM. Assessment of alcohol withdrawal: the revised Clinical Institute Withdrawal Assessment for Alcohol Scale (CIWA-Ar). *Br J Addict*. 1989 Nov;84(11):1353–7.

11. Kessler RC, Chiu WT, Jin R, Ruscio AM, Shear K, Walters EE. The epidemiology of panic attacks, panic disorder, and agoraphobia in the National Comorbidity Survey Replication. *Arch Gen Psychiatry*. 2006 Apr;63(4):415–24.

12. Grant BF, Goldstein RB, Saha TD, Chou SP, Jung J, Zhang H, et al. Epidemiology of DSM-5 alcohol use disorder: results from the National Epidemiologic Survey on Alcohol and Related Conditions III. *JAMA Psychiatry*. 2015 Aug;72(8):757–66.

13. Chamorro AJ, Rosón-Hernández B, Medina-García JA, Muga-Bustamante R, Fernández-Solá J, Martín-González MC, et al. Differences between alcoholic and nonalcoholic patients with Wernicke encephalopathy: a multicenter observational study. *Mayo Clin Proc*. 2017 Jun;92(6):899–907.

14. Prochaska JO, DiClemente CC. Stages and processes of self-change of smoking: toward an integrative model of change. *J Consult Clin Psychol*. 1983;51(3):390–5.

15. Smedslund G, Berg RC, Hammerstrøm KT, Steiro A, Leiknes KA, Dahl HM, et al. Motivational interviewing for substance abuse. *Cochrane Database Syst Rev*. 2011 May 11;2011(5):CD008063.

Case 26: Cannabis Use Disorder

A green trap

Thomas is a 21-year-old university student who uses 'weed' (cannabis) recreationally to relax after studying.

- **Question 1: What are the acute intoxication symptoms of cannabis use?**

- **Question 2: What are the acute withdrawal symptoms of cannabis use?**

- **Question 3: What is the typical timeframe for a positive urine assay with acute and chronic exposure to cannabis?**

Answers to Case 26

Question 1

What are the acute intoxication symptoms of cannabis use?

	Psychological effects	Physical effects
Acute intoxication symptoms	Euphoria Anxiety Sensation of slowed time Impaired judgement Social withdrawal	Impaired motor coordination Conjunctival injection Increased appetite Dry mouth Tachycardia

Answer

Explanation

Cannabis is produced from the dried leaves, flowers, stems and seeds of the weed *Cannabis sativa*. Delta-9-tetrahydrocannabinol (THC) is the most important active cannabinoid compound in cannabis and responsible for its euphorigenic, sedative and analgesic properties [1]. Cannabis can be smoked alone, mixed with tobacco or consumed orally. As cannabis is often smoked together with tobacco, the harmful effects of tobacco are to be considered as well.

In addition to its association with the development of psychotic disorders, acute intoxication of cannabis can also result in paranoia.

Exam Essentials

- Cannabis use is associated with the development of psychotic disorders and educational underachievement [2]

- Symptoms of cannabis intoxication – **DIRT**

  ○ **D**ry mouth
  ○ **I**ncreased appetite
  ○ **R**ed eye
  ○ **T**achycardia

- Ask for the mode of drug administration, which can have health risk implications

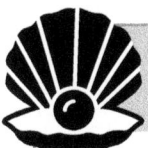

Clinical Pearls

- After alcohol and tobacco, cannabis is the third most commonly used substance

Question 2
What are the acute withdrawal symptoms of cannabis use?

Answer

	Psychological effects	**Physical effects**
Withdrawal symptoms within one week of cessation	Irritability, anger, or aggression Nervousness or anxiety Sleep difficulty (e.g., insomnia, disturbing dreams) Restlessness Depressed mood	Decreased appetite or weight loss

Explanation

While cannabis is not usually associated with physical dependency, there is a mild but characteristic withdrawal syndrome in heavy regular users who stop using suddenly, consisting of insomnia, anxiety and irritability. Withdrawal symptoms appear 24 to 72 hours after cessation, peak over the first week and largely resolve after one to two weeks. Risk factors for psychosis in cannabis use include [3]:

- Early onset of drug use

- Regular high doses of drug use

- Homozygous CC genotype variant of the *AKT1* gene

- One or two copies of the Val variant of the *COMT* gene

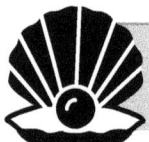 **Clinical Pearls**

- Withdrawal symptoms appear within one to two weeks of cessation [1]

Question 3
What is the typical timeframe for a positive urine assay with acute and chronic exposure to cannabis?

Answer
One to three days with acute exposure
Up to one month with heavy use [4]

Explanation
Second-hand smoke exposure is considered unlikely or impossible to cause false-positive urine testing. A positive test is also unlikely from solely consuming hemp-containing foods.

Diving Deep …

'Amotivational syndrome' [5] is a controversial phenomenon describing apathy developed through the depletion of motivation-based constructs such as self-efficacy from chronic cannabis use. Cannabinoid hyperemesis syndrome has been described. The triad is characterised by chronic marijuana use, cyclical vomiting and compulsive bathing.

The use of medical marijuana is growing and medical cannabis products are typically labelled with a specific ratio of THC and cannabidiol content. Dronabinol is a synthetic form of THC and was approved by the United States Food and Drug Administration (FDA) in 1985 for the treatment of anorexia-associated weight loss in HIV. Dronabinol and nabilone are licensed for use in chemotherapy-associated nausea and vomiting. The use of medical marijuana in chronic pain has garnered significant interest although most studies are of low or moderate quality due to small sample size, short follow-up periods and non-blinded or unrandomised study design [6, 7].

References

1. Boland RJ, Verduin ML, Ruiz P, Shah A, Sadock BJ, editors. *Kaplan & Sadock's synopsis of psychiatry*, 12th edition. Philadelphia: Wolters Kluwer; 2022.
2. Hall WD. Cannabis use and the mental health of young people. *Aust N Z J Psychiatry*. 2006 Feb;40(2):105–13.
3. Carvalho C, Vieira-Coelho MA. Cannabis induced psychosis: a systematic review on the role of genetic polymorphisms. *Pharmacol Res*. 2022 Jul;181:106258.
4. Robert J Hoffman. Testing for drugs of abuse (DOAs). UpToDate, Wolters Kluwer. Available from: www.uptodate.com/contents/testing-for-drugs-of-abuse
5. Lac A, Luk JW. Testing the amotivational syndrome: marijuana use longitudinally predicts lower self-efficacy even after controlling for demographics, personality, and alcohol and cigarette use. *Prev Sci*. 2018 Feb;19(2):117–26.
6. McDonagh MS, Morasco BJ, Wagner J, Ahmed AY, Fu R, Kansagara D, et al. Cannabis-based products for chronic pain: a systematic review. *Ann Intern Med*. 2022 Aug;175(8):1143–53.
7. Whiting PF, Wolff RF, Deshpande S, Di Nisio M, Duffy S, Hernandez AV, et al. Cannabinoids for medical use: a systematic review and meta-analysis. *JAMA*. 2015 Jun 23;313(24):2456–73.

Case 27: Stimulant Use Disorder

High on Ice

Rachel is a 23-year-old woman who was admitted to accident and emergency after collapsing at a club. Her friends said she had taken 'ice' (methamphetamine) before partying.

- **Question 1: What are the acute intoxication symptoms of methamphetamine?**

- **Question 2: What are the acute withdrawal symptoms of methamphetamine?**

- **Question 3: What is the typical timeframe for a positive urine assay with acute and chronic exposure to stimulants?**

- **Question 4: What is the characteristic feature of stimulant-induced psychotic disorder?**

- **Question 5: Does stimulant detoxification require inpatient treatment?**

Answers to Case 27

Question 1
What are the acute intoxication symptoms of methamphetamine?

Answer
Methamphetamine is a type of psychostimulant.

	Psychological effects	Physical effects
Acute intoxication symptoms	Euphoria or affect blunting Changes in sociability and increased libido Hypervigilance Interpersonal sensitivity Anxiety Tension Anger Stereotyped behaviours Impaired judgement	Tachycardia or bradycardia Pupillary dilation Blood pressure changes Perspiration or chills Nausea or vomiting Weight loss Psychomotor changes Muscular weakness, respiratory depression, chest pain or cardiac arrhythmias Confusion, seizures or coma

Explanation

Methamphetamines are psychostimulants; the group includes other substances such as cocaine, amphetamines, 3, 4-methylenedioxymethamphetamine (MDMA or ecstasy) and caffeine. These drugs cause the release and block the reuptake of monoamine neurotransmitters, including dopamine, noradrenaline and serotonin, resulting in increased cortical excitability, producing effects of increased alertness and endurance, insomnia and a subjective sense of well-being. Psychotic symptoms are seen during acute intoxication.

Psychostimulants are most often smoked and snorted but can also be injected or ingested orally. Cardiovascular complications, such as malignant hypertension and arrhythmias, are known to cause death among users [1]. MDMA has both hallucinogenic and stimulant properties. MDMA is known to cause serotonin syndrome, cardiovascular complications, hyperthermia, hyponatraemia and hepatotoxicity. Cocaine is often snorted or injected. Specific chronic harmful effects of cocaine include necrosis of the nasal septum, teratogenic effects, panic and anxiety disorders, persecutory delusions and psychosis.

Exam Essentials

- MDMA has both hallucinogenic and stimulant properties. It is characterised by a feeling of increased camaraderie and 'closeness' to others

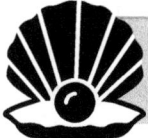

Clinical Pearls

- MDMA affects libido and is a commonly used drug in chemsex

Question 2
What are the acute withdrawal symptoms of methamphetamine?

Answer

	Psychological effects	Physical effects
Withdrawal symptoms within a few hours to several days	Vivid, unpleasant dreams Insomnia or hypersomnia	Fatigue Increased appetite Psychomotor retardation or agitation

Explanation

Withdrawal symptoms typically reach their peak within two to four days and resolve within a week [2]. The most severe symptom is depression, which can be especially intense following prolonged high-dose stimulant use and may be linked to suicidal thoughts or behaviours.

Exam Essentials

- Anxiety and depressive symptoms are frequently seen in users, especially during 'crashes'

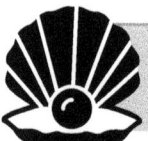

Clinical Pearls

- Punding is a compulsive repetitive behaviour (e.g., collecting or sorting objects), which is associated with chronic methamphetamine use

Question 3
What is the typical timeframe for a positive urine assay with acute and chronic exposure to stimulants?

Answer

For amphetamines:

- One to two days with acute exposure

- Two to four days with heavy use [3]

Explanation

False positives occur more frequently with amphetamine assays, which often lack specificity due to the structural similarities between amphetamines and many other drugs and medications (such as nasal decongestants containing ephedrine)

Question 4

What is the characteristic feature of stimulant-induced psychotic disorder?

Answer

Paranoid delusions and hallucinations

Explanation

Paranoid delusions and hallucinations occur in up to 50% of individuals who misuse stimulants [2]. While auditory hallucinations are common, visual and tactile hallucinations are less frequent than paranoid delusions.

Exam Essentials

- 'Formication' refers to the sensation of bugs crawling under the skin, arising from cocaine use

Question 5

Does stimulant detoxification require inpatient treatment?

Answer

No

Explanation

The physiological effects of stimulant withdrawal are generally not severe enough to necessitate inpatient or residential care. Outpatient withdrawal can be attempted instead. No pharmacological treatments reliably alleviate the intensity of withdrawal. Recovery typically occurs within one to two weeks without major complications. However, it may take longer for sleep, mood and cognitive functions to fully recover.

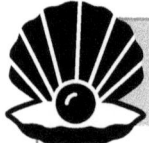

Clinical Pearls

• Stimulant withdrawal is usually mild and not fatal

Diving Deep ...

'Khat' is a plant from eastern Africa and southern Arabia that is chewed like tobacco and contains the stimulants cathinone and cathine. Synthetic cathinones were developed in the mid-2000s and were known as 'bath salts'.

Stimulant-induced psychotic disorder is characterised by the presence of delusions and hallucinations in patients who misuse stimulants. This occurs in up to 50% of stimulant users [2]. Auditory hallucinations and paranoid delusions are most common, with some users also experiencing tactile and visual hallucinations. Cocaine is associated with the phenomenon of formication, where the user experiences the sensation of bugs crawling beneath the skin. Patients with stimulant-induced psychotic disorder are typically treated with short-term antipsychotics (e.g., haloperidol).

References

1. Dominic P, Ahmad J, Awwab H, Bhuiyan MS, Kevil CG, Goeders NE, et al. Stimulant drugs of abuse and cardiac arrhythmias. *Circ Arrhythm Electrophysiol*. 2022 Jan;15(1):e010273.
2. Boland RJ, Verduin ML, Ruiz P, Shah A, Sadock BJ, editors. *Kaplan & Sadock's synopsis of psychiatry*, 12th edition. Philadelphia: Wolters Kluwer; 2022.
3. Robert J Hoffman. Testing for drugs of abuse (DOAs). UpToDate, Wolters Kluwer. Available from: www.uptodate.com/contents/testing-for-drugs-of-abuse

Case 28: Opioid Use Disorder

Chasing the Dragon

Blake is a 45-year-old man who has been visiting his general practitioner weekly for cough and asks specifically for cough syrups containing codeine. When offered alternatives, he becomes agitated and refuses to leave the clinic until his prescription is filled.

- **Question 1: What are the acute intoxication symptoms of opioids?**

- **Question 2: What are the acute withdrawal symptoms of opioids?**

- **Question 3: What is the typical timeframe for a positive urine assay with acute and chronic exposure to opioids?**

- **Question 4: What pharmacological treatment options are available in the treatment of a patient with opioid use disorder?**

Answers to Case 28

Question 1
What are the acute intoxication symptoms of opioids?

Answer

	Psychological effects	Physical effects
Acute intoxication symptoms	Euphoria followed by apathy Dysphoria Impaired judgement Impairment in attention or memory	Psychomotor agitation or retardation Pupillary constriction (or dilation due to anoxia from severe overdose) Drowsiness or coma Slurred speech

Explanation

Opiates are derived from the opium poppy (*Papaver somniferum*) and opioids are its synthetic counterparts. They have potent analgesic properties and are widely used in medical treatment. However, they are also prone to abuse for their euphoric and anxiolytic properties. Heroin is the most frequently abused opiate, it is commonly inhaled (also known as 'chasing the dragon') but can also be taken through snorting and parenteral routes. Codeine is a prodrug of morphine; it is a common active compound in cough mixtures, making it prone to abuse.

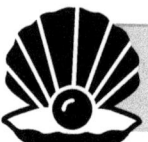 **Clinical Pearls**

- Normal pupil examination does NOT exclude opioid toxicity. The best indication of **opioid toxicity is a respiratory rate** of **< 12 breaths per minute** [1].

Question 2

What are the acute withdrawal symptoms of opioids?

Answer

	Psychological effects	Physical effects
Withdrawal symptoms within minutes to several days	Dysphoric mood Insomnia	Nausea or vomiting Muscle aches Lacrimation or rhinorrhoea Pupillary dilation, piloerection or sweating Diarrhoea Yawning Fever

Explanation

Opioid withdrawal occurs after the cessation or reduction of heavy and prolonged opioid use. It can also be triggered by administering an opioid partial agonist, such as buprenorphine, or an opioid antagonist, like naloxone or naltrexone, to a patient who regularly uses opioid agonists.

Exam Essentials

- Opioid withdrawal is not usually fatal unless individuals have a severe pre-existing physical illness, such as cardiac disease [2]

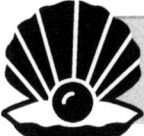

Clinical Pearls

- The use of opioid agonists (e.g., naloxone) in patients on chronic opioid medications for chronic pain can precipitate withdrawal symptoms

Question 3
What is the typical timeframe for a positive urine assay with acute and chronic exposure to opioids?

Answer
One to three days

Methadone has a highly variable but long half-life, permitting detection for 3–10 days [3]

Explanation
Routine opiate screening does not detect synthetic opioids, such as buprenorphine, fentanyl, methadone, meperidine, pentazocine, propoxyphene, tramadol and loperamide.

Question 4
What pharmacological treatment options are available in the treatment of a patient with opioid use disorder?

Answer
Opioid substitutes such as methadone or buprenorphine are used for detoxification and maintenance.

Opioid antagonists such as naltrexone are used in maintenance.

Explanation
Methadone is a synthetic opioid that substitutes for heroin and is a full mu-opioid receptor agonist. It is given to suppress symptoms of withdrawal and aid in detoxification.

Buprenorphine is a partial mu-opioid receptor agonist and can similarly be used to suppress symptoms of withdrawal and aid in detoxification.

Naltrexone is a long-acting opioid antagonist, which is used after detoxification to prevent recurrent physiological dependence and relapse. Naloxone is a short-acting opioid antagonist which is used to reverse the effects of an opioid overdose.

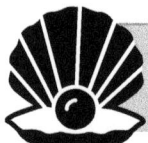

Clinical Pearls

- **Naloxone** is a short-acting opioid antagonist, given intravenously in the **treatment of an acute opioid overdose.** However, it also carries the risk of inducing withdrawal symptoms in chronically dependent users

Diving Deep …

If the route of substance misuse is via injections, special attention should be paid to local and systemic complications. Examples include local abscesses, cellulitis, osteomyelitis, bacterial endocarditis, septicaemia and the transmission of viral infections (e.g., HIV). Track marks (scars running the length of the vein) are suggestive of chronic injection drug use.

Illicit opioid use during pregnancy has adverse effects on both mother and child (although it has not been associated with any specific teratogenic effects), with complications such as infections, preeclampsia, miscarriages, premature rupture of membranes, pre-term birth, infant of low birth weight and neonatal opioid withdrawal syndrome. Detoxification is a stressful process and medically assisted opioid withdrawal is safest in the second trimester. However, because of the complications of illicit opioid use, medically assisted opioid withdrawal should be offered and can take place in any trimester of pregnancy.

References

1. Hoffman JR, Schriger DL, Luo JS. The empiric use of naloxone in patients with altered mental status: a reappraisal. *Ann Emerg Med.* 1991 Mar;20(3):246–52.
2. Boland RJ, Verduin ML, Ruiz P, Shah A, Sadock BJ, editors. *Kaplan & Sadock's synopsis of psychiatry*, 12th edition. Philadelphia: Wolters Kluwer; 2022.
3. Robert J Hoffman. Testing for drugs of abuse (DOAs). UpToDate, Wolters Kluwer. Available from: www.uptodate.com/contents/testing-for-drugs-of-abuse

Case 29: Hallucinogen Use Disorder

What a colourful world!

Tyler is a 25-year-old man who was brought to the emergency room by his friend after he had fallen out of his window (from the second floor) and was found to be talking incoherently. On physical examination he was noted to be confused, dysarthric and had horizontal nystagmus, hypertension and tachycardia. His friend admitted they had been taking phencyclidine (PCP) before the accident.

- **Question 1: What are the acute intoxication symptoms of PCP?**

- **Question 2: What is the typical timeframe for a positive urine assay with acute exposure to ketamine, lysergic acid diethylamide (LSD) and PCP?**

One year later, Tyler returns with complaints of visual disturbances. He has been having geometric hallucinations, flashes of colour and halo effects, which are reminiscent of his previous hallucinogenic symptoms when he took LSD. These episodes are intermittent, each one lasting for a few minutes before resolving on its own. This occurs despite him having been abstinent from using LSD over the past few months.

- **Question 3: What is the diagnosis for the above phenomenon?**

Answers to Case 29

Question 1
What are the acute intoxication symptoms of PCP?

Answer

	Psychological effects	Physical effects
Acute PCP intoxication symptoms	Belligerence Assaultiveness Impulsiveness Unpredictability Impaired judgement	Agitation Vertical or horizontal nystagmus Hypertension or tachycardia Numbness Diminished pain response Ataxia Dysarthria Muscle rigidity Seizures or coma Hyperacusis
Other hallucinogen acute intoxication	Perceptual changes occurring in a state of full alertness (e.g., subjective intensification of perceptions, depersonalisation, derealisation, illusions, hallucinations, synaesthesia)	
	Marked anxiety or depression Ideas of reference Fear of 'losing one's mind' Paranoid ideation Impaired judgement	Pupillary dilation Tachycardia Sweating Palpitations Blurring of vision Tremors Incoordination
Withdrawal symptoms	Classically not associated with any recognised withdrawal syndrome	

Explanation

Hallucinogens (also known as psychedelics) produce altered sensory and perceptual experiences. Examples include LSD, PCP, magic mushrooms and ketamine. At higher doses, PCP can cause disorientation, severe agitation, violent behaviour, auditory hallucinations and catatonic stupor.

LSD is known to cause behavioural toxicity (i.e., harm related to acting on beliefs such as having the ability to fly) and 'bad trips' (i.e., dissociation, fear of incipient madness, frightening perceptions). With chronic use, there is a risk of flashbacks for years after consumption and post-hallucinogenic perceptual disorder. Ketamine is structurally similar to PCP and is used as an anaesthetic and sedative agent in clinical practice. In higher doses, it can lead to LSD-like synaesthesia and hallucinations, associated with nausea, ataxia and slurred speech. Ketamine and its enantiomer (esketamine) are used in clinical practice for treatment-resistant depression.

Exam Essentials

- Hallucinogens do not have a recognised withdrawal syndrome

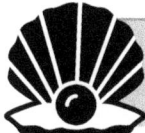

Clinical Pearls

- PCP intoxication is characterised by bizarre or violent behaviour, nystagmus (vertical and horizontal) and incoordination
- Chronic ketamine use can lead to '**ketamine bladder syndrome**', which includes painful urination, frequency, incontinence, haematuria and cystitis [1]

Question 2
What is the typical timeframe for a positive urine assay with acute exposure to ketamine, LSD and PCP?

Answer
   Ketamine: one to three days with acute exposure
   LSD: one to three days with acute exposure
   PCP: four to seven days with acute exposure [2]

Explanation
False-positive PCP results can arise from over-the-counter cold medications (e.g., doxylamine, dextromethorphan) or commonly used analgesics (e.g., tramadol).

Question 3
What is the diagnosis for the above phenomenon?

Answer
Hallucinogen-persisting perception disorder

Explanation

Diagnosis of hallucinogen-persisting perception disorder [3]

1. After discontinuing the use of a hallucinogen, the recurrence of one or more perceptual symptoms previously experienced during intoxication with the hallucinogen

2. There is clinically significant functional impairment from the recurrence of perceptual symptoms

Long after ingesting a hallucinogen, a person can continue to have flashbacks of the hallucinogenic symptoms. Fifteen to eighty per cent of users of hallucinogens develop hallucinogen-persisting perception disorder, which is typically triggered by emotional stress, sensory deprivation or the use of a psychoactive substance such as alcohol [4]. ICD-11 does not have specific criteria for hallucinogen-persisting perception disorder.

Diving Deep …

Tolerance to hallucinogens develops rapidly and occurs after three to four days of continuous use. The treatment of hallucinogen intoxication involves reassurance and supportive care in a quiet environment. Benzodiazepines (e.g. diazepam) can be used to provide more rapid relief. Haemodialysis is not effective in treating PCP intoxication due to the substantial volume of distribution [4].

References

1. Srirangam S, Mercer J. Ketamine bladder syndrome: an important differential diagnosis when assessing a patient with persistent lower urinary tract symptoms. *Case Reports*. 2012 Sep 30;2012(sep26 1):bcr2012006447–bcr2012006447.

2. Robert J Hoffman. Testing for drugs of abuse (DOAs). UpToDate, Wolters Kluwer. Available from: www.uptodate.com/contents/testing-for-drugs-of-abuse

3. American Psychiatric Association. *Diagnostic and statistical manual of mental disorders*, 5th edition, text revision (DSM-5-TR). Washington, DC: American Psychiatric Association Publishing; 2022. Available from: www.psychiatry.org/psychiatrists/practice/dsm

4. Boland RJ, Verduin ML, Ruiz P, Shah A, Sadock BJ, editors. *Kaplan & Sadock's synopsis of psychiatry*, 12th edition. Philadelphia: Wolters Kluwer; 2022.

Case 30: Gambling Disorder

Chance and Control

Mr Hunter is a 38-year-old male who presents to your clinic with worsening low mood over the past month. On further probing, he reveals to you that he is currently in debt after losing his savings to gambling. Over the past year, he has spent an increasing amount of time gambling at the local casino. It started with small amounts initially, but as his losses accrued, he found himself gambling away larger amounts to chase after the losses. His wife had begged him to stop but he has been unsuccessful in cutting down on his gambling habits. This in turn has been a source of friction in his relationship with his family and he often lies to his wife about the extent of his gambling. Things worsened over the past month after he was fired from his job after making frequent mistakes and being late to work.

- **Question 1: What is the diagnosis?**

- **Question 2: What are the risk factors for gambling disorder?**

Apart from low mood, Mr Hunter also had poor sleep and appetite. His concentration was poor, and he no longer enjoys exercising. With his difficulty in repaying his mortgage and continued strained relationship with his wife, he admits to having thoughts of suicide. You diagnosed him with major depressive disorder as a co-morbid condition.

- **Question 3: What other co-morbidities are common in patients with gambling disorder?**

- **Question 4: How is gambling disorder managed?**

Answers to Case 30

Question 1
What is the diagnosis?

Answer
Gambling disorder

Explanation
Gambling disorder is characterised by persistent and recurrent maladaptive patterns of gambling behaviour that lead to significant personal, family and occupational difficulties.

Diagnosis of gambling disorder [1]

1. A persistent pattern of gambling behaviour – which may be predominantly online (i.e., over the internet or similar electronic networks) or offline – is required for diagnosis, manifested in all of the following:

    - Impaired control over gambling behaviour (e.g., onset, frequency, intensity, duration, termination, context)

    - Increasing priority given to gambling behaviour to the extent that gambling takes precedence over other life interests and daily activities

    - Continuation or escalation of gambling behaviour despite negative consequences (e.g., marital conflict due to gambling behaviour, repeated and substantial financial losses, negative impact on health)

2. The pattern of gambling behaviour may be continuous or episodic and recurrent, but is manifested over an extended period of time (e.g., 12 months)

2. The gambling behaviour is not better accounted for by another mental disorder (e.g., a manic episode) and is not due to the effects of a substance or medication

4. The pattern of gambling behaviour results in significant distress or impairment in personal, family, social, educational, occupational or other important areas of functioning

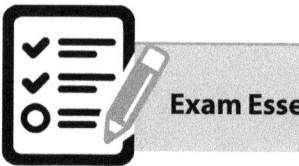

Exam Essentials

- Remember to rule out mania as the cause of gambling behaviour

Question 2
What are the risk factors for gambling disorder?

Answer
Age: children, adolescents and senior citizens
Male gender
Adults undergoing mental health treatment
Nicotine or substance abuse: alcohol, marijuana, inhalants, illegal steroids
Positive family history
Childhood abuse and child neglect
Lower socioeconomic status
Being a witness to trauma or being a victim of a physical attack
Weapon possession or being involved in a fight

Explanation
The prevalence of pathological and problem gambling in men is two to three times higher than in women [2]. Common genetic vulnerability for pathological gambling and alcohol abuse has been reported among twins [3].

Exam Essentials

- Attention deficit hyperactivity disorder (ADHD) and anxiety disorders are linked to a higher risk of developing gambling disorder in individuals who gamble and contribute to the ongoing presence of gambling disorder symptoms over time [4].

Question 3
What other co-morbidities are common in patients with gambling disorder?

Answer
Bipolar disorder
Psychotic disorder
Anxiety disorders
Personality disorder (in particular, cluster B)
Substance misuse disorders (including alcohol and tobacco)
ADHD
Parkinson's disease

Explanation
Seventy-six per cent of pathological gamblers suffer from major depressive disorder at some point in their lives and recurrent depressive episodes occur in 28% [5]. In heavy

281

drinkers, 12.9% had one or more gambling-related problems compared with 5% of non-drinkers [6]. Gambling disorder has been observed more frequently in patients with Parkinson's disorder than in the general population.

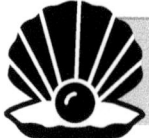

Clinical Pearls

- Half of the individuals undergoing treatment for gambling disorder reported experiencing suicidal thoughts, and approximately 17% reported having attempted suicide [4, 7]

- Patients with Parkinson's disease are at an increased risk of developing impulse-control disorders, such as compulsive gambling, shopping, hoarding or hypersexuality. These behaviours are often linked to Parkinson's medications, particularly dopamine agonists

Question 4
How is gambling disorder managed?

Answer

Psychoeducation and involving family members in treatment

Joining support groups, such as Gamblers Anonymous

Psychotherapy using cognitive behavioural interventions

Pharmacotherapy: selective serotonin reuptake inhibitors (SSRIs; e.g., fluvoxamine, fluoxetine)

Other pharmacotherapy with more limited evidence includes lithium, clomipramine and naltrexone

Explanation

Involving family members can help encourage the patient to follow through with treatment recommendations. The patient and family members should be provided with support resources, such as hotlines or Gamblers Anonymous chapters and meetings.

There is a modest to moderate benefit for behavioural techniques (imaginal desensitisation) and cognitive behavioural interventions [8–10]. Cognitive interventions can target errors in thinking; for example, some problem gamblers have the illusion of control over chance events and believe they can control them by relying on superstitious behaviour or methods. Behavioural therapy targets the learned gambling behaviour and relies on techniques such as systematic exposure or desensitisation and skill development (e.g., relaxation techniques and improving social skills) [11].

Traditionally, pharmacotherapy is used in the treatment of psychiatric co-morbidities such as depression. However, recent studies [12] have shown that SSRIs may help reduce gambling behaviours independent of their effect on mood and anxiety disorders. Treatment with fluvoxamine resulted in a significantly greater percentage improvement in overall gambling severity on the Pathological Gambling Clinical Global Impression scale [13]. Other SSRIs, including citalopram and fluoxetine, have been found to be effective for treating non-depressed pathological gamblers in open-label studies.

Diving Deep ...

There are various hypotheses underlying the pathophysiology of gambling disorder. The DSM-5-TR classifies gambling disorder as a non-substance-related and addictive disorder with overlapping features of tolerance, withdrawal, anticipatory craving and a chronic relapsing course. There is also a common genetic vulnerability for pathological gambling and alcohol misuse reported in twin studies. The other school of thought classifies gambling disorder under impulse-control disorders due to similar changes in serotonin metabolites in both pathological gamblers and patients with impulse-control disorders. Biochemically, dysregulation of dopaminergic tone is also suspected. Evidence for this includes patients with Parkinson's disease developing gambling disorder after being started on dopaminergic therapy.

The number of people with gambling problems is increasing. The disorder is believed to start in adolescents, with 4–7% prevalence. Prevalence in adults is reported to be around 1–3% [14]. Pathological and problem gamblers in the United States cost society approximately $5 billion annually and an additional $40 billion in lifetime costs for productivity reductions, social services and creditor losses [15].

The Lie/Bet Questionnaire is a useful screening tool for pathological gamblers (99% sensitivity, 91% specificity) [16]:

1. 'Have you ever had to lie to people important to you about how much you gambled?'

2. 'Have you ever felt a need to bet more money?'

A 'Yes' answer to either question suggests the need to investigate the presence of additional criteria for gambling disorder.

Based on the lessons learned from addressing tobacco availability and addiction, a public health approach to control problem gambling includes:
- Institute moratoriums on building new casinos and decrease available gambling locations

- Strictly enforce the legal age for gambling

- Ban advertising for gambling activities

- Plain package gambling products, and add warning labels with the risk of problem gambling

- Keep lottery tickets out of sight

- Regulate or ban instant play/reward games (immediate gratification may exacerbate gambling behaviour)

References

1. World Health Organization. *International classification of diseases*, 11th edition (ICD-11). Geneva: World Health Organization; 2024. Available from: https://icd.who.int/en

2. Husky MM, Michel G, Richard JB, Guignard R, Beck F. Gender differences in the associations of gambling activities and suicidal behaviors with problem gambling in a nationally representative French sample. *Addict Behav.* 2015 Jun;45:45–50.

3. Slutske WS, Ellingson JM, Richmond-Rakerd LS, Zhu G, Martin NG. Shared genetic vulnerability for disordered gambling and alcohol use disorder in men and women: evidence from a national community-based Australian twin study. *Twin Res Hum Genet.* 2013 Apr;16(2):525–34.

4. American Psychiatric Association. *Diagnostic and statistical manual of mental disorders*, 5th edition, text revision (DSM-5-TR). Washington, DC: American Psychiatric Association Publishing; 2022. Available from: www.psychiatry.org/psychiatrists/practice/dsm

5. Becona E, Del Carmen Lorenzo M, Fuentes MJ. Pathological gambling and depression. *Psychol Rep.* 1996 Apr;78(2):635–40.

6. Bray RM, Kroutil LA, Luckey JW, Wheeless SC, Iannacchione VG. *1992 Worldwide survey of substance abuse and health behaviors among military personnel*. Defense Technical Information Center; 1992.

7. Petry NM, Kiluk BD. Suicidal ideation and suicide attempts in treatment-seeking pathological gamblers. *J Nerv Ment Dis.* 2002;190:462–9.

8. Oakley-Browne MA, Adams P, Mobberley PM. Interventions for pathological gambling. *Cochrane Database Syst Rev.* 2000;2000(2):CD001521.

9. Echeburúa E, Báez C, Fernández-Montalvo J. Comparative effectiveness of three therapeutic modalities in the psychological treatment of pathological gambling: long-term outcome. *Behav Cogn Psychother.* 1996 Jan;24(1):51–72.

10. Pasche SC, Sinclair H, Collins P, Pretorius A, Grant JE, Stein DJ. The effectiveness of a cognitive-behavioral intervention for pathological gambling: a country-wide study. *Ann Clin Psychiatry.* 2013 Nov;25(4):250–6.

11. McConaghy N, Armstrong MS, Blaszczynski A, Allcock C. Behavior completion versus stimulus control in compulsive gambling. Implications for behavioral assessment. *Behav Modif.* 1988 Jul;12(3):371–84.

12. Zimmerman M, Breen RB, Posternak MA. An open-label study of citalopram in the treatment of pathological gambling. *J Clin Psychiatry.* 2002 Jan;63(1):44–8.

13. Hollander E, DeCaria CM, Finkell JN, Begaz T, Wong CM, Cartwright C. A randomized double-blind fluvoxamine/placebo crossover trial in pathologic gambling. *Biol Psychiatry.* 2000 May 1;47(9):813–7.

14. Shaffer HJ, Hall MN, Vander Bilt J. Estimating the prevalence of disordered gambling behavior in the United States and Canada: a research synthesis. *Am J Public Health.* 1999 Sep;89(9):1369–76.

15. Fong TW. The biopsychosocial consequences of pathological gambling. *Psychiatry (Edgmont).* 2005 Mar;2(3):22–30.

16. Johnson EE, Hamer R, Nora RM, Tan B, Eisenstein N, Engelhart C. The Lie/Bet Questionnaire for screening pathological gamblers. *Psychol Rep.* 1997 Feb;80(1):83–8.

Case 31: Borderline Personality Disorder

Emotional turmoil

Kacey is a 32-year-old lady who comes in for a deep cut on her left wrist. This is not her first admission to the emergency department. She has cut herself since the age of 15 and had two suicide attempts over the past 10 years. She often feels there is no meaning in life and that her existence is 'hollow'. This episode of self-harm was triggered by finding out that her husband was having an extramarital affair, and a sense of abandonment led her to slash her wrist. She feels that she must be unworthy, as she had multiple failed relationships, and this was her third marriage. She mentions that her husband means the world to her, and if threatening to die was the only way he would stay right by her side, she would.

- **Question 1: What is the most likely diagnosis?**

- **Question 2: What are the risk factors for developing borderline personality disorder?**

- **Question 3: What are common co-morbidities in borderline personality disorder?**

- **Question 4: How would you manage Kacey's borderline personality disorder?**

Answers to Case 31

Question 1
What is the most likely diagnosis?

Answer
Personality disorder with borderline pattern (ICD-11)/borderline personality disorder (DSM-5-TR) [1, 2]

Explanation

Diagnosis of personality disorder with borderline pattern specifier [1]

The borderline pattern specifier may be applied to individuals whose pattern of personality disturbance is characterised by a pervasive pattern of instability of interpersonal relationships, self-image and affects, and marked impulsivity, as indicated by five (or more) of the following:

1. Frantic efforts to avoid real or imagined abandonment

2. A pattern of unstable and intense interpersonal relationships, which may be characterised by vacillations between idealisation and devaluation, typically associated with both strong desire for and fear of closeness and intimacy

3. Identity disturbance, manifested in markedly and persistently unstable self-image or sense of self

4. A tendency to act rashly in states of high negative affect, leading to potentially self-damaging behaviours (e.g., risky sexual behaviour, reckless driving, excessive alcohol or substance use, binge eating)

5. Recurrent episodes of self-harm (e.g., suicide attempts or gestures, self-mutilation)

6. Emotional instability due to marked reactivity of mood – fluctuations of mood that may be triggered either internally (e.g., by one's own thoughts) or by external events, as a consequence of which the individual experiences intense dysphoric mood states, which typically last for a few hours but may last for up to several days

7. Chronic feelings of emptiness

8. Inappropriate intense anger or difficulty controlling anger, manifested in frequent displays of temper (e.g., yelling or screaming, throwing or breaking things, getting into physical fights)

9. Transient dissociative symptoms or psychotic-like features (e.g., brief hallucinations, paranoia) in situations of high affective arousal

 **Exam Essentials**

- Symptoms of borderline personality disorder – **DESPAIRER**
  - **D**isturbed identity
  - **E**motionally labile

- ◦ **S**uicidal thinking/self-harm recurrent
- ◦ **P**aranoia transient/severe dissociations
- ◦ **A**bandonment
- ◦ **I**mpulsivity in two areas (exclude suicidal/self-harm thoughts)
- ◦ **R**elationship instability
- ◦ **E**mptiness
- ◦ **R**age inappropriate

- There are some differences in the presentation of bipolar disorder and borderline personality disorder. Refer to Case 6 for more information.

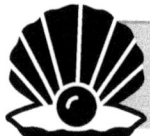

Clinical Pearls

- Borderline personality disorder presentations vary with the development of one's personality over time. Presentation at the adolescent stage is more likely to present with executive symptoms (i.e., self-harm, impulse-control issues), whilst adults present with enduring symptoms (i.e., unstable relationships)

- Core symptoms include **affective dysregulation, interpersonal disturbance** and **impulsivity**

Question 2
What are the risk factors for developing borderline personality disorder?

Answer
Modifiable: Lower socioeconomic status, maladaptive parenting, trauma
Non-modifiable: Genetic predisposition (oxytocin receptor gene AA/AG), significant maternal psychiatric history

Explanation
Maladaptive parenting includes low warmth, rejection, hostility and discipline/punishment, which often leads children to feel abandoned leading to a higher risk of borderline personality disorder. Certain psychiatric disorders in mothers including conduct disorder, oppositional defiant disorder, attention deficit hyperactivity disorder, self-harm behaviours and substance use disorder were also risk factors for their children developing borderline personality disorder. Maternal borderline personality disorder is consistently found to be a predictor of adolescent (15 years old) and early adulthood (24 years old) onset of borderline personality disorder [3].

Trauma, including verbal, emotional and physical/sexual abuse, is often a trigger for the development of borderline personality disorder traits such as affect instability and self-harm. Borderline personality disorder may be modulated by the oxytocinergic system.

Question 3
What are common co-morbidities in borderline personality disorder?

Answer
Mood disorders: major depressive disorder, bipolar disorder, dysthymia
Anxiety spectrum disorders: generalised anxiety disorder, panic disorder, social phobia, obsessive–compulsive disorder, post-traumatic stress disorder (PTSD)
Eating disorders: anorexia nervosa, bulimia nervosa
Others: substance use disorder, suicidality

Explanation
Mood disorders are the most common co-morbidity in borderline personality disorder, with a lifetime prevalence of 85% [4]. Prevalence of co-morbid depression is reported at 71–83%; anxiety spectrum, 88%; PTSD, 47–56%; and any eating disorders, 7–26% [5]. The prevalence of substance use disorder as a co-morbidity is at a rate of 78% [6]. Suicide rates in borderline personality disorder patients are at 8–12% [7, 8].

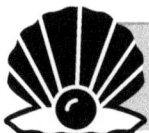

Clinical Pearls

- The presence of a personality disorder may affect the prognosis of a co-morbidity due to possible interference in treatment due to:

    - More sensitive to psychosocial stressors
    - More self-harm and negative self-perception
    - Transference and counter-transference issues (refer to the Diving Deep section)

Question 4
How would you manage Kacey's borderline personality disorder?

Answer
Psychotherapy: dialectical behaviour therapy (DBT), mentalisation-based therapy (MBT), transference-focused psychotherapy (TFP)
Social: art therapies
Biological agents (to treat co-morbidities): selective serotonin reuptake inhibitors (SSRIs), antipsychotics, anxiolytics, mood stabilisers

Explanation

DBT is a borderline personality disorder-specific intervention which addresses interpersonal difficulties, and application to borderline problems through theoretical and practical attention as well as functional analysis. The four primary modes of treatment in DBT include group skill training, individual therapy, phone consultation and consultation team. Patients are typically seen weekly and learn to improve interpersonal skills and decrease self-harm behaviours.

MBT focuses on mentalisation as a social construct that allows a person to be attentive to the mental state of oneself and others. It is hypothesised that patients with borderline personality disorder have deficits in mentalisation, which lead to difficulty in regulating emotions and managing impulsivity. Thus, teaching mentalisation techniques allows patients to build relationship skills and regulate their emotions better, reducing interpersonal conflicts.

TFP is a form of psychodynamic therapy which is grounded in object relations theory. Object relations theory centres around theories of stages of ego development arising from the infant's relationship with the mother and ensuing personality development. In TFP, the therapist uses clarification to analyse transference more directly such that the patient becomes quickly aware of his or her distortions about the therapist. Confrontation is a technique where the therapist points out how transference distorts the patient's view on interpersonal relations with others (objects). Therefore, with therapy, 'good objects' and 'bad objects' are seen with more ambiguity and splitting diminishes in patients.

Art therapy aims to use art media as a primary mode of communication to express thoughts and emotions.

The pharmacological agents are mainly to treat the high prevalence of co-morbidities and trait- and state-related symptoms of borderline personality disorder, such as transient stress-related psychotic symptoms and affect instability.

Exam Essentials

- The four sets of specific skills taught in DBT – **DICE**
    - **D**istress tolerance
    - **I**nterpersonal effectiveness
    - **C**ore mindfulness
    - **E**motion regulation

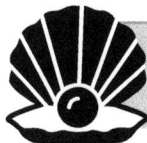

Clinical Pearls

- When managing patients with borderline personality disorder, it is crucial for clinicians to set clear boundaries and remain mindful of transference and countertransference dynamics

- Patients may occasionally exhibit '**splitting**'. This is a psychological mechanism that allows the individual to bear overwhelming emotions by perceiving others as either good or bad (idealised or devalued). Therefore, clinicians should always consult with other healthcare team members to ensure that everyone is on the same page

Diving Deep ...

Defence mechanisms are the automatic psychological responses that individuals use in response to anxiety and internal or external stress and conflict. Managing individuals with borderline personality disorder can be challenging at times; with frequent manifestations of emotion dysregulation, the use of primitive defences like splitting (cognitive and affective disturbances which typically manifest as shifts of emotional perception of objects, other persons and the self with typical fluctuations between idealisation and devaluation), relational disruptions and difficulties in maintaining boundaries in the therapeutic interaction. Other defence mechanisms include projection (displacing unacceptable psychological impulses and traits in oneself onto others) and reaction formation (externally expressing attitudes and behaviours which are the opposite of the unacceptable internal impulses).

Transference is the unconscious development in the patient of feelings, thoughts, attitudes and patterns of behaviour towards the therapist which recapitulate earlier life relationships. Countertransference refers to unconscious, conflict-based responses to the patient's transference, and therapists unconsciously displace feelings from their past into analytical situations. Current perspectives on countertransference suggest that the reasons for these reactions are not necessarily located only within the client, and could also stem from aspects of the therapist or the therapy situation, such as termination of the sessions.

References

1. World Health Organization. *International classification of diseases*, 11th edition (ICD-11). Geneva: World Health Organization; 2024. Available from: https://icd.who.int/en

2. American Psychiatric Association. *Diagnostic and statistical manual of mental disorders*, 5th edition, text revision (DSM-5-TR). Washington, DC: American Psychiatric Association Publishing; 2022. Available from: www.psychiatry.org/psychiatrists/practice/dsm

3. Bozzatello P, Bellino S, Bosia M, Rocca P. Early detection and outcome in borderline personality disorder. *Front Psychiatry*. 2019;10:710.

4. Lenzenweger MF, Lane MC, Loranger AW, Kessler RC. DSM-IV personality disorders in the National Comorbidity Survey Replication. *Biol Psychiatry*. 2007 Sep 15;62(6):553–64.

5. Biskin RS, Paris J. Comorbidities in borderline personality disorder: real-world issues and treatment implications. *Psychiatric Times*. 2013;30. Available from: link.gale.com/apps/doc/A316796600/AONE?u=googlescholar&sid=googleScholar&xid=5e549b37

6. Kienast T, Stoffers J, Bermpohl F, Lieb K. Borderline personality disorder and comorbid addiction. *Deutsches Ärzteblatt*. 2014 Apr 18. Available from: www.aerzteblatt.de/10.3238/arztebl.2014.0280

7. Pompili M, Girardi P, Ruberto A, Tatarelli R. Suicide in borderline personality disorder: a meta-analysis. *Nord J Psychiatry*. 2005;59(5):319–24.

8. Paris J. Implications of long-term outcome research for the management of patients with borderline personality disorder. *Harv Rev Psychiatry*. 2002;10(6):315–23.

Case 32: Antisocial Personality Disorder

A void of empathy

George is a single 39-year-old gentleman currently warded for treatment of his leg cellulitis. He has been displaying difficult behaviour in the ward, requesting to go down to the car park to smoke and does not comply with his doctor's instructions to elevate his leg to reduce leg swelling. He shouted at the nurses when his food was not warm enough and hurled vulgarities toward the registrar in charge for not prescribing diazepam. His sister revealed that he has had such challenging behaviours since the age of 13. He would pick-pocket others as a 'thrill-seeking' behaviour and has been convicted twice for armed robbery and arson. His relationship with his father is estranged, as he previously verbally abused and punched his father after his father stopped giving him a financial allowance. He has been unable to hold a job for longer than a few months. He does not appear to be remorseful over his past behaviour or present issues with the medical staff.

- **Question 1: What is the most likely diagnosis?**

- **Question 2: Does George fulfil the criteria for conduct–dissocial disorder as well?**

- **Question 3: What are the risk factors that may predict the development of antisocial personality disorder?**

- **Question 4: What are the common co-morbidities with antisocial personality disorder?**

- **Question 5: What are the management principles for antisocial personality disorder?**

> • **Question 6: What immediate advice can we provide for the nursing staff member, who is understandably stressed from George's behaviour?**

Answers to Case 32

Question 1
What is the most likely diagnosis?

Answer

Antisocial personality disorder (DSM-5-TR)/personality disorder with dissociality (ICD-11)

Explanation

Diagnosis of antisocial personality disorder [1]

1. A pervasive pattern of disregard for the rights of others since the age of 15 years. Three or more of the following symptoms:

    •   Failure to conform to social norms with repeated acts of breaking the law
    •   Deceitfulness and cheating of others for personal profit or pleasure
    •   Acting impulsively or failing to plan ahead
    •   Frequent displays of irritability and aggressiveness, often demonstrated through repeated physical fights or assaults
    •   Demonstrating reckless disregard for the safety of oneself or others
    •   Consistent irresponsibility, as evidenced by repeated failure to sustain stable work behaviour or fulfil financial obligations
    •   Lack of remorse

2. The individual is at least age 18 years

3. There is evidence of conduct–dissocial disorder with onset before age 15 years

The DSM and ICD use two different approaches when it comes to the diagnosis of personality disorders. The DSM-5-TR employs a categorical approach, by providing more detailed and specific criteria for diagnosing each personality disorder type [1]. Instead, the ICD-11 focuses on broader personality functioning impairment levels and the use of trait domain specifiers to describe personality features with dysfunction [2]. The trait domain of dissociality consists of the core features of disregard for the rights and feelings of others, encompassing both self-centredness and lack of empathy.

Exam Essentials

- Symptoms of antisocial personality disorder – **ACID SIR**
    - **A**ggression
    - **C**annot conform
    - **I**mpulsivity
    - **D**eceitful
    - **S**afety disregard
    - **I**rresponsible
    - **R**emorse lacking

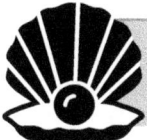

Clinical Pearls

- A diagnosis of a personality disorder should only be made when a longitudinal review of the patient's personality traits has been made, and not based on solely one encounter

Question 2
Does George fulfil the criteria for conduct–dissocial disorder as well?

Answer
Yes. However, conduct–dissocial disorder is not the primary diagnosis for him currently.

Explanation
George displayed early symptoms of deceitfulness (theft), damage of property (arson) and aggression towards others (armed robbery) for a minimum duration of one year. Hence, he did fulfil the criteria for conduct–dissocial disorder when he was young. Other symptoms of conduct–dissocial disorder include the violation of rules by an individual, such as running away from home or playing truant.

Diagnosis of conduct–dissocial disorder

1. A repetitive and persistent pattern of behaviour in which the basic rights of others or major age-appropriate social or cultural norms, rules or laws are violated is required for diagnosis. Typically, multiple behaviours are involved, including one or more of the following:

295

- Aggression to people and animals, such as bullying, threatening or intimidating others, instigating physical fights, using weapons that can cause serious physical harm to others (such as a brick, broken bottle, knife or gun), physical cruelty to people, physical cruelty to animals, aggressive forms of stealing (e.g., mugging, purse snatching, extortion) or forcing someone into sexual activity
- Destruction of property, such as deliberate fire setting to cause serious damage or deliberate destruction of others' property (e.g., purposely breaking other children's toys, breaking windows, scratching cars, slashing tires)
- Deceitfulness or theft, such as stealing items of value (e.g., shoplifting, forgery), lying to obtain goods or favours or to avoid obligations (e.g., 'conning' others) or breaking into someone's house, building or car
- Serious violations of rules, such as children or adolescents repeatedly staying out all night despite parental prohibitions, repeatedly running away from home or often skipping school or work without permission

2. The pattern of behaviour must be persistent and recurrent, including multiple incidents of the types of behaviours described above over an extended period of time (e.g., at least one year). The mere commission of one or more delinquent acts is not sufficient for the diagnosis

3. The behaviour pattern results in significant impairment in personal, family, social, educational, occupational or other important areas of functioning

Specifiers:

- Childhood onset: One or more features of the disorder have clearly been present and persistent during childhood prior to adolescence (e.g., before 10 years of age)

- Adolescent onset: none of the features of the disorder were present prior to adolescence (e.g., before 10 years of age)

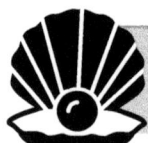

Clinical Pearls

- Conduct–dissocial disorder is a diagnosis that is only made in childhood and adolescence, and not adulthood

Question 3
What are the risk factors that may predict the development of antisocial personality disorder?

Answer
Attention deficit hyperactivity disorder (ADHD), difficult infant temperament, harsh and inconsistent parenting styles, history of substance use disorder and history of conduct–dissocial disorder.

Explanation
Children with ADHD have four times the risk of developing antisocial personality disorder [3]. Difficult infant temperament and harsh and inconsistent parenting styles may be related to conduct–dissocial disorder and may therefore be related to later antisocial personality disorder. The association between a history of substance use disorder and antisocial behaviour is well documented, and past substance use disorder before the age of 25 also predicts antisocial behaviours [4].

Question 4
What are the common co-morbidities with antisocial personality disorder?

Answer
    Substance use disorder: illicit drug use is the most common
    Suicidal ideations
    Mood disorder

Explanation
Among individuals with antisocial personality disorder, 51.4% have a lifetime mood disorder [5] and 54.33% have a lifetime co-morbid anxiety disorder [6], while 77% have a lifetime diagnosis of alcohol use disorder [7] and 90% have a co-occurring substance use disorder [8].

Individuals with antisocial personality disorder are four times more likely to experience a mood disorder, 13 times more likely to also experience a substance use disorder and seven times more likely to have suicidal ideations. Data from waves 1 and 2 of the National Epidemiological Survey on Alcohol and Related Conditions (NESARC) reported that those with antisocial personality disorder were seven to eight times more likely to meet the criteria for alcohol dependence, 15–17 times more likely to meet the criteria for drug dependence and five to six times more likely to be nicotine dependent [9].

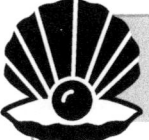

Clinical Pearls

- Clinicians need to have a high suspicion for the presence of co-morbid substance use, especially if patients present with intoxication, withdrawal or signs of intravenous abuse (such as needling marks, infective endocarditis or cellulitis in limbs or groins)

Question 5
What are the management principles for antisocial personality disorder?

Answer
We should offer treatment for co-morbidities. Psychological treatment such as a group based on cognitive and behavioural interventions focuses on reducing offending behaviours. Pharmacological treatment for antisocial personality disorder alone is not recommended.

Explanation
The United Kingdom's National Institute for Health and Care Excellence (NICE) guideline [10] recommends group-based cognitive and behavioural interventions as the mainstay of managing antisocial personality disorder symptoms. Co-morbidities such as substance use disorder should also be the focus of treatment to minimise risks of harm towards self or others.

Question 6
What immediate advice can we provide for the nursing staff member, who is understandably stressed from George's behaviour?

Answer
Working together as a team with the nurses is imperative. Principles such as setting limits and avoiding confrontation may be used. We may also need to consider social, chemical or physical restraints if necessary for safety.

Explanation
The multidisciplinary team members involved in George's care, including the nurses, may be upset, frustrated or distressed by his behaviour. Clinicians need to show support for the nurses and provide advice such as permitting them to say 'no' to patients' unrealistic demands and diminishing guilt by stating that it is not possible to entirely satisfy such patients. Avoid confrontations by tactful redirection of anger towards more productive targets (e.g., away from his refusal to comply with nursing instructions and towards planning for quick recovery and discharge). Lastly, if George shows signs of endangering his or another's safety, social restraints (arranging a security officer or involving the police), chemical and physical restraints may be considered as a last resort.

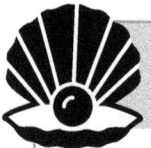 **Clinical Pearls**

- The 1997 United Kingdom Protection from Harassment Act is an Act of the Parliament of the United Kingdom that criminalises harassment, stalking and other antisocial behaviour

- This Act protects healthcare workers from harassment

Diving Deep ...

Personality is an enduring pattern of perceiving, relating to and thinking about the environment and oneself, which is exhibited across numerous social and personal contexts. A personality disorder is diagnosed when personality traits are so inflexible and maladaptive across a wide range of situations that they cause significant distress and impairment of social, occupational and role functioning.

The prevalence of antisocial personality disorder is estimated at 3% for men and 1% for women in the general population [11].

Other diagnoses that may present similarly to antisocial personality disorder include:

- Oppositional defiant disorder, where a spiteful young patient presents with an angry mood and defiant behaviour for at least six months in duration (typically diagnosed before age 12). However, this diagnosis is only made during the childhood and adolescence period and is not as severe compared to conduct–dissocial disorder (e.g., less violence/aggression, symptoms less severe, presence for at least six months compared to one year in conduct–dissocial disorder)

- Intermittent explosive disorder, where an individual is observed to be having recurrent verbal or behavioural outbursts that are grossly out of proportion to provocation, with no intention of a tangible objective to be achieved

References

1. American Psychiatric Association. *Diagnostic and statistical manual of mental disorders*, 5th edition, text revision (DSM-5-TR). Washington, DC: American Psychiatric Association Publishing; 2022. Available from: www.psychiatry.org/psychiatrists/practice/dsm

2. World Health Organization. *International classification of diseases*, 11th edition (ICD-11). Geneva: World Health Organization; 2024. Available from: https://icd.who.int/en

3. Mannuzza S, Klein RG, Bessler A, Malloy P, LaPadula M. Adult psychiatric status of hyperactive boys grown up. *Am J Psychiatry*. 1998 Apr;155(4):493–8.

4. Schoenmacker GH, Sakala K, Franke B, Buitelaar JK, Veidebaum T, Harro J, et al. Identification and validation of risk factors for antisocial behaviour involving police. *Psychiatry Res*. 2020 Sep;291:113208.

5. Goldstein RB, Grant BF. Three-year follow-up of syndromal antisocial behavior in adults: results from the Wave 2 National Epidemiologic Survey on Alcohol and Related Conditions. *J Clin Psychiatry*. 2009 Sep;70(9):1237–49.

6. Goodwin RD, Hamilton SP. Lifetime comorbidity of antisocial personality disorder and anxiety disorders among adults in the community. *Psychiatry Res*. 2003 Feb 15;117(2):159–66.

7. Guy N, Newton-Howes G, Ford H, Williman J, Foulds J. The prevalence of comorbid alcohol use disorder in the presence of personality disorder: systematic review and explanatory modelling. *Personal Ment Health*. 2018 Aug;12(3):216–28.

8. Messina NP, Wish ED, Nemes S. Therapeutic community treatment for substance abusers with antisocial personality disorder. *J Subst Abuse Treat*. 1999 Jul–Sep;17(1–2):121–8.

9. Hasin DS, Grant BF. The National Epidemiologic Survey on Alcohol and Related Conditions (NESARC) Waves 1 and 2: review and summary of findings. *Soc Psychiatry Psychiatr Epidemiol*. 2015 Nov;50(11):1609–40.

10. National Institute for Health and Care Excellence (NICE). Antisocial personality disorder: prevention and management. Clinical guideline [CG77]. NICE; 2009. Available from: www.nice.org.uk/guidance/cg77

11. Boland RJ, Verduin ML, Ruiz P, Shah A, Sadock BJ, editors. *Kaplan & Sadock's synopsis of psychiatry*, 12th edition. Philadelphia: Wolters Kluwer; 2022.

Case 33: Schizoid, Schizotypal and Paranoid Personality Disorder

The loner

Benjamin is a 24-year-old male brought to your clinic by his mother. His mother had urged him to seek help when she noticed he was seemingly unaffected by the recent passing of his father. Corroborative history from his mother reveals Benjamin to be somewhat of a 'loner' growing up. He had few to no friends in his schooling days and never expressed a desire to be in a romantic relationship. Even when teased in school, he would not get angry but merely brushed aside the criticisms. He would spend his free time alone, often playing the same individual computer games, and only left the house when necessary. When asked about his father's passing, he spoke about it in a matter-of-fact manner stating it was regrettable.

- **Question 1: What is the diagnosis?**

- **Question 2: What would you expect of his mental state examination?**

- **Question 3: How is schizoid personality disorder different from paranoid personality disorder?**

His mother also raised concerns over Benjamin's younger brother, Matthew, who had always been a quiet boy as well. His teachers often reported bullying by classmates for being odd and different, with wild conspiracy theories. Matthew was a peculiar child who was often suspicious of the motives of others, frequently believing that others were talking ill about him. He had 'his way of thinking'; for example, he would insist on going to the supermarkets only on Fridays as 'Friday is a good day for going to markets'. His room was always messy, and he was often reprimanded for his poor personal hygiene.

- **Question 4: Which personality disorder is Matthew most likely to have?**

Answers to Case 33

Question 1
What is the diagnosis?

Answer
Schizoid personality disorder (DSM-5-TR))/personality disorder with detachment (ICD-11)

Explanation
Schizoid personality disorder (DSM-5-TR) is a pervasive pattern of detachment from social relationships and a restricted range of expression of emotions in interpersonal settings. This pattern is first apparent in childhood and adolescence, with solitariness, poor peer relationships and underachievement in school. A review of epidemiological studies from several countries found a median prevalence of 1.5% for Cluster A personality disorders [1].

Diagnosis of schizoid personality disorder [2]

A pervasive pattern of detachment from social relationships and a restricted range of expression of emotions in interpersonal settings, beginning by early adulthood and present in a variety of contexts. Four or more of the following symptoms:

1. Does not desire or find joy in intimate connections, including familial bonds

2. Frequently chooses solitary activities

3. Exhibits minimal interest in engaging in sexual experiences with others

4. Derives little, if any, pleasure from various activities

5. Lacks close companions or confidants outside of first-degree relatives

6. Demonstrates indifference to both praise and criticism from others

7. Displays emotional coldness, detachment or flattened affectivity

---

In ICD-11, trait-domain specifiers may be applied to personality disorders to describe the characteristics of the individual's personality that are most prominent and that contribute to personality disturbance [3]. The closest domain trait to schizoid personality disorder would be that of 'detachment'. The detachment trait domain is characterised by the tendency to maintain interpersonal distance (social detachment) and emotional distance (emotional detachment).

Exam Essentials

- Cluster A personality disorders include paranoid, schizoid and schizotypal personality disorders

- Symptoms of schizoid personality disorder – **DISTANT**
    - **D**etachment/flattened affect
    - **I**ndifferent to praises/criticism
    - **S**exual interest lacking
    - **T**asks are done solitarily
    - **A**bsence of close friends/confidants
    - **N**either desire nor enjoy close relationships
    - **T**akes pleasure in few activities only

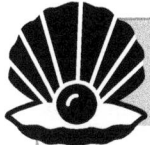

Clinical Pearls

- Autism is a differential diagnosis given the overlapping features of social deficits

Question 2
What would you expect of his mental state examination?

Answer
The patient may display a cold exterior without visible emotional reactivity and rarely reciprocate gestures or facial expressions, such as smiles or nods. A constricted affect may be seen, appearing cold and aloof to the interviewer.

Explanation
Patients with schizoid personality disorder rarely experience strong emotions such as anger and joy. While often appearing detached and cold, there may be rare instances where, in a comfortable social setting, the patient can be forthcoming in acknowledging and expressing their painful feelings.

Question 3
How is schizoid personality disorder different from paranoid personality disorder?

Answer

Patients with paranoid personality disorder are often overly resentful, paranoid and suspicious and can demonstrate explosive anger, whereas those with schizoid personality disorder are aloof and eccentric, and lack paranoid ideation.

Explanation

The essential feature of paranoid personality disorder (DSM-5-TR) is a pattern of pervasive distrust and suspiciousness of others such that their motives are interpreted as malevolent.

Diagnosis of paranoid personality disorder [2]

A pervasive sense of distrust and suspicion towards others, interpreting their motives as malevolent, beginning in early adulthood and evident in various situations. Four or more of the following symptoms:

1. Unfounded suspicion that others are exploiting, harming or deceiving them

2. Preoccupation with unjustified doubts about the loyalty or trustworthiness of friends or associates

3. Reluctance to confide in others due to an unjustified fear of malicious use of information

4. Attributing demeaning or threatening meanings to benign remarks or events

5. Holding persistent grudges, being unforgiving of insults, injuries or slights

6. Perceiving attacks on their character or reputation that are not apparent to others, reacting quickly with anger or counterattack

7. Recurrent suspicions, lacking justification, regarding the fidelity of a spouse or sexual partner

---

The closest domain trait to paranoid personality disorder is that of 'dissociality' and 'disinhibition'. The trait domain of dissociality consists of the core features of disregard for the rights and feelings of others, encompassing both self-centredness and lack of empathy. The trait domain of disinhibition consists of the core features of a tendency to act rashly based on immediate external or internal stimuli (i.e., sensations, emotions, thoughts), without consideration of potential negative consequences.

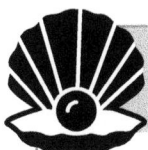

Clinical Pearls

- The tendency for individuals with paranoid personality disorder to react angrily to minor stimuli may similarly be seen in borderline and histrionic personality disorders

Question 4
Which personality disorder is Matthew most likely to have?

Answer
Schizotypal personality disorder

Explanation
Deficits are noted in the three domains typical of schizotypal personality disorder (DSM-5-TR): 'cognitive–perceptual', 'oddness/disorganised' and 'interpersonal'. These deficits should be present since early adulthood.

Diagnosis of schizotypal personality disorder [2]

A pervasive pattern of social and interpersonal challenges characterised by significant discomfort with, and diminished capacity for, close relationships, along with cognitive or perceptual distortions and eccentric behaviors, starting in early adulthood and evident in various contexts. Five or more of the following symptoms:

1. Ideas of reference (excluding delusions of reference)

2. Odd beliefs or magical thinking influencing behaviour, inconsistent with subcultural norms

3. Unusual perceptual encounters, including illusions related to the body

4. Odd thinking and speech

5. Feelings of suspicion or paranoid thoughts

6. Inappropriate or constricted affect

7. Behaviours or appearance that are peculiar or eccentric

8. Lack of close friends or confidants beyond first-degree relatives

9. Excessive social anxiety that remains despite familiarity and is linked to paranoid fears rather than negative self-assessments

Exam Essentials

- Symptoms of schizotypal personality disorder – **OILIES**

  - **O**dd: behaviour, perceptual experience, beliefs, speech
  - **I**deas of reference
  - **L**acks friends
  - **I**nappropriate affect
  - **E**xcessive social anxiety
  - **S**uspiciousness or paranoia

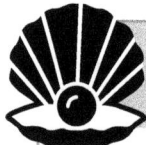

Clinical Pearls

- Ten to twenty per cent of patients with schizotypal personality disorder develop schizophrenia or schizoaffective disorder [4].

- Individuals with schizotypal personality disorder may experience brief psychotic episodes with hallucinations and/or delusions. However, these episodes are not as frequent, prolonged or intense compared to those suffering from schizophrenia.

Diving Deep …

In paranoid personality disorder, exposure to social stressors such as socioeconomic inequality, marginalisation and racism are associated with decreased trust, which in some cases is adaptive. Childhood trauma combined with social stress accounts for the increased prevalence of paranoid symptoms in social groups facing racial discrimination. Relationships are affected by their excessive suspiciousness, and hostility may be expressed as overt argumentativeness, recurrent complaining or by hostile aloofness.

In schizoid personality disorder, relationships are affected because of their detachment and lack of desire for intimacy.

References

1. Huang Y, Kotov R, de Girolamo G, Preti A, Angermeyer M, Benjet C, et al. DSM-IV personality disorders in the WHO World Mental Health Surveys. *Br J Psychiatry*. 2009 Jul;195(1):46–53.

2. American Psychiatric Association. *Diagnostic and statistical manual of mental disorders*, 5th edition, text revision (DSM-5-TR). Washington, DC: American Psychiatric Association Publishing; 2022. Available from: www.psychiatry.org/psychiatrists/practice/dsm

3. World Health Organization. *International classification of diseases*, 11th edition (ICD-11). Geneva: World Health Organization; 2024. Available from: https://icd.who.int/en

4. Asarnow JR. Childhood-onset schizotypal disorder: a follow-up study and comparison with childhood-onset schizophrenia. *J Child Adolesc Psychopharmacol*. 2005 Jun;15(3):395–402.

Case 34: Dependent Personality Disorder

But I need you

Mandy, a 28-year-old female, was referred by the emergency department for a psychiatric evaluation due to a suicide attempt by drug overdose. During the consult, it became apparent that a recent breakup with her boyfriend of four years triggered the attempt. Upon exploring the nature of their relationship, it was revealed that her boyfriend had repeatedly cheated on her with multiple friends throughout their time together and borrowed money from her amounting to £100,000 without repayment. Although her close confidants have repeatedly brought up the undesirable nature of the relationship, she defends him by saying, 'I cannot live without him. He has been very supportive of my decisions. He helps me pick out my clothes daily and affirms my decisions to try out new things'. She reports that her current accountant job was only possible with his encouragement as, initially, she felt inadequate and too incompetent to pursue such a career. She feels disappointed whenever he cheats on her and has self-harmed via cutting. However, she has tried to 'look past' his infidelity. Over the four years, she was constantly worried about him breaking up with her, and to accede to his requests for monetary support has taken a loan of £50,000 from licensed money lenders. She hopes he will return to her, as she is 'lost without him' and cannot carry out her day-to-day life without him.

- **Question 1: What is the diagnosis?**

You diagnosed her with dependent personality disorder. However, a medical student asks if borderline personality disorder should be considered as the patient initially came in for self-harm.

- **Question 2: What are the similarities and differences between borderline personality disorder and dependent personality disorder?**

The medical student also asks 'How about separation anxiety disorder? Since they are both linked to fear of separation'.

- **Question 3: What are the similarities and differences between dependent personality disorder and separation anxiety disorder?**

- **Question 4: How would you manage this patient with a dependent personality disorder?**

Answers to Case 34

Question 1
What is the diagnosis?

Answer
Dependent personality disorder (DSM-5-TR)

Explanation

Diagnosis of dependent personality disorder [1]

A pervasive and intense need to be cared for, resulting in submissive and dependent behaviour and anxieties about separation, starting in early adulthood and evident in various situations. Five or more of the following symptoms:

1. Struggles to make routine decisions without seeking an excessive amount of advice and reassurance from others

2. Depends on others to take on the majority of responsibilities in most important areas of life

3. Finds it challenging to express disagreement with others due to a fear of losing their support or approval. (Note: excludes realistic fears of retribution)

4. Faces difficulty initiating tasks or handling things independently, stemming from a lack of self-confidence in judgement or abilities rather than a lack of motivation or energy

5. Goes to great lengths to secure nurturance and support from others, even volunteering for unpleasant tasks

6. Feels uneasy or helpless when alone, driven by exaggerated fears of being incapable of self-care

7. Urgently seeks a new relationship as a source of care and support when a close relationship comes to an end

8. Harbours unrealistic preoccupations with fears of being left to care for oneself

In ICD-11, trait-domain specifiers may be applied to personality disorders to describe the characteristics of the individual's personality that are most prominent and that contribute to personality disturbance [2]. The closest domain trait to dependent personality disorder would be that of 'negative affectivity'. The negative affectivity trait domain is characterised by the tendency to maintain interpersonal distance (social detachment) and emotional distance (emotional detachment).

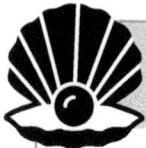

Clinical Pearls

- Age and cultural factors need to be considered in the evaluation of the diagnostic threshold of each criterion

Question 2
What are the similarities and differences between borderline personality disorder and dependent personality disorder?

Answer
Similarity: underlying fear of abandonment
Differences:

Domain	Borderline personality disorder	Dependent personality disorder
Reaction to fear of abandonment	Emotional emptiness, rage and demands	Increasing appeasement and submissiveness
Nature of relationships	Unstable and intense, multiple short relationships in succession	Submissive to abusive relationships, usually long-term relationships

Explanation
Borderline personality disorder is characterised by patterns of instability in interpersonal relationships, self-image and affects and marked impulsivity. Those with the disorder make frantic efforts to avoid abandonment, which could present as self-harm. However, in dependent personality disorder, patients are characterised by the pervasive and excessive need to be taken care of that drives submissive and clingy behaviour and fear of separation. Self-harm is not a hallmark of this disorder, but could be a consequence of the inability to cope with abandonment.

Exam Essentials

- It is important to screen for other personality disorders (borderline, avoidant and histrionic) which are known co-morbidities of dependent personality disorders

Question 3
What are the similarities and differences between dependent personality disorder and separation anxiety disorder?

Answer
Similarity: underlying fear of separation
Differences:

Domain	Separation anxiety disorder	Dependent personality disorder
The patient's underlying concern	Requires proximity with key attachment figures Concerned about well-being and safety	Has an indiscriminate tendency to rely on others
Predominant patient profile	Children	Females > Males

Explanation
Although both disorders are similar in the negative feelings about separation, the key concern in each disorder is markedly different. The essential feature of separation anxiety disorder is excessive fear or anxiety about leaving home or attachment figures. This could cause patients to request reporting of their key attachment's whereabouts and they have a desire for constant contact. There is an underlying worry in such patients about having untoward events occurring to themselves that prevent them from reuniting with their key attachment figures. And as such, they refuse or are reluctant to leave home by themselves.

Dependent personality disorder is characterised by a pattern of submissive and clingy behaviour related to the excessive need to be taken care of. There is a need for reassurance and reliance, which is different from the underlying anxiety seen in separation anxiety disorder. The diagnosis of dependent personality disorder is found more frequently in females than males.

Question 4

How would you manage this patient with a dependent personality disorder?

Answer

As this patient came in for a suicide attempt, it is important to do a suicide risk assessment and determine if there is a need for admission:

- Psychotherapy options: insight-oriented therapies, behavioural therapy, assertiveness training, family therapy and group therapy

- Pharmacological options: antidepressants, benzodiazepines

Explanation

Patients usually respond well to treatment. However, it is important to establish therapist–patient rapport. This is especially so when rendering professional advice about changing the dynamics of the pathological relationship. This could lead to a loss to follow-up, as the patient might become anxious and unable to cooperate with therapy. The distress faced by potential abandonment can overwhelm any therapeutic inroads in the early phases. Therapists have to be versatile to ensure continuity of care. Therapeutic interventions are expected to take time in such patients, with many sessions required to cause an impact on a small number of dysfunctional core beliefs. Therapy needs to end at an agreed point to prevent dependency issues on the therapist from arising.

Insight-oriented therapies help patients to understand the antecedents of their behaviour, and with training become more independent, assertive and self-reliant [3].

Medications are used to treat specific symptoms, such as anxiety and depression. For example, in patients who experience panic attacks or high levels of separation anxiety, antidepressants have been found to be useful.

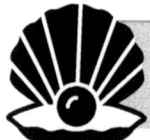

Clinical Pearls

- Therapy needs to end at an agreed point to prevent dependency issues on the therapist from arising

Diving Deep ...

Patients with a dependent personality disorder may be susceptible to shared psychotic disorder (*folie à deux*). *Folie à deux* is a rare disorder characterised by a shared delusion between two or more people in a close relationship. The inducer (primary), who has a psychotic disorder with delusional beliefs, influences another non-psychotic individual (induced, secondary) based on the delusional beliefs. If this happens within a family, it is coined as *folie à famille*.

The risk factors for *folie à deux* include relationship-dependent factors, psychiatric illness-related factors, social environment-related factors and others. Relationship-dependent factors include the length of the relationship and the nature of the relationship. Psychiatric illness-related factors may be untreated mental disorders in the primary and co-morbidity of the secondary, such as personality disorders (dependent, schizoid, schizotypal). Social environment-related factors include social isolation, stressful life events and communication difficulties (leading to a preference for social isolation). Other factors are cognitive impairment in the secondary and female gender.

The increased risk of *folie à deux* [4] in patients with dependent personality disorder arises from their fear of being alone – they tend to seek out others they can depend on. In a shared psychotic disorder, one partner is more dominant, with fixed delusions, while the other tends to have a more dependent personality and is more suggestible (and hence can be induced with the delusional belief).

These cases are difficult to pick up clinically due to the lack of insight within the pair or group. They are usually referred to clinics only when their delusions pose a risk to others. A clear history to establish the temporality of the development of their psychotic disorder will be important to determine the primary and the secondary involved in the shared delusion.

References

1.   American Psychiatric Association. *Diagnostic and statistical manual of mental disorders*, 5th edition, text revision (DSM-5-TR). Washington, DC: American Psychiatric Association Publishing; 2022. Available from: www.psychiatry.org/psychiatrists/practice/dsm.

2.   World Health Organization. *International classification of diseases*, 11th edition (ICD-11). Geneva: World Health Organization; 2024. Available from: https://icd.who.int/en

3.   Boland RJ, Verduin ML, Ruiz P, Shah A, Sadock BJ, editors. *Kaplan & Sadock's synopsis of psychiatry*, 12th edition. Philadelphia: Wolters Kluwer; 2022.

4.   Al Saif F, Al Khalili Y. Shared psychotic disorder. *StatPearls*. Treasure Island, FL: StatPearls Publishing; 2023. Available from: www.ncbi.nlm.nih.gov/books/NBK541211

Case 35: Suicide Risk Assessment

The tipping point

Your emergency department has just received Willy, a 20-year-old foreign student, who his university dormitory mates reported to be unconscious. According to the paramedics, Willy regained consciousness but refused to cooperate with the ambulance transfer initially. One of his dormitory mates found many empty packets of painkillers in the dustbin, which was indicative that Willy took an overdose. However, Willy refused to comply with the paramedics as he did not want to receive help.

- **Question 1: What are the approaches you would undertake during a suicide risk assessment?**

- **Question 2: What are the differences between suicidal ideation, suicidal intent and suicidal plan?**

- **Question 3: What is Willy's level of risk at present?**

Willy was getting restless and agitated in the general ward, and as the nurses were trying to apply physical restraint, they noticed that he has multiple scars from old lacerations on his left wrist.

- **Question 4: What is the clinical significance of his self-harm behaviours for his current suicide attempt?**

Willy reached medical stability in the ward over two days and is medically fit for discharge. However, he is still very guarded and not forthcoming about his suicidal intentions. With his high risk of suicide, your hospital's psychiatrist has advised that he needs inpatient psychiatric care.

- **Question 5: What is the legislation that allows a patient to be involuntarily admitted for safety and further psychiatric treatment?**

Answers to Case 35

Question 1

What are the approaches you would undertake during a suicide risk assessment?

Answer

Assessment of suicidal ideations, intent and behaviour	Pre-planning: research on methods, last acts, etc. Perceived lethality Post-attempt regret Previous attempts
Assessment of factors that contribute to risk of suicide	Risk factors, including impulsivity and substance use Protective factors
Determine level of risk	Low, moderate, high

Explanation

Risk factors may include acute and chronic factors. They may also be categorised into static and dynamic risk factors. It is important to assess impulsivity levels in an individual, both as a distinct component of the suicidal act itself (e.g., loss of control, acting on a whim), and impulsivity as a trait of the individual (e.g., demonstrating inappropriate behaviours such as temper outbursts or sexual indiscretions, using substances exacerbating adverse impulsive behaviours). Of note, **three direct warning signs** are particularly indicative of risk:

- Communicating suicidal thoughts verbally or in writing

- Seeking access to lethal means such as firearms or medications

- Demonstrating preparatory behaviours such as putting affairs in order (e.g., giving away treasured items, writing a will, farewell meetings/messages)

Protective factors include social support, capacities, qualities and environmental and personal resources that increase resilience.

High-risk patients include those with warning signs, serious thoughts of suicide, a plan or intent to engage in lethal self-directed violence, a recent suicide attempt or those with prominent agitation, impulsivity or psychosis. Moderate-risk patients include those patients with suicidal ideation and a plan but with no intent or preparatory behaviour. Low-risk patients include those with recent suicidal ideation who have no specific plans or intent to engage in lethal self-directed violence and have no history of active suicidal behaviour.

Exam Essentials

- In assessing suicide risks, the important 4Ps are:
    - **P**re-planning
    - **P**erceived lethality
    - **P**ost-attempt regret
    - **P**revious attempts

- The best predictor of suicide is a **history of suicide attempts**

- Chronic pain and multiple medical conditions are high-risk factors for suicide

- Be careful of masked depression, especially in the elderly. They may be evasive and mask their suicide intent

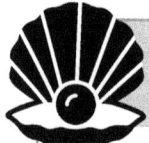

Clinical Pearls

- Structured instruments such as the SAD PERSONS scale (SPS) [1] and the Columbia-Suicide Severity Rating Scale (C-SSRS) [2] are commonly used to augment risk assessments

- The components of the SPS are reflective of some of the static and dynamic risk factors:
    - **S**ex (Male)
    - **A**ge (< 19 or > 45)
    - **D**epression
    - **P**revious attempt
    - **E**xcess alcohol or substance use
    - **R**ational thinking loss
    - **S**ocial supports lacking
    - **O**rganised plan
    - **N**o spouse
    - **S**ickness

Question 2
What are the differences between suicidal ideation, suicidal intent and suicidal plan?

Answer

Suicidal ideation refers to the thought of wishing to die by suicide or thoughts of engaging in suicide-related behaviour.

Suicidal intent refers to implicit or explicit evidence that one wishes to die and has the means to kill oneself.

A suicidal plan refers to the preparatory behaviours that one engages in, for self-directed death (e.g., assembling a method, preparing for one's death via suicide note).

Explanation

You may commonly come across the terms 'passively suicidal' and 'actively suicidal'. A person who is passively suicidal has a general wish to die but does not involve planning for suicide and may include having an indifferent attitude to an accidental demise if steps are not taken to maintain one's life. Those who repeatedly verbalise suicidal ideations could be help-seeking but be aware of patients who have shown escalating means of self-harm. A person who is actively suicidal experiences current and specific suicidal ideation with a constant and ongoing desire to inflict harm via a suicidal plan.

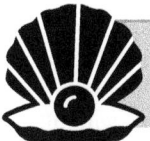 **Clinical Pearls**

- Actively suicidal patients report an ongoing and constant desire to commit a specific suicide act

- Suicide risk is dynamic and time sensitive. Assessment should be done at close intervals especially when the patient is ambivalent or evasive

Question 3

What is Willy's level of risk at present?

Answer

High

Explanation

Willy is of high risk at present as he most likely attempted suicide via overdose and refused to cooperate with medical help. Assessment for other risk factors for Willy is also pertinent, including his current social support, any previous psychiatric history or suicide attempt and any current or past substance use.

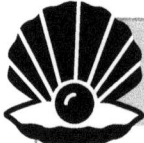

Clinical Pearls

- If the patient is not forthcoming about their symptoms, or details of the attempt, it should be regarded as a reluctance to seek help. This should raise alarm bells

Question 4

What is the clinical significance of his self-harm behaviours for his current suicide attempt?

Answer

The rate of suicide in the self-harm patient population is up to 50–100 times higher than that of the general population [3].

Explanation

Non-suicidal self-directed violence such as cutting is a behaviour that deliberately results in injury or the potential for injury to oneself. Many who engage in such behaviours do so as a coping mechanism in providing temporary relief from psychological distress. It has been reported that one in 25 patients presenting to hospital for self-harm will kill themselves in the next five years [4].

Question 5

What is the legislation that allows a patient to be involuntarily admitted for safety and further psychiatric treatment?

Answer

The United Kingdom Mental Health Act (2007) [5].

Explanation

Clinicians should follow local guidelines concerning the medical detention of patients who may pose a risk to themselves. Where a medical practitioner has under his or her care a person believed to be mentally disordered or to require psychiatric treatment, the medical practitioner may send the person to a designated medical practitioner at a psychiatric institution for treatment.

Diving Deep ...

There are no clear, validated predictive models or risk stratification definitions in a suicide risk assessment. Suicide risk is not static, as many factors influence an individual's risk of suicide at any given point in time. A suicide risk assessment must include the evaluation of the patient's internal experience, thoughts, beliefs and attitudes;

their external world of relationships and stressors; as well as the myriad of factors that increase the likelihood of suicide and those that prevent them from action.

Research studies have shown that 98% of suicide victims have a diagnosable mental health condition [6]. Because of the strong association between mental illness and suicide risk, some research suggests that the effective treatment of mental health conditions (particularly major depression) reduces the risk of suicide and may decrease suicide rates.

Approximately 50% of suicide victims consulted a general practitioner in the one month before suicide, and 75% in the year preceding death. One in five suicide victims saw their psychiatrist in the one month before suicide, and one in three in the year preceding death [7].

References

1. Patterson WM, Dohn HH, Bird J, Patterson GA. Evaluation of suicidal patients: the SAD PERSONS scale. *Psychosomatics*. 1983 Apr;24(4):343–9.

2. Posner K, Brown GK, Stanley B, Brent DA, Yershova KV, Oquendo MA, et al. The Columbia-Suicide Severity Rating Scale: initial validity and internal consistency findings from three multisite studies with adolescents and adults. *Am J Psychiatry*. 2011 Dec;168(12):1266–77.

3. Semple D, Smyth R. *Oxford handbook of psychiatry*, 4th edition. Oxford: Oxford University Press; 2019.

4. Carroll R, Metcalfe C, Gunnell D. Hospital presenting self-harm and risk of fatal and non-fatal repetition: systematic review and meta-analysis. *PLoS One*. 2014;9(2):e89944.

5. Act of the Parliament of the United Kingdom. The Mental Health Act 2007 (c 12). Available from: www.legislation.gov.uk/ukpga/2007/12/contents

6. Bertolote JM, Fleischmann A. Suicide and psychiatric diagnosis: a worldwide perspective. *World Psychiatry*. 2002 Oct;1(3):181–5.

7. Stern TA, editor. *Massachusetts General Hospital handbook of general hospital psychiatry*, 7th edition. Edinburgh: Saunders/Elsevier; 2018.

Case 36: Catatonia and Electroconvulsive Therapy

In stasis

Catherine is a 28-year-old junior lawyer who was previously diagnosed with major depressive disorder. She has been compliant with fluoxetine and lithium, and her condition has been stable during law school and initial entry into the workforce. However, for the past week, after challenges at work, she started to withdraw socially. Her parents noticed she did not speak a single word and would lie in bed all day without changing her posture for hours. She did not wake up to consume any water or food, and when her parents tried to feed her, she grimaced and refused to open her mouth. When her father asked how she was, she only repeated the questions posed to her without any relevant answers. Her parents grew concerned and have now brought her into the emergency department.

- **Question 1: What is the diagnosis?**

- **Question 2: What are the aetiologies of catatonia?**

- **Question 3: What are the differential diagnoses of catatonia?**

- **Question 4: How would you manage Catherine's catatonia?**

- **Question 5: What are some indications which may lead clinicians to consider ECT as an early treatment option in psychiatric conditions?**

- **Question 6: What are some side effects of ECT?**

Catherine's father is particularly concerned about cognitive side effects, and he enquired if there are other methods to reduce such side effects.

- **Question 7: How can one reduce the risk of cognitive side effects from ECT?**

Three years later, she presented with similar symptoms again. She had got married in the past year and is 20 weeks pregnant. Her primary psychiatrist noticed that after changing her medications during pregnancy, the new medications (sertraline) did not help with her underlying condition. She has now stopped eating and drinking for the past week. Her husband enquired if ECT could be considered again, given her previous response to ECT.

- **Question 8: Can ECT be given to pregnant women?**

Answers to Case 36

Question 1
What is the diagnosis?

Answer
Catatonia

Diagnosis of catatonia [1]

1. The presence of three or more of the following symptoms of decreased, increased or abnormal psychomotor activity is required for diagnosis. The three symptoms may come from one or any combination of the following three symptom clusters (note: symptoms that require assessment by physical examination are indicated below):

    - Decreased psychomotor activity:

        ◦ Staring
        ◦ Ambitendency
        ◦ Negativism
        ◦ Stupor
        ◦ Mutism
    - Increased psychomotor activity:

        ◦ Agitation for no reason with non-purposeful movements
        ◦ Uncontrollable, extreme emotional reactions

- ○ Impulsivity (sudden engagement in inappropriate behaviour without provocation)
  - ○ Combativeness

- Abnormal psychomotor activity:

  - ○ Grimacing
  - ○ Mannerism
  - ○ Posturing
  - ○ Stereotypy
  - ○ Rigidity
  - ○ Echopraxia
  - ○ Verbigeration
  - ○ Waxy flexibility
  - ○ Catalepsy

2. The symptoms typically last for at least several hours but can persist much longer. For some severe items (e.g., stupor, catalepsy, mutism, negativism) or if (autonomic) abnormality of vital signs is present, a short duration (e.g., 15 minutes) may be sufficient to be considered a qualifying symptom

3. The symptoms result in significant impairment in daily functioning or are severe enough to cause serious medical complications (e.g., contractures, exhaustion, dehydration, aspiration) or risk of death resulting from autonomic abnormalities or complications (e.g., rigidity leading to renal failure from rhabdomyolysis)

Explanation

It may also be diagnosed independently of any syndromes or medical illness.

There are three types:

- Akinetic catatonia: appears non-responsive, and responses to voice and noxious stimuli are decreased

- Excited catatonia: appears agitated, combative or delirious

- Malignant catatonia: associated with autonomic instability, can evolve rapidly and is potentially lethal; may co-exist with conditions such as neuroleptic malignant syndrome (NMS)

Exam Essentials

- Signs and symptoms of catatonia – **WRENCHES SPMM**
  - **W**axy flexibility
  - **R**igid face (grimacing)
  - **E**cholalia
  - **N**egativism
  - **C**atalepsy
  - **H**yperactivity (agitation)
  - **E**chopraxia
  - **S**tupor
  - **S**tereotypy
  - **P**osturing
  - **M**utism
  - **M**annerism

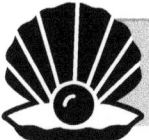

Clinical Pearls

- Catatonia is a constellation of symptoms with a wide symptom variation. Not all patients present as non-responsive

- Rating scales such as the **Bush–Francis catatonia rating scale** [2] may be used

Question 2
What are the aetiologies of catatonia?

Answer
The aetiologies can be broadly divided into psychiatric and organic causes. Some examples include:

- **Psychiatric causes:**
  - Mood disorders (depression or bipolar disorder)
  - Psychotic disorders
  - Obsessive–compulsive disorder

- ○ Autistic spectrum disorder
- ○ Conversion disorders
- ○ Personality disorders

- **Organic causes**:

  - ○ Central nervous system: stroke, seizure disorders, meningitis, encephalitis (especially herpes), lesions involving the thalamus and globus pallidus, multiple sclerosis
  - ○ Infections: acquired immunodeficiency syndrome, bacterial sepsis, tuberculosis, malaria, syphilis, typhoid fever
  - ○ Metabolic disease: Cushing's disease, hyperparathyroidism, Wilson's disease, uraemia, acute intermittent porphyria

Explanation

Approximately 20% of patients with catatonia have a medical cause instead of a psychiatric one [3]. Infectious and autoimmune aetiologies represent 29% of the general medicine cases of catatonia [4]. Meningitis and encephalitis, as well as systemic bacterial, viral or fungal infections, may result in catatonia as well. N-methyl-D-aspartate receptor (NMDAR) encephalitis and systemic lupus erythematosus also have a strong association with catatonia, with NMDAR encephalitis responsible for 72% of all autoimmune cases of catatonia.

Exam Essentials

- • The majority of catatonia cases involve individuals with depressive or bipolar disorders [5]

Question 3
What are the differential diagnoses of catatonia?

Answer
Selective mutism, dissociative stupor, locked-in syndrome, stiff-person syndrome, akinetic parkinsonism, malignant hyperthermia, neuroleptic malignant syndrome, severe psychomotor retardation

Explanation
Most of these differential diagnoses do not respond well to benzodiazepine treatment, which differs them from catatonia

Question 4
How would you manage Catherine's catatonia?

Answer

Investigations should first be performed to rule out organic causes:

- Full history taking

- Physical examination (vitals, eliciting symptoms, checking for signs which may indicate underlying cause and complications of catatonia)

- Biochemical and imaging (not limited to septic workup, brain imaging, EEG, etc.)

Treatment of catatonia includes benzodiazepines and electroconvulsive therapy (ECT). Treatment of the underlying cause is also pertinent. Actively screen for complications of catatonia and aim to reduce the risks of complications developing or treating the complications. Supportive measures including parenteral hydration or nasogastric feeding may be required.

Explanation

When catatonia is suspected, a lorazepam challenge can be performed. This is done by giving a dose of lorazepam, either through the intramuscular or intravenous route, and watching for a positive response (which can be quite rapid). In patients in catatonia who are given a lorazepam challenge, 85.7% respond within two hours [6]. Lorazepam monotherapy produces response in 60–80% of patients with catatonia [7–9].

Benzodiazepines are the first line of treatment for catatonia, and the starting dose of lorazepam is 2–6 mg per day, although lower dosages may be considered in those with concurrent delirium; 6–21 mg a day is effective for most patients, but a dose of 30 mg per day is occasionally necessary [10]. ECT can be a definitive treatment when treatment with benzodiazepines has failed. More than 60% of catatonic patients achieve remission with ECT, including those who do not respond to benzodiazepines [9, 11–13]. Antipsychotics must be used with caution as they can worsen catatonia, or cause a conversion to malignant catatonia.

Complications such as deep venous thrombosis and pulmonary embolism increase substantially due to immobility. Other complications that may occur include malnutrition, infection and muscle contractures.

 **Exam Essentials**

- If the underlying aetiology of catatonia is depression or a psychotic disorder, treatment for the underlying aetiology should still be administered, on top of the benzodiazepine

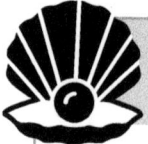

Clinical Pearls

- When giving lorazepam, especially high doses in general wards, monitoring for respiratory depression is imperative

Question 5

What are some indications which may lead clinicians to consider ECT as an early treatment option in psychiatric conditions?

Answer

Indications for early ECT include:

- Significant risk of harm to self (e.g., from suicide) or others (e.g., aggressive or homicidal due to psychosis)

- Food refusal secondary to psychiatric condition or catatonia

- Conditions which require fast resolution and are not responsive to or suitable for medications (e.g., catatonia, NMS, pregnant patients)

- Treatment-resistant depression, bipolar disorder or schizophrenia, where early treatment will assist in reducing risks to self and others

Explanation

ECT involves the induction of seizure via two electrodes by allowing an electrical current to pass into the scalp. ECT works rapidly on suicidal ideations with complete resolution seen in 38% of patients after one week, 61% of patients after two weeks and 81% of patients on completion of ECT [14]. ECT may have a safer profile than antidepressants or antipsychotics in debilitated, elderly, pregnant and breastfeeding patients.

There are no absolute contraindications for ECT. However, raised intracranial pressure, recent stroke, cardiac attacks, unstable medical conditions and anaesthetic risks are relative contraindications. A history of epilepsy is not a contraindication.

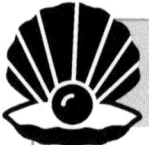

Clinical Pearls

- A review of the medications pre-ECT is important to ensure higher rates of success with treatment (e.g., benzodiazepines, mood stabilisers and hypnotic medications)

- Consider stopping them the night before ECT

- Anti-epileptics can raise the seizure threshold and affect ECT. Discuss with the neurologist if anti-epileptics are indicated, or can be titrated for patients with epileptic disorders

- For patients aged 40 and above (or with suspicion of medical issues), clinicians will need to do baseline blood investigations, chest X-ray and ECG before ECT. Always consult the anaesthetist early if you are worried about complications

Question 6
What are some side effects of ECT?

Answer
Common side effects include muscle aches, headaches and temporary confusion. The more serious side effects include memory loss, such as retrograde amnesia, which is largely temporary but, in rare cases, permanent.

Explanation
ECT is a relatively safe and low-risk procedure. In those with memory loss, 64% have complete resolution of their temporary memory issues post-ECT. The mortality rate of ECT is no greater than for general anaesthesia in minor surgery (2:100,000) [15].

Question 7
How can one reduce the risk of cognitive side effects from ECT?

Answer
Unilateral placement
Reduce the frequency of ECT sessions
Review the electrical dose of ECT
Check if the patient is currently on medications that can worsen cognition (anti-histamines, benzhexol, anticholinergic agents, benzodiazepines, hypnotics, pain-killers such as tramadol, etc.)

Explanation
Bifrontal or bitemporal ECT causes more cognitive impairment than unilateral ECT. Risk factors for cognitive issues post ECT include evidence of unstable or severe cardiovascular disease, a space-occupying intracranial lesion with evidence of elevated intracranial pressure, a history of an acute cerebral haemorrhage or stroke, an unstable vascular aneurysm and severe pulmonary disease. ECT has been shown to improve cognition when the pre-ECT cognitive scores are poorer [16].

Risk factors for cognitive problems post ECT include:

- Baseline cognitive impairment/dementia

- Medications (e.g., antihistamines, benzhexol, anticholinergics)

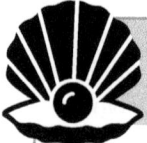

Clinical Pearls

- Always assess for baseline cognition (with the Mini-Mental State Examination or Montreal Cognitive Assessment) before commencing ECT. Monitor cognition periodically during the course of ECT treatments.

- **Lithium** may increase the risk of **post-ictal confusion**, and hence, dosage should be reviewed. Some clinicians may withhold lithium during ECT administration

Question 8
Can ECT be given to pregnant women?

Answer
ECT is indicated and can be prescribed in pregnant patients.

Explanation
ECT is a treatment option due to its rapid action to help with her condition. In her case, she displays risks to herself and her baby as she has now stopped eating and drinking. Hence, early ECT is indicated. However, ECT in the second or third trimester may present with more technical difficulties for the anaesthetist as the risk of aspiration is higher. The patient's obstetrician and anaesthetist should be involved in the preparation of the safe delivery of ECT, including considerations for a higher level of airway monitoring or protecting, and utilising cardiotocography (CTG) to monitor the fetal heart rate and uterine contractions

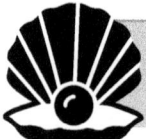

Clinical Pearls

- Sertraline is safe for pregnancy and during breastfeeding. (Refer to Case 52 for more information about the safety of antidepressants in perinatal and post-natal periods)

Diving Deep ...

The Bush–Francis catatonia rating scale overlaps with the DSM-5-TR and ICD-11 criteria, but adds some other presentations, including:

- Ambitendency (appearance of being stuck in indecisive or hesitant movement)

- Automatic obedience (mechanical and reproducible compliance with examiner's request, even if dangerous)

- Autonomic abnormality (diaphoresis, palpitations or abnormal temperature, blood pressure, pulse or respiratory rate), combativeness (striking out against others with or without the potential for injury)

- Gegenhalten (resistance to positioning by the examiner that increases proportionally to the applied force)

- Grasp reflex (strong grasp of any object in proximity of the hand or upon touch)

- Impulsivity (patient suddenly engages in inappropriate behaviour without provocation; afterwards, can give no or only a facile explanation)

- Mitgehen (exaggerated movements in response to light pressure)

- Perseveration (whole or partial repetition of actions or verbal content that is not goal-directed)

- Rigidity (resistance by way of increased muscle tone)

- Staring

- Verbigeration (continuous, directionless repetition of words, phrases or sentences)

- Withdrawal (no eye contact, refusal to take food or drink when offered, or both; turning away from the examiner or social isolation)

ECT for pregnant patients will require inputs from the anaesthetist and obstetrician [17, 18]. In a female with a gestational age > 20 weeks, left lateral uterine displacement is essential to optimize maternal venous return and maintain optimal uterine blood flow. In pregnancies greater than 24 weeks gestation, fetal heart rate and uterine activity via CTG should be measured 30 minutes before and after each treatment by an obstetrician who can manage obstetric and neonatal emergencies [17, 19]. Because pregnant patients are at higher risk for aspiration pneumonitis due to their full stomach status, anticholinergic drugs that reduce lower oesophageal sphincter tone should be avoided, as they can increase reflux.

Other indications for ECT include neurological crises such as extreme parkinsonism symptoms and intractable seizure disorders (ECT acts to raise the seizure threshold).

References

1.   World Health Organization. *International classification of diseases*, 11th edition (ICD-11). Geneva: World Health Organization; 2024. Available from: https://icd.who.int/en

2.   Bush G, Fink M, Petrides G, Dowling F, Francis A. Catatonia. I. Rating scale and standardized examination. *Acta Psychiatr Scand*. 1996 Feb;93(2):129–36.

3. Oldham MA. The probability that catatonia in the hospital has a medical cause and the relative proportions of its causes: a systematic review. *Psychosomatics*. 2018 Jul;59(4):333–40.

4. Rogers JP, Pollak TA, Blackman G, David AS. Catatonia and the immune system: a review. *Lancet Psychiatry*. 2019 Jul;6(7):620–30.

5. American Psychiatric Association. *Diagnostic and statistical manual of mental disorders*, 5th edition, text revision (DSM-5-TR). Washington, DC: American Psychiatric Association Publishing; 2022. Available from: www.psychiatry.org/psychiatrists/practice/dsm

6. Huang TL. Lorazepam and diazepam rapidly relieve catatonic signs in patients with schizophrenia. *Psychiatry Clin Neurosci*. 2005 Feb;59(1):52–5.

7. Northoff G. What catatonia can tell us about "top-down modulation": a neuropsychiatric hypothesis. *Behav Brain Sci*. 2002 Oct;25(5):555–77; discussion 578–604.

8. Fink M, Taylor MA. The many varieties of catatonia. *Eur Arch Psychiatry Clin Neurosci*. 2001;251(Suppl 1):I8-13.

9. Francis A. Catatonia: diagnosis, classification, and treatment. *Curr Psychiatry Rep*. 2010 Jun;12(3):180–5.

10. Fink M, Taylor MA. The catatonia syndrome: forgotten but not gone. *Arch Gen Psychiatry*. 2009 Nov;66(11):1173–7.

11. Falkai P, Wobrock T, Lieberman J, Glenthoj B, Gattaz WF, Möller HJ, et al. World Federation of Societies of Biological Psychiatry (WFSBP) guidelines for biological treatment of schizophrenia, Part 1: acute treatment of schizophrenia. *World J Biol Psychiatry*. 2005;6(3):132–91.

12. Bush G, Fink M, Petrides G, Dowling F, Francis A. Catatonia II. Treatment with lorazepam and electroconvulsive therapy. *Acta Psychiatr Scand*. 1996 Feb;93(2):137–43.

13. Koek RJ, Mervis JR. Treatment-refractory catatonia, ECT, and parenteral lorazepam. *Am J Psychiatry*. 1999 Jan;156(1):160–1; author reply 161.

14. Kellner CH, Fink M, Knapp R, Petrides G, Husain M, Rummans T, et al. Relief of expressed suicidal intent by ECT: a consortium for research in ECT study. *Am J Psychiatry*. 2005 May;162(5):977–82.

15. Semple D, Smyth R. *Oxford handbook of psychiatry*, 4th edition. Oxford: Oxford University Press; 2019.

16. Rajagopalan A, Lim KWK, Tan XW, Martin D, Lee J, Tor PC. Predictors of cognitive changes in patients with schizophrenia undergoing electroconvulsive therapy. *PLoS One*. 2023;18(5):e0284579.

17. Miller LJ. Use of electroconvulsive therapy during pregnancy. *Hosp Community Psychiatry*. 1994 May;45(5):444–50.

18. Stern TA, editor. *Massachusetts General Hospital handbook of general hospital psychiatry*, 7th edition. Edinburgh: Saunders/Elsevier; 2018.

19. Rose S, Dotters-Katz SK, Kuller JA. Electroconvulsive therapy in pregnancy: safety, best practices, and barriers to care. *Obstet Gynecol Surv*. 2020 Mar;75(3):199–203.

Case 37: Neuroleptic Malignant Syndrome and Serotonin Syndrome

A neurochemical catastrophe

Smith is a 32-year-old gentleman, who has a history of major depressive disorder with mood-congruent psychotic features and is currently prescribed haloperidol and sertraline. His brother brought him in after he was found on the floor of his apartment. There were empty medication blister packages by his side. His brother estimated 50 tablets of haloperidol and 15 tablets of sertraline to be missing, and Smith was rushed to the hospital via ambulance.

Vitals recorded at the emergency department:

- Temperature 39.4 °C
- Blood pressure 189/100 mmHg
- Heart rate 126 beats per minute
- Respiratory rate 26 breaths per minute
- Oxygen saturation 97% on room air

Physical examination findings:

- Disorientated and drowsy
- Diaphoretic
- Reduced bowel sounds
- Had bilateral severe rigidity of the upper and lower limbs with tremors observed
- Normal deep tendon reflexes with the absence of clonus
- The rest of the neurological examination is limited by his altered mental state

- **Question 1: What is the most likely diagnosis?**

Serotonin syndrome (SS) is a common differential of neuroleptic malignant syndrome (NMS). In an unconscious patient who may have overdosed on both an antidepressant and antipsychotic, it can be difficult to ascertain the presence of either or both diagnoses.

- **Question 2: How does SS differ from NMS?**

Smith was admitted to the intensive care unit for further evaluation and management.

- **Question 3: What abnormalities will you expect to find in the medical investigations?**

Initial investigations revealed the following:

- Haemoglobin: 16.0 g/dL [13–18 g/dL]

- Total white cells: 17,000/mm³ (↑) [4,000–11,000/mm³]

- Platelets: 250 ×10⁹/L [150–400×10⁹/L]

- Serum creatinine kinase: 16,000 IU/L (↑) [25–195 IU/L]

- Serum lactate dehydrogenase: 530 IU/L (↑) [222 – 454 IU/L]

- Serum sodium: 146 mmol/L (↑) [135–145 mmol/L]

- Serum potassium: 5.3 mmol/L (↑) [3.5–5.0 mmol/L]

- Serum creatinine: 200 mmol/L (↑) [70–150 μmol/L]

Based on the clinical syndrome and investigation findings, you diagnosed Smith with NMS. Smith was admitted to the intensive care unit and haloperidol and sertraline were withheld. Cooling blankets were placed on him with aggressive intravenous hydration initiated and electrolytes were corrected accordingly. Nitroprusside was used to control episodes of hypertension. He was also placed on telemetry to observe for arrhythmias.

- **Question 4: Which specific medications would be appropriate in the treatment of his NMS? How does that differ from the treatment of SS?**

Answers to Case 37

Question 1
What is the most likely diagnosis?

Answer
NMS

Explanation

NMS is a life-threatening neurological emergency associated with the use of anti-psychotic (neuroleptic) agents. It is characterised by a distinctive clinical syndrome of mental status change, rigidity, fever and dysautonomia. In this clinical vignette, Smith presents with a typical tetrad of clinical syndromes (mental status change, muscular rigidity, hyperthermia and autonomic instability).

NMS can occur after a single dose or after treatment with the same agent at the same dose for many years (idiosyncratic) [1]. It can also occur following the cessation of dopamine agonist drugs. It is not a dose-dependent phenomenon, but prescription of higher doses is a risk factor. Other risk factors for NMS include:

- Young age
- Male gender
- Presence of agitation
- Dehydration
- Being antipsychotic naïve
- Use of high-potency typical antipsychotics
- Rapid dose increase or decrease in antipsychotics
- Abrupt withdrawal of anticholinergic drugs

Exam Essentials

- NMS is most often seen in individuals prescribed with high-potency first-generation antipsychotic agents.
- Symptoms of NMS – **FAIR**
  - **F**ever
  - **A**MS
  - **I**nstability of the autonomic nervous system
  - **R**igidity

333

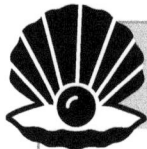

Clinical Pearls

- Rule out other medical causes such as meningitis, encephalitis, septic shock and toxicity due to other drugs

Question 2
How does SS differ from NMS?

Answer

Patients with SS typically have shivering, hyperreflexia, myoclonus, inducible clonus and ataxia, which are not seen in NMS. Nausea, vomiting and diarrhoea are common symptoms of SS, which are rarely seen in NMS. If rigidity and hyperthermia are present in patients with SS, they are less severe than in patients with NMS.

Explanation

SS is a clinical diagnosis, commonly presenting with a triad of mental status changes, autonomic hyperactivity and neuromuscular abnormalities. It can be diagnosed using Hunter toxicity criteria decision rules, which have been proven to be the most accurate diagnostic set.

To fulfil the Hunter Serotonin Toxicity Criteria [2], a patient must have taken a serotonergic agent and meet ONE of the following conditions:

- Spontaneous clonus

- Inducible clonus + agitation or diaphoresis

- Ocular clonus + agitation or diaphoresis

- Tremor + hyperreflexia

- Hypertonia + temperature above 38 °C + ocular clonus or inducible clonus

The following table shows the differences between SS and NMS:

	SS	NMS
	Within 24 hours	Days to weeks
Neuromuscular findings	Neuromuscular hyperreactivity (tremor, clonus, reflexes)	Sluggish neuromuscular responses (bradyreflexia, severe muscular rigidity)

	SS	NMS
Causative agents	Serotonin agonist	Dopamine antagonist
Resolution	Within 24 hours	Days to weeks (most resolve within two weeks)
Common features	Hyperthermia Altered mental status Muscle rigidity	
Investigations	Leucocytosis, elevated creatine phosphokinase, elevated hepatic transaminases, and metabolic acidosis are more commonly seen in NMS than SS	

Exam Essentials

- SS is dose-dependent while NMS can be idiosyncratic
- SS triad:
    - Mental status changes
    - Autonomic hyperactivity
    - Neuromuscular abnormalities
- NMS tetrad:
    - Mental status change
    - Autonomic instability
    - Muscular rigidity
    - Hyperthermia

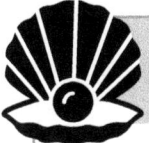

Clinical Pearls

- Selective serotonin reuptake inhibitors (SSRIs) are the most commonly implicated group of medications associated with SS. This is especially so when patients are on high doses and combination psychotropics

- Be careful of unique medication combinations that can precipitate SS:
  - Monoamine oxidase inhibitors (selegiline) with SSRIs, in patients with Parkinson's disease
  - Triptans (sumatriptan) with SSRIs, in patients with migraine
  - Opioid medications (tramadol and fentanyl, but not morphine) with SSRIs, in patients with chronic pain

Question 3
What abnormalities will you expect to find in the medical investigations?

Answer

Investigation	Expected findings [3]
Serum creatinine kinase levels	Raised Typically, more than 1,000 IU/L and can be as high as 100,000 IU/L
White blood cells	Raised White blood cell counts typically 10,000 to 40,000 per mm³ A left shift may be present
Lactate dehydrogenase, alkaline phosphatase and liver transaminases	Raised
Electrolyte abnormalities	Hypocalcaemia, hypomagnesaemia, hypo- and hypernatraemia, hyperkalaemia and metabolic acidosis
Serum creatinine and serum myoglobulin	Myoglobinuric acute renal failure results from rhabdomyolysis
Serum iron concentration	Low Sensitive (92 to 100%) but not a specific marker for NMS among acutely ill psychiatric patients
MRI and CT brain	Typically normal, although diffuse cerebral oedema may be seen in severe metabolic derangements Done to exclude structural brain disease and infection

Investigation	Expected findings [3]
Lumbar puncture	Typically normal, but a non-specific elevation in protein is reported in 37% of cases
EEG	Generalised slow-wave activity may be seen EEG can be done to rule out non-convulsive status epilepticus

Explanation

As NMS is primarily a clinical diagnosis, the role of such investigations is to aid the diagnostic process (to support the diagnosis and exclude differentials), evaluate the severity and rule out any complication.

Exam Essentials

- A common cause of death in NMS is **renal failure secondary to rhabdomyolysis**, leading to a high release of myoglobin that precipitates renal failure [4]

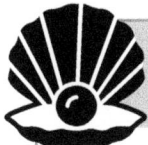

Clinical Pearls

- Extreme rigidity can lead to more profound creatine kinase elevation

- If the patient's symptoms do not seem to be resolving, it is important to do further investigations to rule out superimposed conditions (e.g., infection)

Question 4

Which specific medications would be appropriate in the treatment of his NMS? How does that differ from the treatment of SS?

Answer

First line: benzodiazepines and/or dantrolene
Second line: Add on bromocriptine or amantadine

	SS	NMS
Specific medications	Cyproheptadine	Dantrolene Bromocriptine Amantadine
Common medications	Benzodiazepines	

Explanation

The first step of treatment is to discontinue the offending agent. This is followed by supportive care in managing hypertension, hyperthermia, cardiovascular, respiratory and renal complications. Most episodes resolve within two weeks.

Benzodiazepines and dantrolene are used for symptomatic relief of rigidity, while bromocriptine and amantadine are dopamine agonists that reverse dopamine blockade.

Overlapping management strategies exist in the treatment of SS, including discontinuation of the offending agent (serotonergic antidepressant) and subsequent supportive management. Benzodiazepines are mainly used for their sedative properties, which manage mild increases in blood pressure and heart rate. The key difference in pharmacological agents employed lies in the use of serotonin antagonists (cyproheptadine).

Exam Essentials

- Remember to remove the offending agent when treating patients with NMS or SS

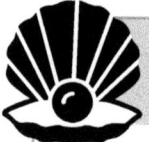

Clinical Pearls

- Mortality rates for NMS vary between 5% and 20%

Diving Deep ...

The tetrad of NMS symptoms typically evolves over one to three days. Each feature is present in 97–100% of patients [5]. Seventy per cent of patients followed a typical course of mental status changes appearing first, followed by rigidity, then hyperthermia and autonomic dysfunction. Symptoms usually develop during the first two weeks of antipsychotic therapy, but the association of the syndrome with drug use is idiosyncratic.

Symptom	Description
Mental status change	The initial symptom in 82% of patients [5]
Muscular rigidity	Generalised and extreme, seen as 'lead pipe rigidity' and 'cogwheel phenomenon' on examination Tremor (45% to 92%) [5, 6] and, less commonly, dystonia, opisthotonos, trismus, chorea and other dyskinesias
Hyperthermia	Temperature > 38 °C seen in 87% of patients Temperature > 40 °C seen in 40% of patients [6]
Autonomic instability	Tachycardia (88%), labile or high blood pressure (61–77%) and tachypnoea (73%) Dysrhythmias and diaphoresis are present as well [7, 8]

A variety of risk factors have emerged from epidemiological and case studies of NMS, which include dehydration, physical exhaustion, exposure to heat, hyponatraemia, iron deficiency, malnutrition, trauma, thyrotoxicosis, alcohol, psychoactive substances and the presence of a structural or functional brain disorder such as encephalitis or dementia.

While the evidence for medication use in the treatment of NMS is conflicting, some studies suggest that it may hasten clinical response (time to recovery) and reduce mortality rates [9]. Dantrolene is a direct-acting skeletal muscle relaxant, which reduces heat production as well as rigidity, and its effects are reported within minutes of administration. Bromocriptine is a dopamine agonist, which restores the lost dopaminergic activity. Amantadine is an alternative to bromocriptine and has both dopaminergic and anticholinergic effects.

Cyproheptadine is a histamine-1 receptor antagonist with non-specific serotonin 1A and 2A antagonistic properties. Bromocriptine and amantadine have serotoninergic activity (in addition to being a dopamine agonist) and may exacerbate SS.

References

1. Pope HG, Aizley HG, Keck PE, McElroy SL. Neuroleptic malignant syndrome: long-term follow-up of 20 cases. *J Clin Psychiatry*. 1991 May;52(5):208–12.

2. Dunkley EJC, Isbister GK, Sibbritt D, Dawson AH, Whyte IM. The Hunter Serotonin Toxicity Criteria: simple and accurate diagnostic decision rules for serotonin toxicity. *QJM*. 2003 Sep 1;96(9):635–42.

3. Semple D, Smyth R. *Oxford handbook of psychiatry*, 4th edition. Oxford: Oxford University Press; 2019.

4. Shalev A, Hermesh H, Munitz H. Mortality from neuroleptic malignant syndrome. *J Clin Psychiatry*. 1989 Jan;50(1):18–25.

5. Velamoor VR, Norman RM, Caroff SN, Mann SC, Sullivan KA, Antelo RE. Progression of symptoms in neuroleptic malignant syndrome. *J Nerv Ment Dis*. 1994 Mar;182(3):168–73.

6. Caroff SN, Mann SC. Neuroleptic malignant syndrome. *Med Clin North Am*. 1993 Jan;77(1):185–202.

7. Levenson JL. Neuroleptic malignant syndrome. *Am J Psychiatry*. 1985 Oct;142(10):1137–45.

8. Rosebush P, Stewart T. A prospective analysis of 24 episodes of neuroleptic malignant syndrome. *Am J Psychiatry*. 1989 Jun;146(6):717–25.

9. Rosenberg MR, Green M. Neuroleptic malignant syndrome. Review of response to therapy. *Arch Intern Med*. 1989 Sep;149(9):1927–31.

Case 38: Insomnia Disorder

The pursuit of sleep

Clement is a 30-year-old sales executive complaining of six months of poor sleep almost every other night. Despite going to bed early, he has problems initiating sleep and wakes up feeling tired, which persists during the day. This has resulted in him having lapses in his work performance. He denies having any issues with his mood or feelings of anxiousness.

- **Question 1: What is the diagnosis?**

- **Question 2: What sleep hygiene advice would you provide Clement?**

Despite employing sleep hygiene advice, Clement continues to have difficulties sleeping.

- **Question 3: What other non-pharmacological treatment options exist in treating primary insomnia?**

- **Question 4: What pharmacological treatment options exist in treating primary insomnia?**

Answers to Case 38

Question 1
What is the diagnosis?

Answer
Insomnia disorder

Explanation

Diagnosis of insomnia disorder [1]

1. Primary dissatisfaction with the quantity or quality of sleep, with one or more of the following symptoms:
   - Difficulty initiating sleep
   - Difficulty maintaining sleep
   - Early-morning awakening with inability to resume sleep

2. The sleep disturbance causes clinically significant functional impairment

3. Symptoms occur at least three nights per week

4. Symptoms for at least three months

5. The sleep difficulty persists despite having sufficient opportunities for sleep

6. The insomnia is not better explained by, and does not exclusively occur during the course of, another sleep–wake disorder

7. The insomnia is not attributed to the physiological effects of a substance

Another differential diagnosis for lethargy could include hypersomnolence disorder; however, patients with this disorder report excessive sleepiness despite having at least seven hours of sleep at least three times per week for at least three months, with at least one of the following:

- Recurrent periods of sleep or lapses into sleep within the same day

- More than nine hours of sleep which is non-restorative

- Difficulty being fully awake after abrupt awakening

Differentials for sleep disturbances include circadian rhythm sleep–wake disorders, primarily due to an altered circadian system or misalignment between the endogenous circadian rhythm and the sleep–wake schedule, causing distress. The different types include:

- Delayed sleep phase type: late sleep onset and wake times

- Advanced sleep phase type: early sleep onset and wake times

- Irregular sleep–wake type: temporally sleep–wake disorganisation

- Non-24-hour sleep–wake type: drift of sleep onset and wake times (usually to later and later)

- Shift-work type: associated with shift-work schedule

Exam Essentials

- Some common issues to rule out in the history:
  - Obstructive sleep apnoea
  - Restless leg syndrome
  - Substance use (caffeine, alcohol, tobacco)
  - Afternoon naps
  - Sleep hygiene
  - Environmental triggers (e.g., non-conducive sleep environment)

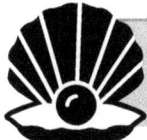

Clinical Pearls

- Causes can be divided into **primary** and **secondary insomnia**
- It is essential to thoroughly screen for secondary causes, such as mental disorders (anxiety, mood disorders, etc.), medical illness, medication or illicit substance-induced states
- Sleep disorders are highly co-morbid with another sleep disorder or mental disorder. Always screen for the use of alcohol and other sedative agents

Question 2
What sleep hygiene advice would you provide Clement?

Answer
These are psychoeducation recommendations you can provide [2]:

- Encourage daily exercise (but not within three hours of bedtime)

- Expose self to bright light during daytime

- Avoid daytime napping

- Avoid caffeinated products (coffee, tea, coke), alcohol and tobacco at bedtime

- Use the bed solely for sleep

- Do not lie in bed unless sleepiness sets in. If one is unable to initiate sleep in bed within 20 minutes, the person should move to another dimly lit room and do light reading or listen to soft music for 30 minutes before attempting to initiate sleep again

343

Explanation

Before pharmacological measures are employed, sleep hygiene advice is an inexpensive way to aid with sleep. As habits can be difficult to change, it will help to focus on one to two behavioural suggestions at a time.

Question 3

What other non-pharmacological treatment options exist in treating primary insomnia?

Answer

Cognitive behavioural therapy for insomnia (CBT-I)

Explanation

In reference to the United Kingdom's National Institute for Health and Care Excellence (NICE) guidelines [3], CBT-I (either face-to-face or digitally) should be offered as the first-line treatment for chronic insomnia in adults of any age.

CBT-I consists of behavioural interventions (e.g., stimulus control and sleep restriction), cognitive therapy and relaxation training. In 2022, NICE also recommended an app-based digital self-help programme called Sleepio, which includes CBT-I [4]. It is a cost-saving option for treating insomnia and insomnia symptoms in primary care.

Question 4

What pharmacological treatment options exist in treating primary insomnia?

Answer

> Melatonin
> Antihistamines (e.g., hydroxyzine)
> A short course of hypnotics (e.g., a benzodiazepine or Z-drug)
> Melatonin receptor agonists (e.g., ramelteon)
> Dual orexin receptor antagonists (DORAs; e.g., suvorexant, lemborexant)
> Histamine receptor antagonists (e.g., low-dose doxepin)

Explanation

In reference to the NICE guidelines [3], for patients over 55 years old with persistent insomnia, modified-release melatonin may be considered. Patients are typically given an initial course of three weeks and, if there is a response to treatment, this can be extended further for 10 weeks only. Melatonin is useful in aligning the circadian rhythm to the desired sleep–wake schedule. The safety of long-term melatonin use has not been established with control studies and common side effects include vivid dreams and nightmares, dizziness and daytime sleepiness.

A short course (less than one week) of hypnotics is considered for patients with severe symptoms or an acute exacerbation of symptoms. It is recommended that hypnotics be given in addition to CBT-I and not alone. Adverse effects of benzodiazepines (e.g., temazepam) include the risk of dependence, ataxia, falls and dizziness. Z-drugs (e.g., zolpidem) have similar effects to benzodiazepines but are less commonly diverted for recreational use.

Ramelton has agonist activity at the melatonin MT1 and MT2 receptors and helps with sleep onset. Common side effects include somnolence, dizziness, fatigue, nausea and, paradoxically, exacerbation of insomnia.

DORAs have antagonist activity at both orexin (OX1 and OX2) receptors, which helps with sleep onset and/or sleep maintenance by decreasing the wake drive. The most common side effect of DORAs is somnolence. The presence of narcolepsy is a contraindication.

Doxepin is a tricyclic antidepressant medication that also has a high selectivity and antagonistic effect on the post-synaptic histamine H1 receptor, which produces sedation and enhances sleep maintenance. When treating insomnia, it is used at a much lower starting dose of 6 mg (3 mg for the elderly). The most common side effects are somnolence, sedation and nausea.

Exam Essentials

- As pharmacological therapy is not without adverse effects (including the risk of hypnotic dependence), it should be avoided in the long-term management of insomnia

- **DORAS are contraindicated in narcolepsy**

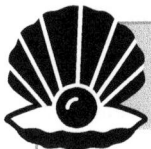

Clinical Pearls

- Other medications to consider if those in Question 4 fail include:
  - Low-dose sedating antidepressant (e.g., mirtazapine, trazodone, amitriptyline), low potency antipsychotic (quetiapine) or pregabalin
- Avoid prescribing benzodiazepines and Z-drugs for prolonged durations due to the risk of:
  - Dependency
  - Cognitive impairment
  - Falls
  - Respiratory depression (especially in the elderly and those with respiratory disease)
- Sudden withdrawal from benzodiazepines can lead to seizures. Tapering should be done gradually, especially in chronic users

Diving Deep …

Medications approved for the treatment of insomnia carry an adverse depressant effect on the central nervous system (CNS), including impaired alertness, motor inco-ordination and next-morning impairment. This risk is highest for benzodiazepine use and especially when combined with other CNS depressant medications (e.g., gabapentin or opioids) or alcohol. Avoid prescribing benzodiazepines to patients taking opioids due to the risk of respiratory depression. Patients prescribed opioids in the past three months have an increased risk of drug overdose among young adults prescribed benzodiazepines for sleep disorders [5]. For patients on opioid medications, preferred choices include DORAs, doxepin and ramelteon.

References

1. American Psychiatric Association. *Diagnostic and statistical manual of mental disorders*, 5th edition, text revision (DSM-5-TR). Washington, DC: American Psychiatric Association Publishing; 2022. Available from: www.psychiatry.org/psychiatrists/practice/dsm

2. Boland RJ, Verduin ML, Ruiz P, Shah A, Sadock BJ, editors. *Kaplan & Sadock's synopsis of psychiatry*, 12th edition. Philadelphia: Wolters Kluwer; 2022.

3. National Institute for Health and Care Excellence (NICE). Insomnia scenario: managing short-term insomnia (less than 3 months duration). NICE; 2022. Available from: https://cks.nice.org.uk/topics/insomnia/management/managing-insomnia

4. NICE. Sleepio to treat insomnia and insomnia symptoms. Medical technologies guidance [MTG70]. NICE; 2022. Available from: www.nice.org.uk/guidance/mtg70/chapter/1-Recommendations

5. Bushnell GA, Gerhard T, Keyes K, Hasin D, Cerdá M, Olfson M. Association of benzodiazepine treatment for sleep disorders with drug overdose risk among young people. *JAMA Netw Open*. 2022 Nov 1;5(11):e2243215.

Case 39: Narcolepsy Disorder

Sleep attacks

Zoe is an 18-year-old girl who comes to your clinic reporting recurrent episodes of falling asleep uncontrollably once a day. These episodes have occurred at unpredictable times daily for the past year and happen in different settings, for instance while watching movies or during school lessons. Her friends teased her as the 'drop monster' as she frequently dropped to the ground while laughing or joking with friends. She is highly embarrassed by the symptoms and is keen for treatment.

- **Question 1: What is the diagnosis?**

- **Question 2: According to the ICD-11 classification, what is the difference between type 1 and type 2 narcolepsy?**

- **Question 3: How will you treat Zoe's narcolepsy?**

Answers to Case 39

Question 1
What is the diagnosis?

Answer
Narcolepsy

Explanation

Diagnosis of narcolepsy [1]

1. Recurrent periods of an irrepressible need to sleep, lapsing into sleep or napping occurring within the same day. These must have been occurring at least three times per week over the past three months.

2. One or more of the following symptoms:

- Episodes of cataplexy, either (a) or (b), occurring at least a few times per month:

    a. In individuals with a prolonged illness, short episodes (lasting seconds to minutes), triggered by laughter or joking, of abrupt bilateral loss of muscle tone while remaining conscious

    b. In children or individuals within six months of onset, spontaneous grimaces or jaw-opening episodes accompanied by tongue thrusting or overall reduced muscle tone, without clear emotional triggers

- Hypocretin deficiency: cerebrospinal fluid (CSF) hypocretin-1 immunoreactivity values ≤ 1/3 of values obtained in healthy subjects tested using the same assay, or ≤ 110 pg/mL. (Exclusion criteria: low CSF levels of hypocretin-1 in the context of acute brain injury, inflammation or infection)

- Nocturnal sleep polysomnography showing rapid eye movement (REM) sleep latency ≤ 15 minutes, or a multiple sleep latency test showing a mean sleep latency ≤ 8 minutes and two or more sleep-onset REM periods

The severity of narcolepsy is dependent on the need for naps and the number of cataplexy attacks. As her episodes of cataplexy occur daily, her narcolepsy would be classified as moderate.

Severity	Nap symptoms	Cataplexy symptoms
Mild	Need for naps only once or twice per day Sleep disturbance is mild	Infrequent (occurring less than once per week)
Moderate	Need for multiple naps daily Sleep is moderately disturbed	Occurs daily or every few days
Severe	Nearly constant sleepiness and, often, highly disturbed nocturnal sleep	Drug-resistant, with multiple attacks daily

Exam Essentials

- Cataplexy is defined as brief episodes of sudden, bilateral loss of muscle tone, with maintained consciousness, which are precipitated by sudden strong emotions such as fear, stress or excitement

- **Cataplexy** should not be confused with **catalepsy** (muscle rigidity – a symptom seen in catatonia)

- Symptoms of narcolepsy: **CHESS**

  ◦ Cataplexy
  ◦ Hallucinations (hypnogogic and hypnopompic)
  ◦ Excessive daytime sleepiness
  ◦ Sleep paralysis
  ◦ Sleep disruption

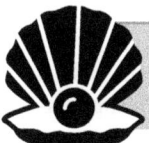

Clinical Pearls

- Rating scales such as the self-rated **Epworth Sleepiness Scale** [2] may be used to assess daytime sleepiness

- Narcolepsy is considered an REM sleep disorder

- Rule out seizures as a differential diagnosis

Question 2
According to the ICD-11 classification, what is the difference between type 1 and type 2 narcolepsy?

Answer
According to the ICD-11 classification [3], type 2 narcolepsy must not have signs of cataplexy or a deficiency in CSF hypocretin (if tested).

Explanation
Type 2 narcolepsy is similar to type 1 narcolepsy in that there is excessive sleepiness characterised by daily periods of irrepressible need to sleep or daytime lapses into sleep and abnormal manifestations of REM sleep as demonstrated by Multiple Sleep Latency

Test/polysomnography findings. However, in type 2 narcolepsy, patients have normal hypothalamic hypocretin (orexin) signalling, with CSF hypocretin determinations > 110 picograms per millilitre. Cataplexy is not present either.

Question 3
How will you treat Zoe's narcolepsy?

Answer
For daytime somnolence: modafinil, sodium oxybate
For cataplexy: sodium oxybate, antidepressants
For REM-related symptoms: sodium oxybate
Non-pharmacological methods: cognitive behaviour therapy (CBT)

Explanation
It is hypothesised that sodium oxybate acts through gamma-aminobutyric acid B (GABA-B) receptors to treat cataplexy, excessive daytime somnolence and disturbed nocturnal sleep. The most common side effects include nausea, dizziness, confusion, weight loss, enuresis, anxiety and low mood.

Modafinil improved excessive daytime somnolence by increasing dopaminergic signalling by blocking dopamine reuptake. Compared with other stimulants, modafinil has less abuse potential and is generally well tolerated. Typical side effects are headache, nausea and anxiety.

Antidepressants that increase noradrenergic and serotonergic neurotransmitters such as venlafaxine, fluoxetine, citalopram and clomipramine may be considered, with suppression of REM sleep, which may help with cataplexy.

CBT is aimed at identifying and possibly modifying dysfunctional cognitions and treatment adherence, including maintaining good sleep hygiene and taking scheduled naps.

Diving Deep

Narcolepsy type 1 (narcolepsy with cataplexy) is estimated to affect 25–50 per 100,000 people, with an incidence of 0.74 per 100,000 person-years [4–6]. This condition occurs equally in males and females [7]. It typically starts in the teens or early twenties but can sometimes begin as early as age five or after age 40. The prevalence of type 2 narcolepsy (narcolepsy without cataplexy) is less certain due to it being less studied and harder to diagnose, but estimates range from 20 to 34 per 100,000 people [8, 9]. Narcolepsy is associated with the human leucocyte antigen (HLA) DQB1*0602 haplotype, which is present in 95% of patients with cataplexy and 96% of those with orexin deficiency [10–12].

References

1. American Psychiatric Association. *Diagnostic and statistical manual of mental disorders*, 5th edition, text revision (DSM-5-TR). Washington, DC: American Psychiatric Association Publishing; 2022. Available from: www.psychiatry.org/psychiatrists/practice/dsm

2. Johns MW. A new method for measuring daytime sleepiness: the Epworth Sleepiness Scale. *Sleep*. 1991 Nov 1;14(6):540–5.

3. World Health Organization. *International classification of diseases*, 11th edition (ICD-11). Geneva: World Health Organization; 2024. Available from: https://icd.who.int/en

4. Longstreth WT, Koepsell TD, Ton TG, Hendrickson AF, van Belle G. The epidemiology of narcolepsy. *Sleep*. 2007 Jan;30(1):13–26.

5. Nohynek H, Jokinen J, Partinen M, Vaarala O, Kirjavainen T, Sundman J, et al. AS03 adjuvanted AH1N1 vaccine associated with an abrupt increase in the incidence of childhood narcolepsy in Finland. *PLoS One*. 2012;7(3):e33536.

6. Partinen M, Saarenpää-Heikkilä O, Ilveskoski I, Hublin C, Linna M, Olsén P, et al. Increased incidence and clinical picture of childhood narcolepsy following the 2009 H1N1 pandemic vaccination campaign in Finland. *PLoS One*. 2012;7(3):e33723.

7. Ohayon MM, Priest RG, Zulley J, Smirne S, Paiva T. Prevalence of narcolepsy symptomatology and diagnosis in the European general population. *Neurology*. 2002 Jun 25;58(12):1826–33.

8. Silber MH, Krahn LE, Olson EJ, Pankratz VS. The epidemiology of narcolepsy in Olmsted County, Minnesota: a population-based study. *Sleep*. 2002 Mar 15;25(2):197–202.

9. Shin YK, Yoon IY, Han EK, No YM, Hong MC, Yun YD, et al. Prevalence of narcolepsy-cataplexy in Korean adolescents. *Acta Neurol Scand*. 2008 Apr;117(4):273–8.

10. Mahlios J, De la Herrán-Arita AK, Mignot E. The autoimmune basis of narcolepsy. *Curr Opin Neurobiol*. 2013 Oct;23(5):767–73.

11. Mignot E, Lammers GJ, Ripley B, Okun M, Nevsimalova S, Overeem S, et al. The role of cerebrospinal fluid hypocretin measurement in the diagnosis of narcolepsy and other hypersomnias. *Arch Neurol*. 2002 Oct;59(10):1553–62.

12. Mignot E, Hayduk R, Black J, Grumet FC, Guilleminault C. HLA DQB1*0602 is associated with cataplexy in 509 narcoleptic patients. *Sleep*. 1997 Nov;20(11):1012–20.

Case 40: Breathing-Related Sleep Disorders

You snore too loudly

Sean is a 40-year-old gentleman seeking help for snoring after his wife complained that he snores loudly at night. His wife also notices episodes where he appears to stop breathing for a minute throughout the night. Sean wakes up tired in the daytime. Polysomnography was performed, which showed multiple episodes of apnoea despite the respiratory effort observed.

- **Question 1: What is the likely diagnosis?**

- **Question 2: Central sleep apnoea (CSA) is a differential diagnosis to obstructive sleep apnoea (OSA), how is CSA diagnosed?**

Answers to Case 40

Question 1
What is the likely diagnosis?

Answer
Obstructive sleep apnoea (OSA)
Central sleep apnoea (CSA)

Explanation

Diagnosis of OSA [1]

OSA is characterised by repetitive episodes of apnoea or hypopnoea that are caused by upper airway obstruction occurring during sleep. The disorder may also be diagnosed when any of the following is fulfilled:

1. In adults (> 18 years), when the frequency of obstructive events (apnoeas, hypopnoeas or respiratory event-related arousals) is greater than 15 per hour

2.   Five or more obstructive apnoeas or hypopnoeas per hour of sleep as evidenced by polysomnography and either of the following sleep symptoms:

- Symptoms attributable to the disorder (e.g., sleepiness or sleep disruption) are present
- Nocturnal respiratory distress or observed apnoea/habitual snoring are reported
- When hypertension, a mood disorder, cognitive dysfunction, coronary artery disease, stroke, congestive heart failure, atrial fibrillation, or type 2 diabetes mellitus are present

3.   In children, the disorder is diagnosed when the frequency of obstructive events is greater than one per hour, accompanied by signs or symptoms related to the breathing disorder

Note: A definitive diagnosis requires objective evidence based on polysomnography.

OSA is characterised by recurring episodes of cessation (apnoea) or reduction (hypopnoea) in airflow during sleep caused by obstruction of the upper airway. Patients with OSA report daytime sleepiness, and a greater proportion report unrefreshing sleep or fatigue. Other symptoms include frequent nocturnal waking due to choking or gasping, morning headaches, poor concentration, irritability and erectile dysfunction. Features on physical examination include signs of central obesity (e.g., increased waist circumference, increased neck circumference), nasal septal deviation or turbinate hypertrophy, crowding of the posterior oropharynx as estimated by the Mallampati or Friedman score or retrognathia. Polysomnography should be ordered to confirm the diagnosis of OSA. Treatment options include continuous positive airway pressure (CPAP) prescribed by a certified practitioner, an oral appliance custom-fitted by a dentist and maxillomandibular advancement surgery.

Exam Essentials

- **Polysomnography** should be ordered to confirm the diagnosis of OSA
- Psychiatric complications of OSA include:
  - insomnia
  - depression
  - anxiety
  - irritability
  - cognitive impairment

- Severity according to the DSM-5-TR [2]:
  - Mild: apnoea hypopnoea index < 15
  - Moderate: apnoea hypopnoea index = 15–30
  - Severe: apnoea hypopnoea index > 30

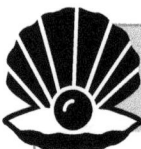

Clinical Pearls

- Rating scales such as **STOP-Bang** [3] may be used to identify patients with OSA

- A Cheyne–Stokes breathing pattern is common in patients with heart failure and might be a prognostic indicator of poor outcome

Question 2
CSA is a differential diagnosis to OSA, how is CSA diagnosed?

Answer

Diagnosis of CSA [2]

1. Five or more central apnoeas per hour of sleep as evidenced by polysomnography

2. The disorder is not better accounted for by another current sleep disorder

Explanation

CSA is characterised by recurrent apnoea during sleep with no associated respiratory effort, which can lead to important co-morbidity and increased risk of adverse cardiovascular outcomes. There are several manifestations of CSA, including high-altitude-induced periodic breathing, idiopathic CSA, narcotic-induced CSA, obesity hypoventilation syndrome and Cheyne–Stokes breathing.

Symptoms of CSA include sleep fragmentation, insomnia and daytime hypersomnolence, which is usually not as severe as in OSA. Adaptive servo-ventilation is a promising treatment modality, which might improve cardiac function, improve sleep quality and possibly confer a survival benefit.

Exam Essentials

- CSA can be distinguished from OSA by the presence of repetitive apnoeas or hypopnoeas due to the reduction or absence of respiratory effort on the polysomnographic recording

Diving Deep …

In the United Kingdom, it is estimated that 4% of middle-aged men and 2% of middle-aged women have OSA [4]. The use of polysomnography provides quantitative data on the frequency of sleep-related respiratory disturbances and associated changes in oxygen saturation and sleep continuity. Other common symptoms include early morning headaches, heartburn, nocturia, dry mouth, erectile dysfunction and reduced libido. Approximately 50–60% of patients with OSA have hypertension [5].

References

1. World Health Organization. *International classification of diseases*, 11th edition (ICD-11). Geneva: World Health Organization; 2024. Available from: https://icd.who.int/en

2. American Psychiatric Association. *Diagnostic and statistical manual of mental disorders*, 5th edition, text revision (DSM-5-TR). Washington, DC: American Psychiatric Association Publishing; 2022. Available from: www.psychiatry.org/psychiatrists/practice/dsm

3. Chung F, Abdullah HR, Liao P. STOP-Bang questionnaire: a practical approach to screen for obstructive sleep apnea. *Chest*. 2016 Mar;149(3):631–8.

4. Young T, Palta M, Dempsey J, Skatrud J, Weber S, Badr S. The occurrence of sleep-disordered breathing among middle-aged adults. *N Engl J Med*. 1993 Apr 29;328(17):1230–5.

5. Chaudhary SC, Gupta P, Sawlani KK, Gupta KK, Singh A, Usman K, et al. Obstructive sleep apnea in hypertension. *Cureus*. 2023 Apr;15(4):e38229.

Case 41: Non-Rapid Eye Movement Sleep Arousal Disorder

Answers to Case 41

Question 1
What is James' diagnosis?

Answer
Sleep terrors

Explanation

Diagnosis of non-rapid eye movement (NREM) sleep arousal disorder [1]

1. Recurrent instances of incomplete awakening from sleep, typically happening in the initial third of the major sleep episode, accompanied by either:

   - Sleepwalking: repeated incidents of getting out of bed during sleep and walking around. While sleepwalking, the person exhibits a blank, staring expression, is relatively unresponsive to attempts by others to communicate and can be roused only with great difficulty

- Sleep terrors: repeated episodes of sudden, intense terror arousal from sleep, usually starting with a panicky scream. Each episode involves intense fear and signs of autonomic arousal, such as dilated pupils, rapid heart rate, quick breathing and sweating. The individual is relatively unresponsive to attempts by others to offer comfort during these episodes

2. Little or no dream imagery is remembered (e.g., only a single visual scene)

3. Amnesia for the episodes is present

4. The episodes cause clinically significant distress or functional impairment

Sleep terrors are classified under the NREM sleep arousal disorder, whereby the patient will present with recurrent episodes of abrupt terror arousals from sleep, usually starting with a panicky scream. There is intense fear and signs of autonomic arousal (tachycardia, high respiratory rate and sweating) during these episodes, and the patient is relatively unresponsiveness to the efforts of others to comfort. NREM disorders typically arise from incomplete arousals from deep NREM (N3) sleep, with an exception being sleep-related eating disorder, which has been observed to arise during all stages of non-REM sleep [2].

Exam Essentials

- For patients with **NREM sleep disorders**, one distinct characteristic is **amnesia** of the episodes, with the absence of dream imagery

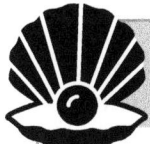

Clinical Pearls

- Night terrors are most common in children around three to four years of age. They can occur up to around 12 years old. Most children outgrow sleep terrors by their teenage years
- Sleepwalking can occur in the presence of Z-drugs such as zolpidem

Question 2
How can sleepwalking be managed?

Answer
Non-pharmacological management:

- The child's environment should be secured.

Pharmacological management [3]:

- A low dose of a benzodiazepine (e.g., clonazepam at bedtime)
- Tricyclic antidepressants
- Melatonin
- Selective serotonin reuptake inhibitors

Explanation
Sleepwalkers may interact with their environment inappropriately, resulting in injury, such as stepping out of an upstairs window or leaving the house.

Environmental changes include:

- Clear the bedroom of obstructions
- Lock doors and windows
- Place the mattress on the floor
- Consider sleeping on the ground floor to avoid falling down stairs
- Cover windows with heavy curtains to reduce light that may cause awakenings

If no specific underlying triggers are found and the NREM parasomnias remain problematic, the above psychotropics can be trialled.

Diving Deep …

Sleep comprises three stages of NREM sleep (N1, N2, N3) and REM sleep. As one progresses from N1 to N2 to N3, there is a progressive slowing of the electroencephalographic background with a gradual drop in muscle tone and a loss of eye movements. Each cycle consists of a period of NREM sleep followed by REM sleep, lasting about 90–120 minutes. Typically, one enters NREM sleep and experiences a sequence of 'descending' stages and then an 'ascent' (indicating greater brain activation levels) with an entry into REM sleep.

Sleepwalking episodes include a variety of behaviours from simple movements such as sitting up in bed, looking around or picking at the blanket to walking out of the room, talking or even eating. Sexsomnia refers to an individual's engagement in varying degrees of sexual activity (e.g., masturbation and sexual intercourse etc.) during sleep without conscious awareness. Sexsomnia may result in medicolegal consequences and serious interpersonal relationship problems. Isolated or infrequent NREM sleep arousal behaviors are common in the general population with 10–30% of children having had at least one episode of sleepwalking [1].

References

1. American Psychiatric Association. *Diagnostic and statistical manual of mental disorders, 5th edition, text revision (DSM-5-TR)*. Washington, DC: American Psychiatric Association Publishing; 2022. Available from: www.psychiatry.org/psychiatrists/practice/dsm

2. World Health Organization. *International classification of diseases*, 11th edition (ICD-11). Geneva: World Health Organization; 2024. Available from: https://icd.who.int/en

3. Drakatos P, Marples L, Muza R, Higgins S, Gildeh N, Macavei R, et al. NREM parasomnias: a treatment approach based upon a retrospective case series of 512 patients. *Sleep Med*. 2019 Jan;53:181–8.

Case 42: Rapid Eye Movement Sleep Behaviour Disorder

Dream Enactments

Harry is a 67-year-old gentleman with a history of Parkinson's disease who presents with movement issues during sleep. Harry thrashes in his sleep and frequently injures his wife, who shares the bed with him at night. He often wakes up complaining of nightmares as well.

- **Question 1: What do you think is the likely diagnosis?**

Harry's daughter is a 46-year-old lady who complains of the intense need to move her legs when she is lying in bed. The urge is usually worse at night, affecting her sleep and is relieved by shaking her legs. This has been going on for the past six months. She denies any symptoms of anxiety or the use of illicit substances or chronic medications. She is worried she may have rapid eye movement (REM) sleep behaviour disorder as well.

- **Question 2: What is her diagnosis?**

Answers to Case 42

Question 1
What do you think is the likely diagnosis?

Answer
Harry most likely suffers from REM sleep behaviour disorder, which is associated with neurodegenerative diseases such as Parkinson's disease.

Explanation

Diagnosis of REM sleep behaviour disorder [1]

1. REM sleep behaviour disorder is characterised by repeated episodes of sleep-related vocalisation or complex motor behaviours that are either documented by polysomnography to occur during REM sleep or are presumed to occur during REM sleep due to a clinical history of dream enactment

2. Polysomnographic recording (when performed) demonstrates REM sleep without atonia

3. The disorder may occur as an isolated, idiopathic form but is frequently associated with latent or manifest disease of the nervous system, especially alpha-synucleinopathies

Note: a provisional diagnosis may be established on clinical grounds but definitive diagnosis requires polysomnographic demonstration of REM sleep without atonia.

REM sleep behaviour disorder is a parasomnia that is characterised by a loss of muscle atonia and abnormal behaviours occurring during REM sleep. It often presents as dream enactments 90 minutes after sleep onset and is more frequent during the later sleep periods. REM sleep behaviour disorder can be categorised into idiopathic and secondary forms. Clonazepam and melatonin may be useful for treatment.

An important differential for REM sleep behaviour disorder is nocturnal frontal lobe epilepsy. In frontal lobe epilepsy, stereotypical behaviours occur several times in the night for short durations. It can happen regardless of the phase of sleep, and the patient is usually confused on awakening due to a post-ictal confusional state.

Exam Essentials

•   For patients presenting with REM sleep behaviour disorder, always screen for cognitive issues and parkinsonism

•   Longitudinal follow-up is necessary, as REM sleep behaviour disorder may precede the development of a neurodegenerative disease by several years

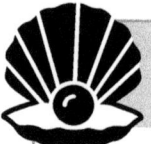

Clinical Pearls

- The secondary causes of REM sleep behaviour disorder are associated with **α-synucleinopathy neurodegenerative diseases** (such as Parkinson's disease, Lewy body dementia and multiple system atrophy)

- **Polysomnography** should be done for a definitive diagnosis of REM sleep behaviour disorder

Question 2

What is her diagnosis?

Answer

Restless leg syndrome

Explanation

Diagnosis of restless legs syndrome [2]

1. An urge to move the legs accompanied with uncomfortable and unpleasant sensations in the legs. It is characterised by all of the following:

    - Periods of rest or inactivity worsen the urge to move the legs
    - Movement partially or completely relieves the urge to move the legs
    - The urge to move the legs is worse or occurs exclusively in the evening or at night

2. The above symptoms occur at least three times per week and last for at least three months

3. Symptoms should not be caused by physiological effects of a drug or medication (e.g., akathisia) or another mental or medical condition

Restless legs syndrome, also known as Willis–Ekbom disease, is a sensorimotor disorder where there is an urge to move the legs due to an uncomfortable sensation for at least three times per week for at least three months.

The aetiology of restless legs syndrome can be categorised as primary or secondary. Reversible causes include iron deficiency anaemia, vitamin B12 and folate deficiency, pregnancy and end-stage renal disease. Other secondary causes include peripheral neuropathy (associated with diabetes mellitus), rheumatoid arthritis, spinal disorders such as spinal nerve root irritation, Parkinson's disease, fibromyalgia, spinocerebellar ataxia and Charcot–Marie–Tooth disease.

Non-pharmacological interventions involve lifestyle changes (avoid caffeine or alcohol before bedtime) and sleep hygiene. Advice for behavioural strategies, such as walking and stretching, massaging the affected limbs, bathing in hot or cold water, relaxation exercises (biofeedback or yoga) and distracting the mind, may also be incorporated. Medications such as ropinirole or pramipraxole may be considered.

Exam Essentials

- Rule out iron and vitamin B12/folate deficiency if restless legs syndrome is suspected

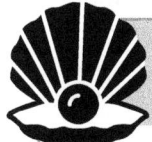

Clinical Pearls

- Akathisia should be a differential diagnosis, especially if the patient is on antipsychotics
- Medications such as antidepressants, antipsychotics and antinausea drugs can also cause restless legs syndrome

Diving Deep ...

Melatonin is a hormone produced by the pineal gland that has multiple effects, including somnolence, and is believed to play a role in regulating the sleep–wake cycle [3]. Melatonin supplements may be prescribed for jet lag, insomnia (short-term treatment of primary insomnia characterised by poor sleep quality in patients aged 55 or over), shift-work disorder, circadian rhythm disorders and sleep–wake cycle disturbances in children and adolescents with mental retardation and autism. Side effects of the medication melatonin include headaches and increased dreams.

In patients with idiopathic REM sleep behaviour disorder, 75% develop a defined neurodegenerative disease, most often a synucleinopathy (i.e., Parkinson's disease, major or mild neurocognitive disorder with Lewy bodies or multiple system atrophy within 10–15 years following diagnosis [2]. The annualised risk is approximately 6–7% per year. Therefore, patients with idiopathic REM sleep behaviour disorder should be closely monitored for neurological symptoms.

Nightmare disorder [1] is an REM sleep disorder characterised by recurrent, vivid and highly dysphoric dreams, often involving threat to the individual, which generally occur during REM sleep and often result in awakening with anxiety. The person is rapidly oriented and alert upon awakening. Nightmares are relatively common in childhood, affecting about 1–5% of children [2]. They often start between the ages of three and six years, reaching their highest frequency and severity during late adolescence or early adulthood. Polysomnographic studies reveal abrupt awakenings from REM sleep, typically occurring in the second half of the night, just before a nightmare is recalled. Before waking, there may be an increase in heart rate, breathing rate and eye movement variability. Nightmares triggered by traumatic events can sometimes replicate the traumatic experience ('replicative nightmares') but most do not. Factors like sleep disruption, deprivation, jet lag or certain medications that increase early-night REM sleep intensity can provoke nightmares earlier in the night, even at sleep onset. When nightmares occur during sleep-onset REM periods (hypnagogic), they are frequently accompanied by sleep paralysis, a state where one feels awake but is unable to move, which can also happen without a prior dream or nightmare. Mild physiological responses, such as sweating, tachycardia and tachypnoea, may be present, although body movements and vocalisations are uncommon due to REM sleep-related muscle paralysis.

References

1. World Health Organization. *International classification of diseases*, 11th edition (ICD-11). Geneva: World Health Organization; 2024. Available from: https://icd.who.int/en

2. American Psychiatric Association. *Diagnostic and statistical manual of mental disorders*, 5th edition, text revision (DSM-5-TR). Washington, DC: American Psychiatric Association Publishing; 2022. Available from: www.psychiatry.org/psychiatrists/practice/dsm

3. Boland RJ, Verduin ML, Ruiz P, Shah A, Sadock BJ, editors. *Kaplan & Sadock's synopsis of psychiatry*, 12th edition. Philadelphia: Wolters Kluwer; 2022.

Case 43: Dissociative Amnesia and Dissociative Identity Disorder

Who Am I?

Kevin is an 18-year-old male who was brought to the clinic by his mother, after she noticed unusual shifts in his behaviour and 'personality'. Kevin was initially guarded about his experiences, but after rapport was built, he described two other 'alters' that emerged over the past few years that 'control' his body at different times. Kevin first became aware of these alters when his peers at work would claim to have conversations with him that he did not recall. His friends also remarked a change in voice and behaviour when these alters dominate. The first one, 'Harry', is a 6-year-old boy who gets moody and throws tantrums. The second alter, 'Brad', is more physically aggressive and drinks alcohol frequently. Kevin's memory is patchy, and he has difficulty recalling events that occurred when these alters emerged. He often 'wakes up' to find self-harm cut marks over his right forearm. Kevin notices that these alters dominate when he is under significant emotional stress. During subsequent sessions he revealed a traumatic past in which he had suffered through chronic sexual assaults by a family member from a young age. Having recently found a new job, he has been under increased pressure, and his transitions to these states have become more frequent. He experiences difficulties fulfilling his work obligations and has trouble keeping his job. His friends and family have expressed concerns over the recent deterioration of his condition, and his mood has been affected.

- **Question 1: What is dissociation?**

Kevin describes moments where he appears to float out of his body and he can observe the actions of the alters from a distance. He feels numb and detached during these episodes. At other times the world around him appears to be 'foggy' and he feels like he is in a dream. During these episodes, he maintains awareness that these experiences are unusual and cause him distress.

- **Question 2: What are the two phenomena described above?**

- **Question 3: What is Kevin's diagnosis?**

Kevin mentions that his uncle, Mr White, may have suffered from a similar condition. Mr White was brought to the emergency department five years ago after he found himself in a different city with no recollection of how he got there. Kevin recalls that his uncle had no memory of how and why he had travelled and appeared bewildered. This event happened soon after Kevin's grandmother passed away. Investigations were normal and did not reveal any abnormalities or substance use.

- **Question 4: What is Mr White's diagnosis?**

Answers to Case 43

Question 1
What is dissociation?

Answer
Dissociation is the separation of unpleasant emotions and memories from conscious awareness, with subsequent disruption to the normal integrated function of consciousness and memory.

Explanation
Dissociative symptoms can be conceptualised as 'positive' and 'negative' symptoms. Positive dissociative symptoms are intrusions into the individual's awareness and behaviour resulting in a loss of continuity in subjective experience, such as the division of identity, depersonalisation and derealisation. Negative dissociation symptoms result in the inability to access information or normal mental functions, for example amnesia [1].

Question 2
What are the two phenomena described above?

Answer
Depersonalisation and derealisation.

Explanation
Episodes of depersonalisation and derealisation are characterised by a feeling of unreality or detachment from one's mind, self or body and/or one's surroundings. Individuals with this disorder can have depersonalisation, derealisation or both.

Diagnosis of depersonalisation/derealisation disorder [2]

1. Persistent or recurrent experiences of either depersonalisation or derealisation, or of both symptoms, are required for diagnosis

   - **Depersonalisation**: is characterised by experiencing the self as strange or unreal, or by feeling detached from – or as though one were an outside observer of – one's thoughts, feelings, sensations, body or actions. Depersonalisation may take the form of emotional and/or physical numbing, a sense of watching oneself from a distance or 'being in a play', or perceptual alterations (e.g., a distorted sense of time)

   - **Derealisation**: is characterised by experiencing other people, objects or the world as strange or unreal (e.g., dreamlike, distant, foggy, lifeless, colourless or visually distorted), or by feeling detached from one's surroundings

2. During experiences of depersonalisation or derealisation, reality testing remains intact. The experiences are not associated with delusions or beliefs that the individual is being controlled by external people or forces

3. The symptoms are not better accounted for by another mental disorder (e.g., post-traumatic stress disorder (PTSD), an anxiety or fear-related disorder, another dissociative disorder, personality disorder)

4. The symptoms are not due to the effects of a substance or medication on the central nervous system (including withdrawal effects) and are not due to a disease of the nervous system (e.g., temporal lobe epilepsy), head trauma or another medical condition

5. The symptoms result in significant distress or significant impairment in personal, family, social, educational, occupational or other important areas of functioning. If functioning is maintained, it is only through significant additional effort

A commonly associated symptom is a subjectively altered sense of time (i.e., too fast or too slow), as well as a subjective difficulty in vividly recalling memories and owning them as personal and emotional.

Exam Essentials

- Depersonalisation and derealisation can occur in the context of other psychiatric conditions (e.g., PTSD)

Question 3
What is Kevin's diagnosis?

Answer
Dissociative identity disorder

Explanation
The defining feature of dissociative identity disorder is the presence of two or more distinct personality states or an experience of possession and recurrent episodes of dissociative amnesia.

The primary identity is the patient's original identity that carries their given name and is passive, dependent and may struggle with guilt and depression. The alternate personality states are referred to as alters and, when in control, have a distinct history and identity from their primary identity.

Patients with dissociative identity disorder experience recurrent, inexplicable intrusions into their conscious functioning and sense of self (e.g., voices; dissociated actions and speech; intrusive thoughts, emotions and impulses). There may be alterations of their sense of self (e.g., attitudes, preferences and feeling like their body or actions are not their own), odd changes of perception (e.g., depersonalisation or derealisation) and intermittent functional neurological symptoms.

Diagnosis of dissociative identity disorder [2]

1. Disruption of identity characterised by the presence of two or more distinct personality states (dissociative identities), involving marked discontinuities in the sense of self and agency, is required for diagnosis. Each personality state includes its own pattern of experiencing, perceiving, conceiving and relating to self, the body and the environment

2. At least two distinct personality states recurrently take executive control of the individual's consciousness and functioning in interacting with others or with the environment, such as in the performance of specific aspects of daily life (e.g., parenting, work), or in response to specific situations (e.g., those that are perceived as threatening)

3. Changes in personality state are accompanied by related alterations in sensation, perception, affect, cognition, memory, motor control and behaviour. There are typically episodes of amnesia inconsistent with ordinary forgetting, which may be severe

4. The symptoms are not better accounted for by another mental disorder (e.g., schizophrenia or another primary psychotic disorder)

5. The symptoms are not due to the effects of a substance or medication on the central nervous system – including withdrawal effects – (e.g., blackouts or

chaotic behaviour during substance intoxication), and are not due to a disease of the nervous system (e.g., complex partial seizures) or to a sleep–wake disorder (e.g., symptoms occur during hypnagogic or hypnopompic states)

6. The symptoms result in significant impairment in personal, family, social, educational, occupational or other important areas of functioning. If functioning is maintained, it is only through significant additional effort

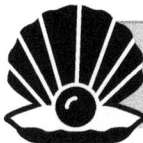

Clinical Pearls

- Stress often produces transient exacerbation of dissociative symptoms that makes them more evident

Question 4
What is Mr White's diagnosis?

Answer
Dissociative amnesia with dissociative fugue

Explanation
The defining characteristic of dissociative amnesia is an inability to recall important autobiographical information that should be successfully stored in memory and ordinarily would be freely recollected.

Diagnosis of dissociative amnesia [2]

1. Inability to recall important autobiographical memories – typically of recent traumatic or stressful events – that is inconsistent with ordinary forgetting is required for diagnosis

2. The memory loss does not occur exclusively during episodes of trance disorder, possession trance disorder, dissociative identity disorder or partial dissociative identity disorder, and is not better accounted for by another mental disorder (e.g., PTSD, complex PTSD, a neurocognitive disorder such as dementia)

3. The symptoms are not due to the effects of a substance or medication on the central nervous system (e.g., alcohol) – including withdrawal effects – and are not due to a disease of the nervous system (e.g., temporal lobe epilepsy), another medical condition (e.g., a brain tumour) or head trauma

4. The memory loss results in significant impairment in personal, family, social, educational, occupational or other important areas of functioning

The most common form of dissociative amnesia is localised while generalised dissociative amnesia is rare. Localised amnesia refers to a failure to recall events during a circumscribed period of time. Generalised amnesia refers to a complete loss of memory for most or all of the individual's life history.

Dissociative fugue refers to a form of dissociative amnesia where there is apparently purposeful travel/wandering that is associated with amnesia of self-identity or loss of other important autobiographical information.

Exam Essentials

- Dissociative amnesia is conceptualised as a potentially reversible memory retrieval deficit
- We need to rule out medical causes of episodic amnesia:
  - Transient epileptic amnesia
  - Transient global amnesia
  - Syncopal attack

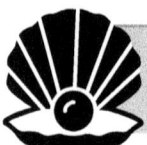

Clinical Pearls

- Dissociative amnesia is usually retrograde and, except in rare cases, is not associated with ongoing amnesia for contemporary life events
- Factors that favour amnesia of dissociation over amnesia of dementia:
  - Loss or alteration of identity
  - Usually retrograde amnesia
  - Isolated to personal information
  - Associated with traumatic or emotionally charged events

Diving Deep ...

Most individuals with dissociative disorders are initially unaware of their amnesia or minimise or rationalise the deficits. Awareness of amnesia occurs when they realise that they do not recall their personal identity or when circumstances make these individuals aware that important autobiographical information is missing (e.g., when they are told of past events that they cannot recall).

The fragmentation of identity may vary across circumstances and cultural contexts (e.g., possession–form presentations). Therefore, individuals may experience discontinuities in identity and memory that may not be immediately evident to others or are obscured by attempts to hide dysfunction.

A history of psychological trauma is common in patients with dissociative disorders. Various types of trauma have been identified as risk factors: earlier onset; neglect and sexual, physical and emotional abuse by parents; cumulative early life trauma and adversities; and repeated sustained trauma or torture associated with captivity (e.g., experienced by prisoners of war, victims of trafficking) [1]. Other risk factors include a lack of secure attachment to caregivers, a lack of comfort following overwhelming experiences and genetic predisposition [3, 4]. These factors lead to a lack of integration of identity across contexts and states.

Dissociative identity disorder is exceedingly rare; however, in recent times there appears to be a rise in patients presenting with a self-diagnosis of this disorder based on information from literature and the internet [5]. With this rise in self-diagnosis, an accurate diagnosis and identification of false-positive and imitated dissociative identity disorder is crucial in rendering the most appropriate form of treatment. Pietkiewicz et al. [6] found the following five themes from an interpretative phenomenological analysis after interviewing women whose earlier dissociative identity disorder diagnosis was disconfirmed:

- Theme 1: endorsement and identification with the diagnosis
- Theme 2: using the notion of dissociative parts to justify identity confusion and conflicting ego-states
- Theme 3: gaining knowledge about dissociative identity disorder affects the clinical presentation
- Theme 4: fragmented personality becomes an important discussion topic with others
- Theme 5: ruling out dissociative identity disorder leads to disappointment or anger

The following list is taken from the paper by Pietkiewicz et al. [6], and highlights the red flags for identifying false-positive or imitated dissociative identity disorder.

Red flags for identifying false-positive or imitated dissociative identity disorder [6]

1. Directly or indirectly expects to confirm self-diagnosed dissociative identity disorder

2. Dissociative identity disorder previously suggested by someone (friend, psychologist or doctor) without thorough clinical assessment

3. Keen on dissociative identity disorder diagnosis and familiarised with symptoms: read books, watched videos, talked to other patients, participated in a support group for dissociative patients

4. Uses clinical jargon: parts, alters, dissociating, switch, depersonalisation, etc.

5. Reveals little avoidance: eagerly talks about painful experiences and dissociation, no indicators for genuine shame or inner conflicts associated with disclosing symptoms or parts

6. Readily justifies losing control of emotions and unacceptable or shameful behavior in terms of not being oneself or being influenced by an alternative personality

7. No evidence for the intrusions of unwanted and avoided traumatic memories or re-experiencing them in the present

8. Denies having ego-dystonic thoughts or voices, especially starting in early childhood and child-like voices. (Note: dissociative patients may be afraid, ashamed, or feel it is forbidden to talk about the voices)

9. No evidence of amnesia for neutral or pleasant everyday activities, e.g., working, doing shopping, socialising, playing with children

10. Tries to control the interview and provide evidence for having dissociative identity disorder (e.g., eagerly reports dissociative symptoms without being asked about them)

11. Announces and performs a switch between personalities during clinical assessment, especially before a good relationship with the clinician and trust has been established

12. Finds apparent gains associated with having dissociative identity disorder: receives special interest from family and friends with whom symptoms and personalities are eagerly discussed, runs support groups, blogs or video channels for people with dissociative disorders

13. Gets upset or disappointed when dissociative identity disorder is not confirmed, for example demands re-evaluation, excuses oneself for not being accurate enough in giving right answers, wants to provide more evidence

References

1. American Psychiatric Association. *Diagnostic and statistical manual of mental disorders*, 5th edition, text revision (DSM-5-TR). Washington, DC: American Psychiatric Association Publishing; 2022. Available from: www.psychiatry.org/psychiatrists/practice/dsm

2. World Health Organization. *International classification of diseases*, 11th edition (ICD-11). Geneva: World Health Organization; 2024. Available from: https://icd.who.int/en

3. Savitz JB, van der Merwe L, Newman TK, Solms M, Stein DJ, Ramesar RS. The relationship between childhood abuse and dissociation. Is it influenced by catechol-O-methyltransferase (COMT) activity? *Int J Neuropsychopharmacol*. 2008 Mar;11(2):149–61.

4. Becker-Blease KA, Deater-Deckard K, Eley T, Freyd JJ, Stevenson J, Plomin R. A genetic analysis of individual differences in dissociative behaviors in childhood and adolescence. *J Child Psychol Psychiatry*. 2004 Mar;45(3):522–32.

5. SA Boon PD. *Screening en diagnostiek van dissociatieve stoornissen*. 1995; Lisse: Swets & Zeitlinger.

6. Pietkiewicz IJ, Bańbura-Nowak A, Tomalski R, Boon S. Revisiting false-positive and imitated dissociative identity disorder. *Front Psychol*. 2021 May 6;12:637929.

Case 44: Voyeuristic, Exhibitionistic, Frotteuristic and Sexual Masochism and Sadism Disorders

Forbidden fascinations

Tyler is a 25-year-old male who was brought to the clinic after he was caught by the police for taking upskirt photos of a woman in a public bathroom stall. Police investigations revealed multiple indecent photos of other women dating many years ago. Tyler admits to hiding in public bathrooms to take these unsuspected photos and says it gives him sexual arousal watching these women disrobe themselves. He is aware that such acts are illegal but has trouble controlling these urges. He feels ashamed of his behaviour and asks you for help.

- **Question 1: What is the diagnosis?**

- **Question 2: What is the difference between voyeuristic disorder and exhibitionistic disorder?**

In subsequent interviews, Tyler revealed that he was previously caught rubbing his penis against another girl on the bus. It causes sexual arousal within him whenever he performs the act. He has committed similar acts in the past year. He was conscious of the fact and felt guilty about what he was doing but had difficulty controlling the urges.

- **Question 3: What is the co-morbid diagnosis?**

Years later, Tyler returns to the clinic together with his girlfriend Jenny to seek help regarding their sexual practices in bondage and discipline, dominance and submission, and sadism and masochism (BDSM). They are concerned about their current practices as it has led to multiple clinic visits for Jenny.

Tyler prefers watching pornography where one of the parties is humiliated and bound. After entering a relationship with Jenny, he brought up these fantasies to her and she expressed a willingness to enact them. Tyler would often tie her up in ropes and use derogatory language on her during intercourse. However, there have been instances where the ropes were tied too tightly, leading to rope burns as well as an emergency department visit for asphyxiation. Jenny acknowledges that she is sexually aroused when being humiliated and bound and assures you that these sexual acts with Tyler are consensual. However, with the repeated clinic visits and injuries sustained, she has become increasingly worried that such sexual inclinations could be physically detrimental and is keen to seek further treatment if required.

- **Question 4: Does Tyler qualify for a co-morbid diagnosis of coercive sexual sadism disorder?**

- **Question 5: What is the diagnosis for Jenny?**

Answers to Case 44

Question 1
What is the diagnosis?

Answer
Voyeuristic disorder

Explanation

> ### Diagnosis of voyeuristic disorder [1]
>
> 1. A sustained, focused and intense pattern of sexual arousal – as manifested in persistent sexual thoughts, fantasies, urges or behaviours – that involves observing an unsuspecting person who is naked, in the process of disrobing or engaging in sexual activity, is required for diagnosis
>
> 2. The individual must have acted on these thoughts, fantasies or urges, or be markedly distressed by them

If individuals report distress (e.g., anxiety, obsessions, guilt or shame) or psychosocial problems because of their voyeuristic sexual preferences, they could be diagnosed with voyeuristic disorder. However, if individuals do not declare any distress, have no impairment in other important areas of functioning and no significant psychiatric or legal histories relating to it, they could be ascertained as having voyeuristic sexual interest but should not be diagnosed with voyeuristic disorder.

375

Even if individuals adopt a non-disclosing stance (e.g., denial of sexual arousal, fantasies, impulses, etc.) they can still be diagnosed with voyeuristic disorder. The diagnosis can be made if there is evidence of recurrent voyeurism and this paraphilia-motivated behaviour is causing harm to others.

Exam Essentials

- According to the DSM-5-TR [2] diagnostic criteria, the **minimum age for the diagnosis of voyeuristic disorder is 18 years**. While ICD-11 does not include an age cutoff, it is written that voyeuristic disorder should not be diagnosed among children, and is not typically diagnosed among adolescents [1]

Question 2
What is the difference between voyeuristic disorder and exhibitionistic disorder?

Answer
In exhibitionistic disorder, patients often feel a sense of inner tension and have a sudden urge to undress and expose themselves. Voyeuristic disorder requires a minimum age of 18 years old while exhibitionistic disorder does not require a minimum age for diagnosis.

Both disorders require a minimum duration of at least six months for diagnosis. Victims are usually non-consenting individuals.

Explanation

Diagnosis of exhibitionistic disorder [1]

1. A sustained, focused and intense pattern of sexual arousal – as manifested in persistent sexual thoughts, fantasies, urges or behaviours – that involves exposing one's genitals to an unsuspecting person in public places, usually without inviting or intending closer contact, is required for diagnosis

2. The individual must have acted on these thoughts, fantasies or urges, or be markedly distressed by them

The subtypes are based on the age or physical maturity of the non-consenting persons to whom the individual prefers to expose his or her genitals, such as prepubertal children, physically mature individuals or both. Similarly, if an individual reports distress or adopts a non-disclosing stance, they can still be diagnosed with exhibitionistic disorder.

Exam Essentials

- Exhibitionistic disorder is the most commonly reported of all sex offences

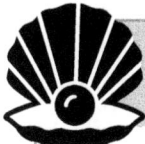

Clinical Pearls

- If the victim is of a younger age, we will need to evaluate for the presence of a co-occurring paedophilic disorder
- Non-disclosing individuals may deny such sexual behaviour or report that known episodes of exposure were all accidental and non-sexual

Question 3
What is the co-morbid diagnosis?

Answer
Frotteuristic disorder

Explanation
In frotteurism, the preferred form of sexual excitement is by rubbing the male genitalia against another person, or by fondling the breasts of an unwilling participant, who is usually a stranger, generally in a crowded place.

Diagnosis of frotteuristic disorder [1]

1. A sustained, focused and intense pattern of sexual arousal – as manifested in persistent sexual thoughts, fantasies, urges or behaviours – that involves touching or rubbing against a non-consenting person is required for diagnosis

2. The individual must have acted on these thoughts, fantasies or urges, or be markedly distressed by them

Similarly, if an individual reports distress or adopts a non-disclosing stance, they can still be diagnosed with frotteuristic disorder.

Question 4
Does Tyler qualify for a co-morbid diagnosis of coercive sexual sadism disorder?

Answer
No, he does not have coercive sexual sadism disorder. While there is a pattern of sexual arousal from acts of sadism, Tyler's actions are directed towards a consenting person (Jenny). Hence, he does not fulfil the criteria for a disorder.

Explanation

Diagnosis of coercive sexual sadism disorder [1]

1. A sustained, focused and intense pattern of sexual arousal – as manifested in persistent sexual thoughts, fantasies, urges or behaviours – that involves the infliction of physical or psychological suffering on a non-consenting person is required for diagnosis

2. The individual must have acted on these thoughts, fantasies or urges, or be markedly distressed by them

BDSM refers to a wide range of behaviours that individuals with sexual masochism and/or sexual sadism engage in, such as roleplaying involving bondage, discipline, submission and dominance, sadomasochism, etc.

While some individuals may be non-disclosing, the presence of recurrent sexual sadism involving multiple non-consenting victims increases the confidence in the clinical inference that the individual is motivated by coercive sexual sadism disorder. Coercive sexual sadism disorder can also be inferred if there are multiple instances of infliction of pain and suffering on the same victim. One-third of individuals who have committed sexually motivated homicides display sexually sadistic behaviour [2].

Question 5
What is the diagnosis for Jenny?

Answer
Sexual masochism disorder

Explanation

Diagnosis of sexual masochism disorder [2]

1. For at least six months, recurrent and intense sexual arousal from being humiliated, beaten, bound or otherwise subjected to suffering, as evidenced by fantasies, urges or behaviours

2. The individual has acted on these sexual urges with a person who did not consent, or it has caused significant functional impairment in other areas of life

In asphyxiophilia, the individual restricts breathing to achieve sexual arousal. Individuals reporting sexual interest in asphyxiophilia seem to experience more sexual distress and psychological maladjustment than the general population and are at risk of accidental death when practising asphyxiophilia.

There is insufficient evidence to support the association that individuals with masochistic sexual interests have a history of childhood sexual abuse [2].

Diving Deep ...

Paraphilias are characterised by any intense and persistent sexual interest in activities or targets other than sexual interest in genital stimulation or fondling with phenotypically normal, physically mature, human partners who can give consent.

Some paraphilias primarily concern the individual's erotic activities and others concern primarily the individual's erotic targets. An individual's pattern of paraphilic interests is often reflected in their choice of pornography.

Paraphilias are revised into a disorder when they cause distress or impairment to the individual or a paraphilia whose satisfaction has entailed personal harm, or risk of harm, to others. A paraphilia by itself does not necessarily justify or require clinical intervention. It is not rare for an individual to manifest two or more paraphilias.

The lifetime prevalence of voyeurism disorder is estimated to be as high as 12% in males and 4% in females [1]. Voyeurism is usually accompanied by or followed by masturbation.

The prevalence of exhibitionistic behaviour is estimated at 2–4% in the general population [3]. Almost all patients are male, and adolescents account for approximately 10% of exhibitionistic offences. Over a five-year follow-up, 5–10% of exhibitionistic perpetrators had escalated to contact sexual offending and approximately 25% recidivated with a subsequent exhibitionistic offence [4]. The strongest risk factor for escalation was a general clustering of antisocial behaviour, including a history of sexual and non-sexual convictions. Sexual reoffending recidivists were less educated and had more prior sexual and criminal offences.

Frotteuristic activity usually starts in adolescence, with onset usually occurring between the ages of 15 and 25 years. Prevalence estimates suggest that 30% of adult men in the US and Canadian general population have committed frotteuristic acts. However, the prevalence of frotteuristic disorder is much lower at 3.8% for 'intense desire' and 0.7% for 'persistent behaviour' [2].

Treatment of paraphilias is challenging given that the majority of patients rarely seek treatment voluntarily. However, if a patient is willing to receive treatment, psychotherapy may be helpful and has been shown to reduce reoffending [5–7].

Amongst psychotherapies, cognitive behavioral therapy is the most prominent and commonly employed therapy with some effectiveness [8–10].

Possible pharmacological treatments include selective serotonin reuptake inhibitors (SSRIs), synthetic steroidal analogues and anti-androgens [11]. SSRIs increase serotonin levels and this may decrease sexual desire and fantasy, potentially reducing unwanted sexual urges associated with paraphilic disorders [2, 3]. Anti-androgens, particularly gonadotropin-releasing hormone analogues, greatly decrease the severity and occurrence of abnormal sexual arousal and behaviour, but obtaining informed consent is essential in every instance [14].

References

1. World Health Organization. *International classification of diseases*, 11th edition (ICD-11). Geneva: World Health Organization; 2024. Available from: https://icd.who.int/en

2. American Psychiatric Association. *Diagnostic and statistical manual of mental disorders*, 5th edition, text revision (DSM-5-TR). Washington, DC: American Psychiatric Association Publishing; 2022. Available from: www.psychiatry.org/psychiatrists/practice/dsm

3. Seeman MV. Portrait of an exhibitionist. *Psychiatr Q*. 2020 Dec;91(4):1249–63.

4. Greenberg SRR, Firestone P, Bradford JM, Greenberg DM. Prediction of recidivism in exhibitionists: psychological, phallometric, and offense factors. *Sex Abuse*. 2002 Oct;14(4):329–47.

5. Hanson RK, Gordon A, Harris AJ, Marques JK, Murphy W, Quinsey VL, Seto MC. First report of the collaborative outcome data project on the effectiveness of psychological treatment for sex offenders. *Sex Abuse*. 2002 Apr;14(2):169–94; discussion 195–7.

6. Schmucker M, Lösel F. Does sexual offender treatment work? A systematic review of outcome evaluations. *Psicothema*. 2008 Feb;20(1):10-9.

7. Marshall WL, Marshall LE. Psychological treatment of the paraphilias: a review and an appraisal of effectiveness. *Curr Psychiatry Rep*. 2015 Jun;17(6):47.

8. Kaplan MS, Krueger RB. Cognitive–behavioral treatment of the paraphilias. *Isr J Psychiatry Relat Sci*. 2012;49(4):291–6.

9. Laws DR, Marshall WL. A brief history of behavioral and cognitive behavioral approaches to sexual offenders: Part 1. Early developments. *Sex Abuse*. 2003 Apr;15(2):75–92.

10. Marshall WL, Laws DR. A brief history of behavioral and cognitive behavioral approaches to sexual offender treatment: Part 2. The modern era. *Sex Abuse*. 2003;15(2):93–120.

11. Culos C, Di Grazia M, Meneguzzo P. Pharmacological interventions in paraphilic disorders: systematic review and insights. *J Clin Med*, 2024;13(6):1524.

12. Greenberg DM, Bradford JMW, Curry S, O'Rourke A. A comparison of treatment of paraphilias with three serotonin reuptake inhibitors: a retrospective study. *Bull Am Acad Psychiatry Law*. 1996;24(4):525–32.

13. Winder B, Lievesley R, Elliott H, Hocken K, Faulkner J, Norman C, et al. Evaluation of the use of pharmacological treatment with prisoners experiencing high levels of hypersexual disorder. *J Forensic Psychiatry Psychol*. 2018;29(1):53–71.

14. Thibaut F. Pharmacological treatment of paraphilias. *Isr J Psychiatry Relat Sci*. 2012;49(4):297–305.

Case 45: Paedophilic Disorder

Disturbed desires

Simmons is a 43-year-old man who was brought to the clinic by the police after he had allegedly molested Jacob, an 11-year-old boy. During the police investigation, it was revealed that Simmons had first met Jacob online before meeting in person. He then asked Jacob for sexual favours and to keep it a secret. However, Jacob grew increasingly uncomfortable and eventually told his parents about it, which led to police investigations being initiated. After building rapport, Simmons admitted to feeling sexually attracted to children and had previously committed similar acts with his niece, aged 8. The police had raided his home and found child pornography in his possession.

- **Question 1: What is the diagnosis?**

When asked about his attraction towards children, Simmons describes his preference towards social interactions with children over adults. He feels that he has more in common with children than adults. This is one of the reasons why he chooses to work as a primary school teacher.

- **Question 2: What is the phenomenon described?**

- **Question 3: What are the risk factors for paedophilic disorder?**

- **Question 4: How are patients with paedophilic disorder managed?**

- **Question 5: What is the risk of sexual recidivism for child molesters?**

Answers to Case 46

Question 1
What is the diagnosis?

Answer
Paedophilic disorder

Explanation
Individuals with paedophilia have an intense sexual interest in children greater than or equal to sexual interest in physically mature persons. They may be diagnosed with pae-dophilic disorder if it causes marked distress or psychosocial difficulties. Strong evidence for paedophilic disorder includes a self-reported interest in children, use of child por-nography, a history of multiple child victims, boy victims and unrelated child victims.

Diagnosis of paedophilic disorder [1]

1. A sustained, focused and intense pattern of sexual arousal – as manifested in persistent sexual thoughts, fantasies, urges or behaviours – involving prepubertal children is required for diagnosis

2. The individual must have acted on these thoughts, fantasies or urges, or be markedly distressed by them

3. The diagnosis does not apply to sexual arousal and accompanying behaviour between pre- or postpubertal children who are close in age

---

The DSM-5-TR [2] age guideline of 13 or younger is only approximate because the onset of puberty varies from person to person. The average age at onset of puberty has been declining over time and differs across ethnicities and cultures.

If individuals report distress or adopt a non-disclosing stance they can still be diagnosed with paedophilic disorder.

The use of sexually explicit content depicting prepubescent children alone in the absence of the individual's sexual interactions is insufficient to diagnose paedophilic disorder, although possession of such materials violates the law.

 **Exam Essentials**

- The victimised child may be of the opposite sex (heterosexual paedophilia) or the same sex (homosexual paedophilia)

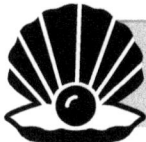

Clinical Pearls

- During the assessment, take a detailed sexual and personal history, such as:
  - Sexual encounters, fantasies and deviant behaviour including other paraphilic disorders
  - Romantic relationships
  - History of abuse
- **Ascertain any risks** (e.g., access to children)

Question 2
What is the phenomenon described?

Answer
Emotional congruence

Explanation
The tendency of some children sexual offenders to display an exaggerated cognitive and emotional affiliation with childhood is known as 'emotional congruence' [3]. This phenomenon is more closely associated with homosexual paedophiles. Emotional congruence with children is related to paedophilic sexual interest and the likelihood of sexually reoffending among individuals who have sexually offended.

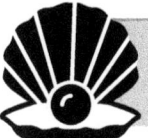

Clinical Pearls

- Emotional congruence with children is a risk factor for sexual offending against children [2]

Question 3
What are the risk factors for paedophilic disorder?

Answer
Antisocial personality traits (e.g., callousness, impulsivity) and a willingness to take risks without adequate regard for the consequences. Other factors include:

- History of childhood emotional and sexual abuse [4]
- History of family dysfunction
- Genetics

Explanation

Men with antisocial personality traits and paedophilic disorders are more likely to commit sexual acts with children and thus qualify for a diagnosis of paedophilic disorder [2].

A history of sexual abuse as children is common in adult men with paedophilia. It is unclear, however, whether this correlation reflects a causal influence of childhood sexual abuse on adult paedophilia. Childhood emotional abuse and family dysfunction (as defined by poor parental care, family adaptability, childhood emotional abuse, parental control, family problems and childhood physical abuse) were also found to be common developmental risk factors for paedophilia [4].

While the literature on genetic influences in the development of paedophilia is limited, some studies show familial aggregation in individuals with paedophilic disorder.

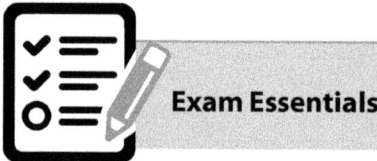

Exam Essentials

- Antisocial personality traits are a risk factor for paedophilic disorder

Question 4

How are patients with paedophilic disorder managed?

Answer

Psychotherapy: cognitive behavioural therapy (CBT) or psychodynamic therapy
Pharmacotherapy (e.g., anti-androgens)
Treat associated psychiatric disorders

Explanation

Direct treatment of paedophilic disorder is challenging. Group therapy held jointly by mental health and probation services in the community and in prison may be helpful, as is individual and group support provided by some charities. A recent systematic review [5] has shown that group CBT may reduce reoffending at one year, but, despite enormous investment in prison services, strong evidence of the effect is lacking.

Anti-androgens such as cyproterone and medroxyprogesterone have been used, but their use is associated with many adverse effects and ethical issues. There are social concerns that chemical castration may violate human rights for involuntary cases performed without the informed consent of the sexual offender [6–8]. Medical concerns include a significant decline in serum testosterone and oestradiol, leading to depression, osteoporosis, cardiovascular disease and impaired glucose and lipid metabolism.

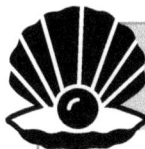

Clinical Pearls

- The use of anti-androgens in the treatment of paedophilic disorder is contentious with ethical concerns

Question 5
What is the risk of sexual recidivism for child molesters?

Answer
The recidivism rate increased from 15% at 5 years to 27% at 20 years of follow-up [9, 10].

Explanation
Risk factors for recidivism include: paedophiles attracted to boys, psychopathy and anti-social behaviour, denial, low self-esteem, co-morbid addictive disorders (mainly alcoholism or drug abuse) and psychiatric co-morbid disorders.

Diving Deep ...

An estimate of the prevalence of paedophilic disorder is 3% in the male population [2]. It occurs in all ethnic and socioeconomic groups. Paedophiles are rarely mentally ill, though when present, the more common psychiatric co-morbid disorders include personality disorder, paraphilias, alcohol and substance misuse. Intra-familial abuse (incest) is more common than extra-familial abuse. The perpetrators of intra-familial abuse are commonly fathers or stepfathers against daughters. In individuals attracted to minors, there is a distinction between those with a sexual preference for prepubescent minors (paedophilia) and those with a sexual preference for pubescent minors (hebephilia).

In terms of diagnostic markers, penile plethysmography has been researched the most extensively, although the sensitivity and specificity of diagnosis may vary across sites, which frequently use different stimuli, procedures and scoring [11]. Viewing time, using photographs of nude or minimally clothed persons as visual stimuli, is also used to diagnose paedophilic disorder, especially in combination with self-report measures. The diagnostic marker used is a relative sexual response to stimuli depicting children compared with stimuli depicting adults, rather than an absolute response to child stimuli.

References

1. World Health Organization. *International classification of diseases*, 11th edition (ICD-11). Geneva: World Health Organization; 2024. Available from: https://icd.who.int/en

2. American Psychiatric Association. *Diagnostic and statistical manual of mental disorders*, 5th edition, text revision (DSM-5-TR). Washington, DC: American Psychiatric Association Publishing; 2022. Available from: www.psychiatry.org/psychiatrists/practice/dsm

3. Wilson RJ. Emotional congruence in sexual offenders against children. *Sex Abuse*. 1999 Jan;11(1):33–47.

4. Lee JKP, Jackson HJ, Pattison P, Ward T. Developmental risk factors for sexual offending. *Child Abuse Negl*. 2002 Jan;26(1):73–92.

5. Beaudry G, Yu R, Perry AE, Fazel S. Effectiveness of psychological interventions in prison to reduce recidivism: a systematic review and meta-analysis of randomised controlled trials. *Lancet Psychiatry*. 2021 Sep;8(9):759–73.

6. Lee JY, Cho KS. Chemical castration for sexual offenders: physicians' views. *J Korean Med Sci*. 2013 Feb;28(2):171–2.

7. Gooren LJ. Clinical review: ethical and medical considerations of androgen deprivation treatment of sex offenders. *J Clin Endocrinol Metab*. 2011 Dec;96(12):3628–37.

8. Scott CL, Holmberg T. Castration of sex offenders: prisoners' rights versus public safety. *J Am Acad Psychiatry Law*. 2003;31(4):502–9.

9. Hanson RK, Lee SC, Thornton D. Long term recidivism rates among individuals at high risk to sexually reoffend. *Sex Abuse*. 2022 Nov 16;107906322211391.

10. Helmus L, Hanson RK, Thornton D, Babchishin KM, Harris AJR. Absolute recidivism rates predicted by Static-99R and Static-2002R sex offender risk assessment tools vary across samples: a meta-analysis. *Crim Justice Behav*. 2012 Sep;39(9):1148–71.

11. Boland RJ, Verduin ML, Ruiz P, Shah A, Sadock BJ, editors. *Kaplan & Sadock's synopsis of psychiatry*, 12th edition. Philadelphia: Wolters Kluwer; 2022.

Case 46: Transvestic and Fetishistic Disorders

Whose clothes are those?

Jonathan is an 18-year-old male brought in by his mother due to multiple complaints about sexual misconduct in school. The school reported him for multiple incidents of stealing female students' bras in the hostel he was staying at. When confronted about the reason for his theft, he would often get defensive and have multiple anger outbursts. During the consult, Jonathan revealed that this has been happening for the past four years. He would steal the bras to use them for masturbation. This practice initially stemmed from curiosity; however, as the years progressed, only bras could help him achieve sexual arousal for orgasm.

- **Question 1: What is the diagnosis?**

Upon screening for other psychiatric co-morbid disorders, Jonathan admits to cross-dressing in his sexual encounters as well for the past year. He reports increased sexual gratification when cross-dressed, but post-event often felt guilty for his actions – which he deems to be 'weird and deviant'. However, he does not identify as a woman in these cross-dressing incidents, nor fantasises to be one. He identified as a male and has sexual attraction towards females. He does not engage in other paraphilic behaviours. He does not report intrusive thoughts or any compulsions.

- **Question 2: What is the described co-morbidity?**

Although the action of cross-dressing initially stemmed from curiosity, Jonathan was eventually only sexually stimulated when bras or cross-dressing were involved.

- **Question 3: What does such a phenomenon describe?**

Jonathan recognises that his behaviours have caused much functional impairment – from recurrent reprimands in school to extreme feelings of guilt. He is keen for treatment to change his behaviours and return to a previous sense of normalcy.

- **Question 4: How would you manage Jonathan's conditions?**

Answers to Case 46

Question 1
What is the diagnosis?

Answer

Fetishistic disorder is a disorder where sexual arousal is achieved exclusively by inanimate objects that do not have direct sexual orientations. The most common objects of fetishism include female clothing such as lingerie, high heels, feet, breasts, etc.

Explanation

Diagnosis of fetishistic disorder [1]

1. For at least six months, recurrent and intense sexual arousal from either the use of inanimate objects or a highly specific focus on a non-genital body part(s), as evidenced by fantasies, urges or behaviours

2. The fantasies, sexual urges or behaviours cause clinically significant distress or significant functional impairment in other areas of life

3. The fetish objects extend beyond items such as clothing used in cross-dressing (as seen in transvestic disorder) or devices explicitly created for tactile genital stimulation (e.g., vibrator)

While still present in the DSM-5-TR, fetishism, fetishistic transvestism and sadomasochism were removed from ICD-11 as the Working Group on the Classification of Sexual Disorders and Sexual Health did not consider these arousal patterns to be an appropriate focus of public health surveillance and reporting [2]. It was reasoned that these conditions involve consensual or solitary sexual activities that do not inherently cause harm, are not necessarily distressing to the individual and are not associated with functional impairment.

Exam Essentials

- Screen for other paraphilic disorders, as paraphilic disorders often co-exist

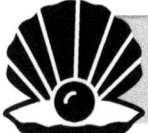

Clinical Pearls

- Obsessive–compulsive disorder is a common co-morbidity

Question 2

What is the described co-morbidity?

Answer

Transvestic disorder

Explanation

Diagnosis of transvestic disorder [1]

1. For at least six months, recurrent and intense sexual arousal from cross-dressing, as evidenced by fantasies, urges or behaviours

2. The fantasies, sexual urges or behaviours cause clinically significant distress or significant functional impairment in other areas of life

If patients present with cross-dressing, gender dysphoria and dual-role transvestism are differentials that should be screened for.

Exam Essentials

- Screen for **gender dysphoria** as a differential or co-morbidity

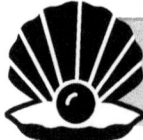

Clinical Pearls

- How patients present to the clinic (e.g., self-referral vs. brought in for forensic assessment) gives a clue to the patient's motivation for treatment

Question 3
What does such a phenomenon describe?

Answer
Classical conditioning

Explanation
Classical conditioning refers to learning when a neutral stimulus becomes associated with a stimulus that naturally produces a behaviour. The neutral stimulus here refers to bras/cross-dressing, with positive feelings that came from sexual gratification from masturbation, which became a learned behaviour – eventually being the sole stimulus for sexual gratification.

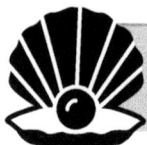

Clinical Pearls

- The conditioning of orgasms to fetishistic/transvestic inclinations or other paraphilias often leads to losing a sense of sexual normalcy

Question 4
How would you manage Jonathan's conditions?

Answer
Multi-modal management would be suitable for him:

- Pharmacological options: selective serotonin reuptake inhibitors (SSRIs) and anti-androgens (e.g., cyproterone acetate and medroxyprogrestrone acetate) [3]

- Cognitive behavioural therapy (CBT)

Explanation
Serotonergic agents have been used with limited success in the treatment of patients with paraphilias. Anti-androgens work by decreasing serum testosterone to subnormal concentrations, which reduces sex drive. The aims of CBT seek to disrupt learned paraphilic

patterns and to couple the fetishistic object with a neutral response rather than a sexual response to lower sexual arousal associated with the object [4].

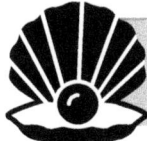

Clinical Pearls

- Pharmacological efficacy in the treatment of paraphilias varies significantly between individuals [4]

Diving Deep …

Paraphilias are usually underlined by fantasies – it has been suggested that fetishes develop towards inanimate objects to overcome feelings of inadequacy [5]. Low self-esteem can cause such individuals to seek alternative expression to mainstream sexuality. Negative self-perceptions could stem from dismissive parenting or rejection by parents at a young age and other negative experiences outside the family context. Patients with paraphilias usually present late to the clinical setting, as they generally adapt to their behaviours and are not distressed by them. They often surface only due to conflict with partners, the law or society at large.

References

1. American Psychiatric Association. *Diagnostic and statistical manual of mental disorders*, 5th edition, text revision (DSM-5-TR). Washington, DC: American Psychiatric Association Publishing; 2022. Available from: www.psychiatry.org/psychiatrists/practice/dsm

2. Krueger RB, Reed GM, First MB, Marais A, Kismodi E, Briken P. Proposals for paraphilic disorders in the international classification of diseases and related health problems, eleventh revision (ICD-11). *Arch Sex Behav.* 2017 Jul;46(5):1529–45.

3. Guay DRP. Drug treatment of paraphilic and nonparaphilic sexual disorders. *Clin Ther.* 2009 Jan;31(1):1–31.

4. Boland RJ, Verduin ML, Ruiz P, Shah A, Sadock BJ, editors. *Kaplan & Sadock's synopsis of psychiatry*, 12th edition. Philadelphia: Wolters Kluwer; 2022.

5. Amber Eagan. Foot obsessed but not necessarily depressed: the relationship between paraphilias and mental health outcomes. Murray State University; 2017. Available from: https://digitalcommons.murraystate.edu/etd/41

Case 47: Gender Dysphoria

A rift between internal and external identities

Nicholas is a 21-year-old male whom his general practitioner referred, as he wanted to be prescribed oestrogen. He introduced himself as "Nicolette" and identified as a female. Nicolette felt like a woman trapped in a man's body since age 6. From a young age, Nicolette would cross-dress and dislike typical masculine clothing. While playing pretend, Nicolette would often adopt female roles e.g. playing a mother or sister. During his schooling years, Nicolette got along better with female classmates and avoided contact sports with the other males in the class, preferring to experiment with makeup. During puberty, Nicolette became increasingly anxious over the development of facial and chest hair, broad shoulders and Adam's apple. Nicolette was disgusted over the growth of his penis and testicles and would bind his penis to make his erections less visible. He desired the development of breasts instead and would practice speaking in a more effeminate manner. Puberty was a turbulent time for Nicolette, who experienced bullying and had trouble with academic work. Nicolette was also worried about acceptance from his parents and confided in friends mainly. After learning more about hormone therapy and gender reassignment surgery, Nicolette decided to visit a general practitioner, leading to your clinic's current visit.

- **Question 1: What is the diagnosis?**

- **Question 2: What are the differential diagnoses of gender dysphoria?**

- **Question 3: What are common co-morbid psychiatric conditions in gender dysphoria?**

- **Question 4: What is the typical course of gender dysphoria?**

- **Question 5: Before starting feminising/masculinising hormone therapy, what criteria should be met?**

Answers to Case 47

Question 1
What is the diagnosis?

Answer
Gender incongruence of adolescence and adulthood (ICD-11) or gender dysphoria (DSM-5-TR)

Explanation
The ICD-11 [1] defines gender incongruence of adolescence and adulthood as: a marked and persistent incongruence between an individual's experienced gender and the assigned sex, which often leads to a desire to 'transition', in order to live and be accepted as a person of the experienced gender, through hormonal treatment, surgery or other healthcare services to make the individual's body align, as much as desired and to the extent possible, with the experienced gender. The diagnosis cannot be assigned prior to the onset of puberty. Gender-variant behaviour and preferences alone are not a basis for assigning the diagnosis.

The equivalent diagnosis in the DSM-5-TR classification is termed 'gender dysphoria'.

Diagnosis of gender dysphoria (DSM-5-TR) [2]

1. For at least six months, there is a marked incongruence between one's experienced/expressed gender and assigned gender. At least two or more of the following symptoms:

    - A significant incongruence between one's experienced/expressed gender and primary and/or secondary sex characteristics
    - In young adolescents, there is incongruence in the anticipated secondary sex characteristics
    - A strong desire to eliminate one's primary and/or secondary sex characteristics due to a significant incongruence with one's experienced or expressed gender. In young adolescents, a desire to prevent the development of anticipated secondary sex characteristics
    - A strong desire for the primary and/or secondary sex characteristics of the other gender
    - A strong desire to be of the other gender

- A strong desire to be treated as the other gender
- A strong conviction that one possesses the typical feelings and responses of the other gender

2. The condition is associated with clinically significant distress or significant functional impairment in major areas of life

Taking reference from the DSM-5-TR [2], the following terms are defined as follows:

- 'Sex' describes the biological characteristics that distinguish male and female – such as in sex chromosomes, gonads, sex hormones and clearly defined internal and external reproductive organs – based on reproductive function

- 'Disorders of sex development or differences of sex development (DSDs)' are terms that encompass what were previously called hermaphroditism and pseudohermaphroditism.

- 'Gender' refers to the publicly recognised and sociocultural role a person lives as – such as boy, girl, man, woman or another gender – often acknowledged legally

- 'Gender identity' is a type of social identity that reflects how a person sees themselves: as male, female, somewhere in between (like gender fluid) or outside the male/female binary (e.g., gender neutral)

- 'Gender assignment' is the process of designating someone as male or female, typically at birth, based on physical sex characteristics, resulting in what's often called the 'birth-assigned gender' or, historically, 'biological sex'

- 'Gender-atypical' describes physical traits or behaviours that are statistically uncommon for people with the same assigned gender in a specific society and time period; other terms include gender non-conforming, gender variant and gender diverse

- 'Transsexual' is an older term for someone who seeks, is in the process of or has completed a social transition from one gender (male to female or female to male) to another

Exam Essentials

- The onset of gender incongruence is divided into **prepubertal** children and **postpubertal** adolescents/adults

Question 2
What are the differential diagnoses of gender dysphoria?

Answer
Transvetism, fetishistic transvestism, dual role transvestism
Body dysmorphic disorder
Schizophrenia

Explanation
Transvestic disorder is characterised by recurrent and intense sexual arousal from cross-dressing, as manifested by fantasies, urges or behaviours. Therefore, when cross-dressing occurs, clarification should be made as to whether their gender is being called into question or otherwise. Cross-dressing with sexual excitement can be a precursor to the diagnosis of gender dysphoria in some cases of postpubertal-onset gender dysphoria in individuals assigned as males at birth who are attracted to women.

In body dysmorphic disorder, the focus of distress is on their physical primary or secondary sexual characteristics, there is no desire to change their gender.

Gender-themed delusions may occur in up to 20% of individuals with schizophrenia [3]. Schizophrenia is usually differentiated from gender dysphoria by the bizarre content as well as a waxing and waning course.

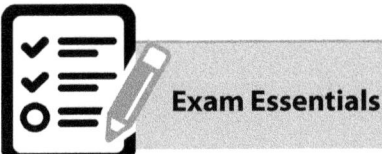

Exam Essentials

- Transvestism must be ruled out as a differential

Question 3
What are common co-morbid psychiatric conditions in gender dysphoria?

Answer
Depression
Anxiety
Impulse-control disorder
Substance misuse
Personality disorder
Autism spectrum disorder

Explanation
Transgender adolescents referred to gender clinics have substantially higher rates of suicidal thoughts and behaviours when compared with non-referred adolescents. The minority stress model predicts increases in mental illness in groups that are stigmatised,

discriminated against, harassed and abused at higher rates than others [4]. Risk factors include past maltreatment, gender victimisation, depression, substance abuse and younger age. Rates of suicidality and suicide attempts for transgender individuals range from 30% to 80% [2].

Another study showed that 38% had a current psychiatric disorder and 69% had a lifetime psychiatric disorder – predominantly mood and anxiety disorders [5].

Autism spectrum disorder is more prevalent in clinically referred adolescents and adults with gender dysphoria than in the general population [2, 6].

Exam Essentials

- Autism spectrum disorder as a co-morbidity is more prevalent in clinically referred adolescents and adults with gender dysphoria than in the general population [2, 6]

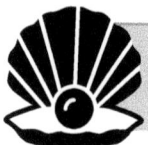

Clinical Pearls

- Among adolescents, the highest rate of suicide attempts comes from transgender young men, followed by those defining themselves as neither male nor female [2]

Question 4
What is the typical course of gender dysphoria?

Answer
In individuals assigned male at birth, studies from North America and the Netherlands found persistence of gender dysphoria ranged from 12% to 39% [7–9]. In individuals assigned female at birth, the persistence of gender dysphoria ranged from 12% to 50% [2].

Explanation
Cross-gender behaviours can be apparent from as young as three years of age, which is the age when children typically begin to develop a sense of their gender identity. The persistence of gender dysphoria is modestly correlated with the severity of symptoms at

the time of childhood baseline assessment. An early social transition may also be a factor in the persistence of gender dysphoria in adolescence. For individuals whose gender dysphoria continues into adolescence and beyond, most self-identify as heterosexual. In those who no longer have gender dysphoria by the time of adolescence, a majority self-identify as gay, lesbian or bisexual [2]. The early/prepubertal-onset group often presents with more intense gender dysphoria than individuals with late/postpubertal-onset gender dysphoria. The early/prepubertal-onset group often presents for clinical, gender-affirming care during childhood, adolescence or young adulthood.

Exam Essentials

- Puberty is a period which can prompt distressing feelings of gender incongruence, which can exacerbate the individual's gender dysphoria

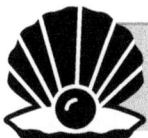

Clinical Pearls

- The majority of patients with gender dysphoria do not have persistent symptoms

Question 5
Before starting feminising/masculinising hormone therapy, what criteria should be met?

Answer
Persistent, well-documented gender dysphoria
Capacity to make a fully informed decision and consent to treatment
Age of maturity in the given country
If significant medical or mental concerns are present, they must be reasonably well controlled

Explanation
The above guidelines are taken with reference to guidelines proposed by the World Professional Association for Transgender Health (WPATH) [10], which is an international, multidisciplinary, professional association for transgender health.

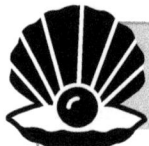

Clinical Pearls

- Check if patients have already started themselves on hormonal treatment obtained from external sources – we need to look for complications if dosages are not prescribed by a medical professional

Diving Deep …

The prevalence of gender dysphoria diagnosis across populations has been assessed to be less than 1/1,000 (i.e., < 0.1%) [2]. In the United Kingdom, male to female (MTF) 1 in 7,500; female to male (FTM) 1 in 31,000. MTF to FTM ratio is approximately 3–4:1.

Management of gender dysphoria remains contentious, with various guidelines suggesting varying treatment modalities. Some of the larger medical professional organisations that have issued guidelines include the WPATH, the Endocrine Society [11] and the American Academy of Child and Adolescent Psychiatry [12]. The choice of treatment modalities varies according to the age at which the patients present. Management of patients with gender dysphoria should be carried out in a multi-disciplinary manner.

In children, treatment of gender dysphoria typically consists of individual, family and group therapy, which guides children in exploring their gendered interests and identities. In adolescents, puberty is a tenuous period, and patients may show intense fear and preoccupation related to the physical changes they anticipate or are developing. In addition to providing psychotherapy, some clinicians may use puberty-blocking medications. Puberty-blocking medications are gonadotropin-releasing hormone (GnRH) agonists, which can be used to temporarily block the release of hormones that lead to secondary sex characteristics and allow for more time for patients to explore their gender identity. GnRH agonists have been used for many years in other populations (e.g., children with precocious puberty) and are felt to be safe. However, puberty blockers still carry the risk of possible reduced adult height, decreased bone mineral density accrual, hot flashes, mood disruption and loss of libido. In adults, psychotherapy is used to explore gender issues and hormonal and surgical treatments are employed for gender affirmation. Gender-affirming treatment often improves coexisting symptoms; however, some individuals continue to experience significant anxiety and affective symptoms and remain at increased risk for suicide. A study of all persons in Sweden who had undergone sex reassignment surgery (cohort size over 300 individuals), showed that their risk for hospitalisation for psychiatric problems remained over double that of controls after surgery, and they were 4.9 times more likely to have made a suicide attempt, and 19 times more likely to have died from suicide [13].

Regret after gender-affirmation surgery and de-transition attempts (to stop or reverse gender transition) have come under increasing spotlight. In February 2022, the Swedish National Board of Health and Welfare (NBHW) [14] issued an update to its healthcare service guidelines for children and younger youth (age < 18 years) with gender dysphoria. The guidance has changed from a previously strong recommendation to treat youth with hormones, to a new caution to avoid hormones except for 'exceptional cases'. The NBHW concluded that the evidence base for hormonal interventions for gender-dysphoric youth is of low quality and that hormonal treatments may carry risks. The NBHW also concluded that the evidence for paediatric transition comes from studies where the population was markedly different from the cases presenting for care today. In addition, the NBHW noted increasing reports of de-transition and transition-related regret among youth who transitioned in recent years. In light of the above limitations in the evidence base, the ongoing identity formation in youth and because gender transition has pervasive and lifelong consequences, the NBHW has concluded that, at present, the risks of hormonal interventions for gender dysphoric youth outweigh the potential benefits.

References

1. World Health Organization. *International classification of diseases*, 11th edition (ICD-11). Geneva: World Health Organization; 2024. Available from: https://icd.who.int/en

2. American Psychiatric Association. *Diagnostic and statistical manual of mental disorders*, 5th edition, text revision (DSM-5-TR). Washington, DC: American Psychiatric Association Publishing; 2022. Available from: www.psychiatry.org/psychiatrists/practice/dsm

3. À Campo J, Nijman H, Merckelbach H, Evers C. Psychiatric comorbidity of gender identity disorders: a survey among Dutch psychiatrists. *AJP*. 2003 Jul;160(7):1332–6.

4. Chodzen G, Hidalgo MA, Chen D, Garofalo R. Minority stress factors associated with depression and anxiety among transgender and gender-nonconforming youth. *J Adolesc Health*. 2019 Apr;64(4):467–71.

5. Zucker KJ, Lawrence AA, Kreukels BPC. Gender dysphoria in adults. *Annu Rev Clin Psychol*. 2016 Mar 28;12(1):217–47.

6. Kahn NF, Sequeira GM, Garrison MM, Orlich F, Christakis DA, Aye T, et al. Co-occurring autism spectrum disorder and gender dysphoria in adolescents. *Pediatrics*. 2023 Aug 1;152(2):e2023061363.

7. Wallien MSC, Cohen-Kettenis PT. Psychosexual outcome of gender-dysphoric children. *J Am Acad Child Adolesc Psychiatry*. 2008 Dec;47(12):1413–23.

8. Singh D, Bradley SJ, Zucker KJ. A follow-up study of boys with gender identity disorder. *Front Psychiatry*. 2021;12:632784.

9. Bradley SJ, Zucker KJ. Gender identity disorder and psychosexual problems in children and adolescents. *Can J Psychiatry*. 1990 Aug;35(6):477–86.

10. Coleman E, Radix AE, Bouman WP, Brown GR, De Vries ALC, Deutsch MB, et al. Standards of care for the health of transgender and gender diverse people, version 8. *Int J Transgend Health*. 2022 Aug 19;23(Suppl 1):S1–259.

11. Hembree WC, Cohen-Kettenis PT, Gooren L, Hannema SE, Meyer WJ, Murad MH, et al. Endocrine treatment of gender-dysphoric/gender-incongruent persons: an Endocrine Society clinical practice guideline. *J Clin Endocrinol Metab*. 2017 Nov 1;102(11):3869–903.

12. Adelson SL, American Academy of Child and Adolescent Psychiatry (AACAP) Committee on Quality Issues (CQI). Practice parameter on gay, lesbian, or bisexual sexual orientation, gender nonconformity, and gender discordance in children and adolescents. *J Am Acad Child Adolesc Psychiatry*. 2012 Sep;51(9):957–74.

13. Dhejne C, Öberg K, Arver S, Landén M. An analysis of all applications for sex reassignment surgery in Sweden, 1960–2010: prevalence, incidence, and regrets. *Arch Sex Behav*. 2014 Nov;43(8):1535–45.

14. Socialstyrensen (The Natioanal Board of Health and Welfare [Sweden]) Uppdaterat Kunskapsstöd för Vård vid Könsdysfori hos Unga (Care of Children and Young People with Gender Dysphoria. National Knowledge Support with Recommendations to the Profession and Decision Makers. 2022. The National Board of Health and Welfare [Sweden]; 2022. Available from: www.socialstyrelsen.se/om-socialstyrelsen/pressrum/press/uppdaterat-kunskapsstod-for-vard-vid-konsdysfori-hos-unga

Case 48: Pyromania

Drawn by the fire

Varen is a 26-year-old volunteer firefighter recently detained for attempting to set fire to a bush by the police. He was referred to the clinic and expressed an internal conflict between his role as a firefighter and his inner desire to set fires. Varen's interest in fires started at a young age, and he would read news articles regarding wildfires and the heroic actions of firefighters who put them out. This led to his eventual interest in volunteering for the fire-fighting corp. Varen admits to fire setting on multiple occasions in the past, but they were usually done in a private setting, for example, he would set papers on fire and quickly extinguish it in his room. Prior to each act, there is a tension which builds up within him and it is released after the act of fire setting. This latest act of fire setting to the bush was done out of a morbid curiosity about the origins of wildfires and he expresses remorse over his actions.

- **Question 1: What is the diagnosis?**

- **Question 2: What other differential diagnoses should be considered?**

- **Question 3: How would you manage Varen's pyromania?**

Answers to Case 48

Question 1
What is the diagnosis?

Answer
Pyromania

Explanation

Diagnosis of pyromania [1]

1. The presentation is characterised by a recurrent failure to control strong impulses to set fires, resulting in multiple acts of, or attempts at, setting fire to property or other objects

2. There is a lack of apparent motive (e.g., monetary gain, revenge, sabotage, political statement, attracting recognition) for the acts of, or attempts at, fire setting

3. The individual exhibits persistent fascination or preoccupation with fire and related stimuli (e.g., watching fires, building fires, fascination with firefighting equipment)

4. The individual experiences increased tension or affective arousal prior to instances of, or attempts at, fire setting

5. The individual experiences pleasure, excitement, relief or gratification during and immediately following the act of setting the fire, and while witnessing its effects or participating in its aftermath

6. Acts of, or attempts at, fire setting are not better accounted for by a disorder of intellectual development, another mental disorder (e.g., a manic episode) or substance intoxication

Exam Essentials

*   Fire setting is a behaviour, whilst arson is a criminal offence, and pyromania is a psychiatric diagnosis

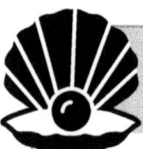

Clinical Pearls

*   Arson is often premeditated and motivated by revenge or financial gain. In pyromania, the acts are performed to achieve gratification, pleasure or relief without secondary gain

Question 2
What other differential diagnoses should be considered?

Answer

> Cognitive disorders: intellectual developmental disorder, major neurocognitive disorder
> Conduct disorder
> Personality disorder: antisocial personality disorder, borderline personality disorder
> Psychotic disorder
> Substance use disorder

Explanation

Fire setting due to other underlying psychiatric diagnoses should be screened for. Co-morbidities associated with pyromania include mood disorders, impulse control-related disorders and substance use disorder. Mood disorders and substance use tend to develop after symptoms of pyromania. Amongst patients suffering from pyromania, a third of patients have contemplated suicide to control their behaviours [2].

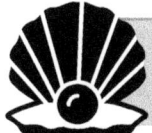

Clinical Pearls

- Pyromania is considered uncommon as compared to fire settings due to other underlying psychiatric diagnoses

Question 3
How would you manage Varen's pyromania?

Answer

> Psychotherapy: cognitive behavioural therapy (CBT), family therapy (in childhood and adolescence)
> Pharmacological options: selective serotonin reuptake inhibitors (SSRIs), atypical antipsychotics, lithium, valproate, carbamazepine or anti-androgens

Explanation

Data on the management of pyromania is limited and the majority of patients with pyromania lack motivation in treatment. Amongst various behavioural approaches, CBT appears to be the most promising [3]. Supervision to prevent a repeated episode of fire setting is often necessary and sometimes incarceration is required after such actions are repeated. Evidence for the choice of pharmacotherapy is limited to case reports.

Diving Deep ...

As fire setting is considered to be a civil crime, the distinction between arson and pyromania is important in the area of forensic psychiatry. Forensic psychiatrists often evaluate the mental state of the culprit by evaluating the motives for fire setting. The success rates of pleading not guilty by reason of insanity (NGRI) in cases of arson seem higher compared to other crimes. Most successful pleads come from offenders impaired by psychotic disorders, such as delusions or command hallucinations influencing their fire-setting behaviour. However, it is difficult for defendants to plead NGRI due to pyromania as the DSM 5-TR criteria state that pyromania is fire setting in the absence of delusional beliefs and impaired judgement. It would therefore be contradictory to plead NGRI secondary to pyromania.

References

1. World Health Organization. *International classification of diseases*, 11th edition (ICD-11). Geneva: World Health Organization; 2024. Available from: https://icd.who.int/en

2. Grant JE, Won Kim S. Clinical characteristics and psychiatric comorbidity of pyromania. *J Clin Psychiatry*. 2007 Nov;68(11):1717–22.

3. Boland RJ, Verduin ML, Ruiz P, Shah A, Sadock BJ, editors. *Kaplan & Sadock's synopsis of psychiatry*, 12th edition. Philadelphia: Wolters Kluwer; 2022.

Case 49: Kleptomania

Caught with your hand in the cookie jar

Savannah is a 25-year-old female who presents to your clinic after receiving a letter of warning from the police as she was caught stealing from a convenience store. She struggles to control her impulses to steal and admits having stolen various items from different shops starting a year ago. She works as a lawyer and recently joined a new firm shortly before these impulses began, and she is now worried that such offences will cause her to lose her job. Before each episode, there is a build-up of tension within her, leading to a feeling of restlessness. This tension is relieved when she pockets an item from a store. Examples of items stolen include an inexpensive pen, a plastic comb and stickers. This puzzles her as she is doing well financially and has no need to steal these items. Nonetheless, these incidents happen fortnightly and allow her to feel a sense of gratification afterwards. She is ashamed of her behaviour and is here to seek help.

- **Question 1: What is the diagnosis?**

- **Question 2: What other differentials should be considered?**

- **Question 3: What are some co-morbidities of kleptomania that you would screen for in Savanah?**

- **Question 4: How would you manage Savanah's kleptomania?**

Answers to Case 49

Question 1
What is the diagnosis?

Answer
Kleptomania

Explanation

Diagnosis of kleptomania [1]

1. The presentation is characterised by a recurrent failure to control strong impulses to steal objects

2. There is a lack of apparent motive for stealing objects (e.g., objects are not acquired for personal use or monetary gain)

3. The individual experiences increased tension or affective arousal prior to instances of theft or attempted theft

4. The individual experiences pleasure, excitement, relief or gratification during and immediately following the act of stealing

5. Acts of theft or attempted theft are not better accounted for by a disorder of intellectual development, another mental disorder (e.g., a manic episode) or substance intoxication

Exam Essentials

- The difference between kleptomania and theft lies in the underlying motivation. Theft is motivated by the item's monetary value and usefulness, whilst kleptomania often aims to relieve a tension build-up within the patient

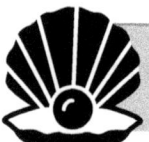

Clinical Pearls

- Kleptomania is difficult to diagnose, and clinicians need to have a high degree of caution in diagnosing it given its legal implications

Question 2
What other differentials should be considered?

Answer
Antisocial personality disorder
Conduct disorder

Mania
Psychotic disorder
Theft

Explanation

In patients with antisocial personality disorder or conduct disorder, there is a lack of guilt and remorse over the offences committed.

In patients with mania, impulsive behaviour is not limited to stealing and is usually accompanied by elevated mood symptoms.

Patients with psychotic disorders may be under the influence of a delusion or command auditory hallucination to steal items, and hence the underlying motivation is different and there is no gratification at the time of committing the theft. It is usually accompanied by other symptoms of psychosis.

In theft, the object stolen is the goal of the act, while in kleptomania, the act of stealing is the goal. In kleptomania, the act of stealing is unplanned, nor does it involve others.

Exam Essentials

- **Rule out the use of substances** that could potentially affect the individual's decision-making ability

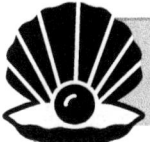

Clinical Pearls

- Individuals diagnosed with kleptomania typically commit multiple thefts. This necessitates a cautious and comprehensive evaluation of each act, as these individuals may also commit thefts that are not kleptomaniac in nature but are instead motivated by their co-morbidities or needs

Question 3

What are some co-morbidities of kleptomania that you would screen for in Savanah?

Answer

Major depressive disorder
Anxiety disorders

Obsessive–compulsive disorder (OCD)
Eating disorders
Gambling disorder
Substance use disorder

Explanation

Mood disorders (the majority being depression) and anxiety disorders are common life-time co-morbidities of patients with kleptomania. Other substance-related and addictive disorders include gambling disorder, substance use disorder (alcoholism) and compulsive shopping. Eating disorders are also a known co-morbid condition of kleptomania and stealing appears to be strongly associated with bulimic symptoms in patients [2].

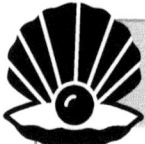

Clinical Pearls

- Individuals with kleptomania are often first referred for their co-morbid conditions rather than stealing

Question 4

How would you manage Savanah's kleptomania?

Answer

Psychotherapy options: insight-oriented psychotherapy, behavioural therapy
Pharmacological options: selective serotonin reuptake inhibitors (SSRIs)

Explanation

The choice of psychotherapy is highly dependent on the patient's motivation to change their behaviour. Insight-oriented psychotherapy targets behavioural change and is more effective in patients who feel guilt and shame over their actions. Behavioural therapy uses systematic desensitisation, aversive conditioning and a combination of aversive conditioning and altered social contingencies and has been reported to be beneficial regardless of patient motivation.

Instead of monotherapy with psychotherapy, combined therapy with pharmacological options is shown to have superior benefits. The use of SSRIs (e.g., fluoxetine and fluvoxamine) is indicated as it is postulated that such actions result from low levels of serotonin in the brain synapses.

Other medications (lithium, anti-epileptics, and naltrexone) and electroconvulsive therapy have been shown in case studies to be possibly useful in treating kleptomania [3, 4]

Diving Deep …

The severity of kleptomania is found to be dependent on two main factors [5]. One of the factors found to predict severe kleptomania included compulsivity, an element commonly seen in individuals who suffer from OCD and anorexia nervosa. The other was the sense of reward from stealing, where it is reported that severe kleptomaniacs tended to steal from family and partners. Such findings have clinical implications on management, as compulsivity could be managed with certain pharmacological agents such as naltrexone which can dampen urges.

References

1. World Health Organization. *International classification of diseases*, 11th edition (ICD-11). Geneva: World Health Organization; 2024. Available from: https://icd.who.int/en
2. Baum A, Goldner EM. The relationship between stealing and eating disorders: a review. *Harv Rev Psychiatry*. 1995 Nov;3(4):210–21.
3. Durst R, Katz G, Teitelbaum A, Zislin J, Dannon PN. Kleptomania: diagnosis and treatment options. *CNS Drugs*. 2001;15(3):185–95.
4. Grant JE. Understanding and treating kleptomania: new models and new treatments. *Isr J Psychiatry Relat Sci*. 2006;43(2):81–7.
5. Grant JE, Chamberlain SR. Symptom severity and its clinical correlates in kleptomania. *Ann Clin Psychiatry*. 2018 May;30(2):97–101.

Case 50: Child and Adolescent Mental Health Services

The growing years

Children and adolescents have different metabolism and social considerations compared to adults. Children are infrequently involved in the early phases of clinical trials because of the unpredictability of new medications and uncertain safety profiles, leading to the paediatric use of medications being inadequately researched and often unlicensed.

- **Question 1: What are the general guiding principles when prescribing medications in childhood and adolescence?**

Jane is a 12-year-old girl who was referred to the psychiatric clinic after her teachers noticed self-harm marks on her left wrist. Over the past two months, the teachers noticed she was withdrawn and quiet in school and no longer hung out with her friends. She has difficulty concentrating in class and struggles to pass her class tests. Jane has trouble falling asleep and feels tired most of the day. When you examine her, she has poor eye contact and appears reticent.

- **Question 2: What are the pharmacological considerations in the treatment of depression in childhood and adolescents?**

Jane was started on fluoxetine in the treatment of her depression and it reached remission. After 12 months, fluoxetine was gradually discontinued. Three years later at age 15, Jane presents to your clinic with a one-week duration of elevated mood, reduced need for sleep, increased energy, talkativeness and distractibility.

- **Question 3: What are the pharmacological considerations in the treatment of bipolar disorder in childhood and adolescents?**

Jane has a friend, Kyle, who was noted to be talking to himself recently. He reported feeling prosecuted by others and carrying a knife to defend himself. His parents have noticed that his room has become increasingly messy and his self-hygiene has been affected as well.

- **Question 4: What are the pharmacological considerations in the treatment of psychotic disorders in childhood and adolescence?**

Fiona is a 16-year-old girl who presents to the clinic with a six-month history of multiple worries concerning her day-to-day life. She finds it hard to control her worries and this leads to difficulties falling asleep. She has trouble concentrating in class and feels tired most of the day. She also complains of neck stiffness and tightness causing her to be irritable.

- **Question 5: What are the pharmacological considerations in the treatment of anxiety disorders in childhood and adolescence?**

Answers to Case 50

Question 1
What are the general guiding principles when prescribing medications in childhood and adolescence?

Answer

Target symptoms, not diagnoses
Informed use of off-label licensed medicine
Start at a low dose and go slow, monitoring for efficacy and adverse reactions
Multiple medications may be required for the severely ill
Allow time for an adequate trial of treatment
Where possible, change one drug at a time
Monitor outcomes in more than one social setting
Patient and family medication education is essential

Explanation

Establishing a diagnosis can be difficult in children, and co-morbidity is very common; therefore, targeting key symptoms should be the treatment aim. Physicians are responsible for ensuring adequate information to support the safety and efficacy of medications before prescribing them to children. Compared to adults, the starting doses for children are usually lower as children are more sensitive to adverse reactions and may achieve therapeutic effects at a lower dose. While monotherapy is ideal, if the childhood-onset illness is severe, it may require treatment with psychosocial approaches combined with more than one medication. Children are generally more ill than adults and often require longer treatment before a response is seen. Medications should be changed one at a time,

411

and attempts to reduce polypharmacy should be made. The expression of symptoms may vary across different social settings (e.g., home and school), so a thorough history should be conducted. Children and their parents should be educated on medications' indications, benefits and side effects to improve adherence and long-term outcomes.

Question 2

What are the pharmacological considerations in the treatment of depression in childhood and adolescents?

Answer

The following pharmacological recommendations are from the Maudsley guidelines [1]:

First line: fluoxetine

Second line: sertraline or citalopram

Third line: escitalopram

Fourth line: augmentation with second-generation antipsychotics (SGAs) or lithium or mirtazapine

Paroxetine and tricyclics are not recommended in child and adolescent mental health services

Explanation

The United Kingdom's National Institute for Health and Care Excellence (NICE) clinical guidelines [2] support the use of selective serotonin reuptake inhibitors (SSRIs) but only in combination with psychological therapy. A Cochrane review in 2012 [3] found limited evidence that combination therapy is more effective than antidepressant medication alone.

Fluoxetine is superior to placebo in children and adolescents and, on its own in addition to routine clinical care, is effective in treating moderate to severe depression. Fluoxetine is initiated at a lower dose of 10 mg daily and can be increased to 20 mg one week later to achieve a minimum effective dosage. Fluoxetine should be continued for at least 6 and up to 12 months to reduce the risk of relapse. Side effects of tricyclic antidepressants in child and adolescent mental health services include relatively increased cardiotoxicity, orthostatic hypotension, vertigo, dry mouth and tremors.

While treatment-emergent suicidal thoughts and acts are possible in adults younger than 25 years [4–7], the risk of untreated depression is greater, with the US Treatment of Adolescents with Depression Study showing combined treatment with fluoxetine and cognitive behavioural therapy (CBT) reduced the risk of suicidal events to the greatest extent [8]. In addition, while increased suicidal ideations were noted, no completed suicides occurred during any of the trials.

Exam Essentials

- When prescribing antidepressants in child and adolescent mental health services, the dose should be increased slowly to minimise the risk of treatment-emergent agitation and suicidal thoughts and acts

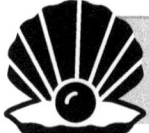

Clinical Pearls

- Between 20% and 40% of children and adolescents treated with antidepressants for depression may develop bipolar affective disorder [9]

- Symptoms suggestive of underlying bipolar disorder in depressed children:
    - Non-episodic, chronic and mixed manic states
    - Hypersomnia
    - May have a co-morbidity of conduct disorder or oppositional defiant disorder
    - Quick initial improvement in symptoms before worsening*
    - Increased irritability*
    - Increased mood lability*
    - Worsening anxiety*

* When on antidepressant.

Question 3
What are the pharmacological considerations in the treatment of bipolar disorder in childhood and adolescents?

Answer
First line: SGAs (e.g., aripiprazole, olanzapine, quetiapine, risperidone, asenapine)

Second line: mood stabilisers (e.g., lithium, can be added after the failure of two trials of an SGA)

In the treatment of bipolar depression, an olanzapine/fluoxetine combination, quetiapine or lurasidone can be used as the first-line treatment

Explanation

The NICE guidelines [10] suggest SGAs as the first-line treatment of hypomania and mania. Height and weight should be measured at each visit and fasting blood tests repeated at three months and subsequently every six months. Most medication trials are between three and five weeks, with a complete absence of response at one to two weeks prompting a switch to another SGA. Children are more sensitive to adverse side effects and SGAs seem to produce significantly greater weight gain and somnolence as compared to adults.

For maintenance treatment, lithium can be initiated early in the course of treatment, either as monotherapy prophylaxis or as an adjunct to a successful acute medication.

Exam Essentials

- The use of structured instrument assessment, such as the Young Mania Rating Scale [11], and mood/sleep diaries can be helpful in diagnosis

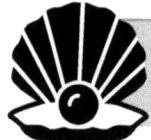

Clinical Pearls

- Valproate should be avoided in females of childbearing age because of the risk of teratogenicity and polycystic ovary syndrome

- Males under age 55 looking to conceive should not be prescribed valproate either! Refer to Case 6 for more elaboration

Question 4
What are the pharmacological considerations in the treatment of psychotic disorders in childhood and adolescence?

Answer
First line: SGAs
First-generation antipsychotics (FGAs) should generally be avoided in children
Medications should be initiated at the lower end of, or below the adult range

Explanation
FGAs should generally be avoided in children because of higher rates of extrapyramidal symptoms, sedation and tardive dyskinesia.

SGAs have been shown to be effective in the treatment of psychosis in early-onset schizophrenia-spectrum disorders.

The NICE guidelines [12] recommend the use of oral antipsychotics with family interventions and individual CBT. All antipsychotics carry a relative increased risk of raised prolactin, sedation, weight gain and metabolic effects in children compared to adults. There is comparable efficacy amongst SGAs except for ziprasidone (inferior efficacy) and asenapine (unclear efficacy). Clozapine is effective in treatment-resistant psychosis in adolescents.

Question 5
What are the pharmacological considerations in the treatment of anxiety disorders in childhood and adolescence?

Answer
  SSRIs are the first-line medications for the treatment of anxiety disorders in children and adolescents
  A different SSRI can be trialled if the first one is ineffective
  Serotonin–noradrenaline reuptake inhibitors are a third-line treatment when two trials of different SSRIs are ineffective
  When prescribing medications, start at the lowest available dose and increase slowly as tolerated

Explanation
There are no significant differences amongst SSRIs in treating anxiety disorders in children and adolescents. The Childhood/Adolescent Anxiety Multimodal Study [13] showed that sertraline monotherapy (55% response) is as effective as CBT (60% response) for anxiety, compared with placebo (24% response). This study also showed that sertraline combined with CBT is most likely to be successful (81% response). If SSRIs are well tolerated, their dose can be increased weekly to the minimal therapeutic dose. A similar dose to adults is required when treating anxiety with SSRIs as there is a faster metabolism in children. A response should appear within six to eight weeks of treatment. Treatment should be continued for at least one year with stable improvement. Buspirone and mirtazapine might be effective in treating young people with anxiety disorders, although this is only based on open-label studies [14, 15].

Baseline severity should be measured with structured interviews or questionnaires before and repeated after starting treatment.

Benzodiazepines should not be routinely prescribed to children. Their use may lead to paradoxical disinhibition in some children in addition to their addictive side effects. However, they are sometimes employed during the initial titration of SSRIs to mitigate adverse effects or to potentiate therapeutic effects.

In preschool children, psychotherapy is the first line of treatment over medications.

Exam Essentials

- Anxiety disorders often begin in childhood and adolescence, and these are the most common psychiatric disorders in this age group

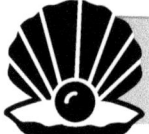

Clinical Pearls

- Exclude mimics of anxiety disorders (e.g., restlessness in attention deficit hyperactivity disorder)
- For children with anxiety, low-dose hydroxyzine may be given at intervals to alleviate anxiety (e.g., 10 mg every eight hours)

Diving Deep ...

In the approach to agitation in children and adolescents, the physician should attempt verbal de-escalation techniques first and oral medications second if these fail. Parenteral treatment such as rapid tranquilisation should be used as a last resort. If required, the NICE guidelines recommend giving intramuscular lorazepam. Care should be taken when giving high-potency antipsychotic medication (such as haloperidol), especially in antipsychotic naïve patients, because of the risks of acute dystonic reactions. If intramuscular haloperidol is given, a parenteral cholinergic medication should be given together, and an ECG performed.

References

1. Taylor DM, Barnes TRE, Young A. *The Maudsley prescribing guidelines in psychiatry*, 14th edition. Chichester Hoboken, NJ: Wiley Blackwell; 2021.

2. National Institute for Health and Care Excellence (NICE). Depression in children and young people: identification and management. Clinical guidance [CG28]. NICE; 2017. Available from: www.nice.org.uk/guidance/CG28

3. Cox GR, Callahan P, Churchill R, Hunot V, Merry SN, Parker AG, et al. Psychological therapies versus antidepressant medication, alone and in combination for depression in children and adolescents. *Cochrane Database Syst Rev.* 2012; CD008324.pub2. Available from: https://doi.wiley.com/10.1002/14651858.CD008324.pub2

4. Healy D. Lines of evidence on the risks of suicide with selective serotonin reuptake inhibitors. *Psychother Psychosom.* 2003;72(2):71–9.

5. Whittington CJ, Kendall T, Fonagy P, Cottrell D, Cotgrove A, Boddington E. Selective serotonin reuptake inhibitors in childhood depression: systematic review of published versus unpublished data. *Lancet.* 2004 Apr 24;363(9418):1341–5.

6. Jureidini JN, Doecke CJ, Mansfield PR, Haby MM, Menkes DB, Tonkin AL. Efficacy and safety of antidepressants for children and adolescents. *BMJ.* 2004 Apr 10;328(7444):879–83.

7. Kafali N, Progovac A, Hou SSY, Cook BL. Long-run trends in antidepressant use among youths after the FDA black box warning. *Psychiatr Serv.* 2018 Apr 1;69(4):389–95.

8. March JS, Silva S, Petrycki S, Curry J, Wells K, Fairbank J, et al. The Treatment for Adolescents With Depression Study (TADS): long-term effectiveness and safety outcomes. *Arch Gen Psychiatry.* 2007 Oct;64(10):1132–43. Erratum in *Arch Gen Psychiatry.* 2008 Jan;65(1):101.

9. Geller B, Fox LW, Clark KA. Rate and predictors of prepubertal bipolarity during follow-up of 6- to 12-year-old depressed children. *J Am Acad Child Adolesc Psychiatry.* 1994 May;33(4):461–8.

10. National Institute for Health and Care Excellence (NICE). Bipolar disorder: assessment and management: Clinical guidance [CG185]. NICE; 2016. Available from: www.nice .org.uk/guidance/cg185

11. Young RC, Biggs JT, Ziegler VE, Meyer DA. A rating scale for mania: reliability, validity and sensitivity. *Br J Psychiatry.* 1978 Nov;133:429–35.

12. NICE. Psychosis and schizophrenia in children and young people: recognition and management. Clinical guidance [CG155]. NICE; 2016. Available from: www.nice.org .uk/guidance/cg155.

13. Compton SN, Walkup JT, Albano AM, Piacentini JC, Birmaher B, Sherrill JT, et al. Child/Adolescent Anxiety Multimodal Study (CAMS): rationale, design, and methods. *Child Adolesc Psychiatry Ment Health.* 2010 Jan 5;4:1.

14. Buitelaar JK, van der Gaag RJ, van der Hoeven J. Buspirone in the management of anxiety and irritability in children with pervasive developmental disorders: results of an open-label study. *J Clin Psychiatry.* 1998 Feb;59(2):56–9.

15. Mrakotsky C, Masek B, Biederman J, Raches D, Hsin O, Forbes P, et al. Prospective open-label pilot trial of mirtazapine in children and adolescents with social phobia. *J Anxiety Disord.* 2008;22(1):88–97.

Case 51: Old Age Psychiatry

The silver years

In the geriatric population, medical and psychiatric conditions often exist concurrently. This results in the possibility of polypharmacy and increased drug interactions. Moreover, the physiological effects of ageing coupled with co-morbid medical conditions result in altered pharmacokinetics and pharmacodynamics of medications.

- **Question 1: What are the general guiding principles when prescribing medications in the older population?**

Robert is a 78-year-old gentleman who is known to the psychiatric clinic for a major neurocognitive disorder secondary to Alzheimer's disease. In the past two months, Robert has been refusing to take his memantine and other medications, such as furosemide for congestive cardiac failure complicated by fluid overload. His wife is concerned over his refusal to take medications and has been secretly putting medications in his food.

- **Question 2: What are the considerations when it comes to covert administration of medicines?**

Apart from a major neurocognitive disorder due to Alzheimer's disease, Robert has multiple other physical medical conditions, including chronic urinary incontinence and back pain.

- **Question 3: What are the pharmacological considerations when treating physical conditions in patients with neurocognitive disorders?**

Robert's wife recounts that before the onset of his dementia, Robert had an episode lasting three months where he was withdrawn, lethargic, had poor sleep, decreased appetite and complained of abdominal pains and headaches.

- **Question 4: How does the presentation of depressive disorder differ in the elderly compared to younger adults?**

Answers to Case 51

Question 1
What are the general guiding principles when prescribing medications in the older population?

Answer
> Due to altered pharmacodynamics, receptors may become more sensitive and elderly patients may be more prone to adverse side effects
> Start with a low dose and titrate upwards slowly
> Therapeutic responses may take longer to achieve as compared to younger adults
> A slower onset of action may occur
> There may be a longer duration of action for some fat-soluble drugs (e.g., diazepam), higher concentrations of some drugs at the site of action (e.g., digoxin) and increased amounts of active 'free drug' normally bound to albumin (e.g., phenytoin)
> Declining hepatic and renal function may affect the clearance of certain drugs in the elderly, and dosages need to be adjusted accordingly
> Aim to reduce polypharmacy and choose better-tolerated alternative medications
> Consider liquid preparations for those who cannot swallow tablets

Explanation
Response to central nervous system-active drugs (e.g., benzodiazepines and opioids) can be exaggerated in the elderly. As gut motility and secretion of gastric acid decrease with age, the absorption rate of drugs slows despite the same amount being taken up. Older adults have more body fat, less body water and less albumin than younger adults. While liver size is reduced in the elderly, metabolic clearance is largely preserved in the absence of hepatic diseases. Renal function declines with age and is affected by co-morbid medical conditions.

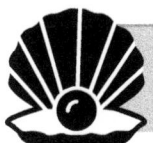

Clinical Pearls

- Start 'low' (dose) and go 'slow' (titrate slowly)

Question 2
What are the considerations when it comes to covert administration of medicines?

Answer
The mental capacity of the patient regarding treatment should first be assessed. If mental capacity is retained, patients have the right to refuse treatment even if it is against medical recommendation. If the patient has been deemed to have no mental capacity, treatment may be given in the patient's best interests after weighing the risk–benefit ratio.

Explanation
Any covert treatment administered must be life-saving, prevent deterioration in health or ensure an improvement in physical or mental health [1]. A best interests meeting should be held between the multidisciplinary team and relatives of the patients, and the outcome clearly documented in the patient's records. A clear management plan should be in place regarding how the covert medication is given and when its use will be next reviewed.

Exam Essentials

- The United Kingdom legal framework covering the covert administration of medications falls under the **Mental Capacity Act** or the **Mental Health Act**

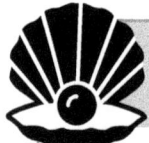

Clinical Pearls

- The relationship between the patient and caregiver may be disrupted if the patient discovers about the covert medicine administration. This is especially so if the patient has underlying paranoia

Question 3
What are the pharmacological considerations when treating physical conditions in patients with neurocognitive disorders?

Answer
As patients with neurocognitive disorder are more prone to cognitive adverse effects, physicians should be mindful of medications that may affect cognition through cholinergic, histaminergic or opioid neurotransmitter pathways. Some medications may also

have drug interactions with existing cognitive-enhancing medications, affecting their metabolism.

Explanation
Anticholinergic drugs can cause sedation, cognitive impairment, delirium and falls. If withdrawal is planned, the medication should be discontinued gradually to avoid rebound (e.g., nausea, diarrhoea, urinary frequency).

Dopamine D2 receptor antagonism (e.g., metoclopramide and prochlorperazine), can produce dystonic reactions or extrapyramidal side effects.

Opiates carry the risk of sedation, falls and delirium. Pethidine is an opiate, and its metabolites have anticholinergic properties, resulting in a high risk of cognitive impairment.

First-generation H1 antihistamines (e.g., hydroxyzine) are non-selective and readily penetrate the blood brain barrier (BBB) leading to impaired cognitive and psychomotor performance and can trigger seizures, dyskinesia, dystonia and hallucinations. Second-generation H1 antihistamines penetrate poorly through the BBB and are a safer alternative.

Exam Essentials

- Refer to Case 21 for elaboration on the **black box warning for antipsychotic use in elderly patients with dementia** [2, 3]. There is a higher risk of mortality and possibly stroke

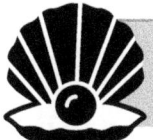

Clinical Pearls

- Always perform a medication reconciliation to identify medications that can potentially cause drug–drug interactions and adverse effects

Question 4
How does the presentation of depressive disorder differ in the elderly compared to younger adults?

Answer
In the elderly, there is an increased emphasis on somatic complaints, anxiety and melancholic features, such as hypochondriasis, low self-esteem, feelings of worthlessness,

guilt, paranoia and suicidal ideations. Psychomotor agitation and neglect may also be seen more commonly in the elderly. Cognitive impairment in depressed elderly patients may be confused with neurocognitive disorders. It is important to ascertain the temporal sequence of symptoms to differentiate the conditions. Delusions of nihilism, poverty and guilt may also be seen in psychotic depression.

Explanation

Risk factors for depression include being widowed and having chronic medical illnesses. Pseudodementia occurs in about 15% of elderly patients with depression and 25–50% of patients with neurocognitive disorders are depressed [4]. Elderly persons are at a higher risk of suicide than other demographic groups, with white men age 85 or older having the highest rate of completed suicide (55 per 100,000 standard population) [5]. Elderly patients with significant medical illnesses or recent losses should be evaluated for depression and suicidal ideations.

A meta-analysis showed a response rate of 51% to antidepressants in older patients, which is similar to that for the adult population [6]. Electroconvulsive therapy is generally safe with no absolute contraindications, even in elderly patients who may have other medical co-morbidity, and it has been shown to improve cognitive outcomes in elderly patients with pseudodementia from depression [7].

Exam Essentials

- Refer to Case 3 on major depressive disorder for differentiating pseudodementia from real dementia

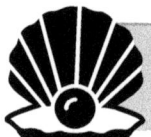

Clinical Pearls

- Elderly patients often complain of constipation and abdominal symptoms. Excessive ruminations regarding these issues may be early signs of depression

- However, if there is severe loss of appetite and weight with multiple physical complaints, it is still paramount to thoroughly investigate and rule out underlying malignancy

Diving Deep …

The National Institute of Mental Health's Epidemiologic Catchment Area study [8] showed that the most common mental disorders in the elderly are cognitive disorders, depressive disorders, phobias and alcohol use disorders. The psychosocial risk factors that predispose the elderly to mental health disorders include loss of social roles, loss of autonomy, loss of friends and family, isolation, chronic medical issues, financial issues and decreased cognitive functioning. Spousal bereavement is a significant life experience, which results in depressive symptoms that peak within the first six months after death but decline after [9].

References

1. Haw C, Stubbs J. Administration of medicines in food and drink: a study of older inpatients with severe mental illness. *Int Psychogeriatr.* 2010 May;22(3):409–16.

2. Kuehn BM. FDA warns antipsychotic drugs may be risky for elderly. *JAMA.* 2005 May 25;293(20):2462.

3. Atypical antipsychotics in the elderly. *Med Lett Drugs Ther.* 2005 Aug 1;47(1214):61–2.

4. Boland RJ, Verduin ML, Ruiz P, Shah A, Sadock BJ, editors. *Kaplan & Sadock's synopsis of psychiatry*, 12th edition. Philadelphia: Wolters Kluwer; 2022.

5. Hoyert DL, Kochanek KD, Murphy SL. Deaths: final data for 1997. *Natl Vital Stat Rep.* 1999 Jun 30;47(19):1–104.

6. Gutsmiedl K, Krause M, Bighelli I, Schneider-Thoma J, Leucht S. How well do elderly patients with major depressive disorder respond to antidepressants: a systematic review and single-group meta-analysis. *BMC Psychiatry.* 2020 Mar 4;20(1):102.

7. Tielkes CEM, Comijs HC, Verwijk E, Stek ML. The effects of ECT on cognitive functioning in the elderly: a review. *Int J Geriatr Psychiatry.* 2008 Aug;23(8):789–95.

8. Eaton WW, Regier DA, Locke BZ, Taube CA. The Epidemiologic Catchment Area Program of the National Institute of Mental Health. *Public Health Rep.* 1981;96(4):319–25.

9. Hung YC, Chen YH, Lee MC, Yeh CJ. Effect of spousal loss on depression in older adults: impacts of time passing, living arrangement, and spouse's health status before death. *Int J Environ Res Public Health.* 2021 Dec 10;18(24):13032.

Case 52: Pregnancy and Breastfeeding

New Beginnings

Pregnancy is an exciting but stressful period of a woman's life, with all mothers hoping for a smooth delivery and birth of a healthy child. However, spontaneous abortions occur in 10–20% of confirmed early pregnancies, and the risk of spontaneous major malformation is 2–3% [1]. Additionally, psychiatric illness during pregnancy is an independent risk factor for congenital malformations, stillbirths and neonatal deaths.

- **Question 1: What are the general guiding principles when prescribing medications to pregnant women?**

Karen is a 28-year-old lady who is currently on sertraline for major depressive disorder. She responded to sertraline and her symptoms began to remit after a few months. On a follow-up visit one year later, Karen presents to you with a positive urine pregnancy test after having missed her period.

- **Question 2: What are the considerations concerning psychotropic use during pregnancy?**

- **Question 3: She expresses concerns over the use of antidepressants during pregnancy. What side effects should be counselled for women taking selective serotonin reuptake inhibitors (SSRIs) during pregnancy?**

After much discussion, Karen decided to stop her sertraline, and it was gradually tapered off. Her pregnancy was uneventful, and she delivered her child with no complications. Four weeks later, she comes for her follow-up appointment and reports persistent daily low mood for the past two weeks. This was associated with poor sleep, loss of appetite and a general lack of energy. This lack of energy is profound, and she reports an inability to find the strength to get out of bed; this can last for hours at a time. Karen breaks down and confesses feelings of inadequacy as a mother. Her husband similarly expresses concerns that her mood has been more labile lately, often finding her in tears.

- **Question 4: What is the likely diagnosis, and what are the differentials?**

Having diagnosed Karen with post-natal depression, you plan to restart her on sertraline. However, she is keen to continue breastfeeding her baby and would like to know how her baby may be affected.

- **Question 5: How would you counsel Karen on the decision to restart sertraline while planning to breastfeed?**

A different pregnant patient, Renée, presents to your clinic. She was noted to have elevated mood, flight of ideas, increased talkativeness, distractibility and grandiose ideas that she has been granted the ability to see the future. Reneé was diagnosed with bipolar disorder.

- **Question 6: What are the general guiding principles when prescribing mood-stabilising medications to pregnant women?**

In selecting a suitable psychotropic for the treatment of her bipolar disorder, Reneé asks about the safety profile of mood stabilisers should she choose to breastfeed post-partum.

- **Question 7: What are the general guiding principles when prescribing mood-stabilising medications to women who are breastfeeding?**

Having considered the potential side effects of mood stabilisers, a joint decision was made to start Reneé on an antipsychotic for its mood-stabilising properties instead of the earlier discussed mood stabilisers.

- **Question 8: What are the general guiding principles when prescribing antipsychotics to women who are pregnant?**

- **Question 9: How would you advise Renée on the use of antipsychotics while breastfeeding?**

Answers to Case 52

Question 1
What are the general guiding principles when prescribing medications to pregnant women?

Answer
First-trimester exposure carries the greatest risk for major malformation
Third-trimester exposure carries the greatest risk for neonatal toxicity
Use the lowest effective dose
Use the medication with the lowest known risk to the mother and fetus
Avoid polypharmacy as much as possible
Doses require adjustment as pregnancy progresses
Manage under specialist perinatal services if possible
Ensure adequate fetal screening
Monitor the neonate for withdrawal effects after birth

Explanation
Due to the nature of pregnancy and the caution surrounding it, there is a dearth of robust, prospective clinical trials, limiting the available data on the safety and efficacy of psychotropic drugs in pregnancy. Organogenesis occurs in the first trimester, which results in a higher risk of malformation when drugs are used. Serum medication levels often decrease in the third trimester as the mother's blood volume expands by around 30% and hepatic enzyme activity increases [2]. Regular plasma level monitoring throughout pregnancy can be helpful in dose titration. The neonate should be monitored for toxicity in the third trimester and withdrawal effects after birth.

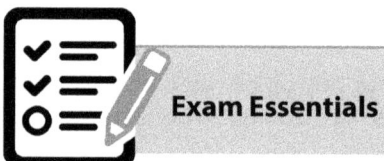

Exam Essentials

• First-trimester exposure carries the greatest risk for major malformation

Question 2
What are the considerations concerning psychotropic use during pregnancy?

Answer
Considerations include:

- Maternal factors

  ◦ Response to non-pharmacological interventions
  ◦ Risk of sudden termination of treatment resulting in a relapse
  ◦ The severity of and risk associated with previous episodes
  ◦ Response to current or past treatments

- Fetal factors

  ° The impact of an untreated mental disorder on the fetus or infant
  ° Risk to the fetus due to direct side effects of medication
  ° Increased risk of harm to the fetus associated with exposure to breastmilk which may contain the drug

Explanation

Major depressive disorder and anxiety are the most common mental health problems during pregnancy, with approximately 12% of women experiencing depression and 13% experiencing anxiety at some point [3]. The use of psychotropics in the first trimester risks major malformation, while use in the third trimester risks neonatal toxicity.

In this case, Karen is already on a regular antidepressant, therefore consideration of her previous episodes and assessment of risk is paramount as abrupt discontinuation of treatment may lead to relapse and more harm than if she were continued on effective drug therapy. One study found that 68% of women who were well on antidepressant treatment and stopped during pregnancy relapsed, compared with 26% who continued antidepressants [4].

If the patient is not keen on pharmacological treatment, psychotherapy (either cognitive behavioural therapy (CBT) or interpersonal psychotherapy) has been proven to be effective in the treatment of perinatal depression.

Exam Essentials

- Major depressive disorder and anxiety are the most common mental health problems during pregnancy

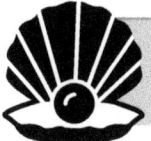

Clinical Pearls

- While mothers may worry about psychotropic use during pregnancy, insufficient medications leading to relapse may ultimately result in poor maternal–baby bonding and more psychotropics being used for stabilisation in future

Question 3

She expresses concerns over the use of antidepressants during pregnancy. What side effects should be counselled for women taking SSRIs during pregnancy?

Answer

Although rare, some side effects include [5]:

- Increased risk of post-partum haemorrhage

- Decreased gestational age (usually a few days)

- Decreased birth weight

- Increased risk of persistent pulmonary hypertension of the newborn when taken in late pregnancy

- Third-trimester use may result in discontinuation symptoms in the neonate, which are usually mild

Explanation

SSRIs are the most commonly prescribed antidepressants in pregnant women. SSRIs appear not to be major teratogens, except for paroxetine [6]. SSRIs do not appear to increase the risk of stillbirth or neonatal mortality. The pregnancy outcomes observed for the different SSRI drugs are comparable, suggesting a class effect of the SSRI drugs.

Treatment of mood disorders with medications may be clinically indicated despite the potential side effects listed, as the risks of untreated post-natal depression outweigh the adverse effects of SSRIs. Untreated post-natal depression increases risks of impaired maternal–infant interactions and suboptimal parenting practices such as reduced talking and reading to children and harsh punishment [7]. It is also associated with cognitive impairment in the infant, including general cognitive performance and executive functioning, intelligence and language development.

Most antidepressants are United States Food and Drug Administration (FDA) pregnancy risk category C, except for paroxetine and nortriptyline, which are in category D.

Exam Essentials

- Sertraline appears to result in the least placental exposure and is a common first-choice medication [8]

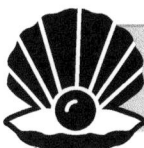

Clinical Pearls

- Paroxetine has been specifically associated with cardiac malformations (ventricular and atrial septal defects) and pulmonary hypertension, and hence should be avoided

Question 4
What is the likely diagnosis, and what are the differentials?

Answer
Post-natal depression (major depressive disorder with peripartum onset)
Differentials include post-natal blues and post-partum psychosis

Explanation
Karen fulfils the criteria for post-natal depression, and the course of illness is consistent with the diagnosis. In post-natal depression (DSM-5-TR: major depressive disorder with peripartum onset), the specifier is given if the onset of mood symptoms occurs during pregnancy or in the four weeks following delivery. Depressive episodes peak three to four weeks post-partum.

Risk factors for post-partum depression include:

- Being single
- Older age
- History of depression
- Family history of depression
- Poor social support
- Other psychosocial stressors

The main differentials to consider are:

- Post-natal blues (baby blues): usually presents with less than two weeks of symptoms
- Post-partum psychosis (puerperal psychosis): although up to 80% of patients present with prominent affective symptoms [9], Karen did not present with any psychotic features, making this diagnosis unlikely

The following psychosocial aspects are important for post-natal issues:

- Planned or unplanned pregnancy
- Number of children and ability to manage

429

- Any problems during pregnancy (e.g., severe morning sickness)
- Complications of pregnancy (use of forceps versus caesarean section, etc.)
- The health of the infant (any illness or malformation)
- Relationship with partner
- Financial issues
- Availability of social support

Risk factors for post-partum psychosis include:

- Personal history of schizophrenia, schizoaffective or bipolar disorder
- Previous post-partum psychosis
- Family history of post-partum psychosis
- Obstetric complications
- Single parenthood
- Poor social support

Unique symptoms of post-partum psychosis include:

- Affective lability
- Perplexity
- Cognitive issues
- Disorientation

Exam Essentials

- Features distinguishing post-natal blues and post-natal depression:
    - Symptoms worsening or persisting beyond two weeks in post-natal depression
    - Presence of suicidal ideations in post-natal depression
    - Functional impairment in post-natal depression

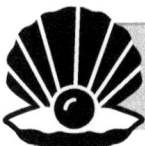

Clinical Pearls

- Always ask about thoughts of self-harm or harm to the baby, especially neglect and abuse of the baby, and possible thoughts of harm to the partner

- Rating scales such as the self-rated Edinburgh Postnatal Depression Scale [10] for post-partum women can be used to screen for post-natal depression

Question 5
How would you counsel Karen on the decision to restart sertraline while planning to breastfeed?

Answer
With some notable exceptions, most psychotropic drugs can be continued in breastfeeding women because of the benefits of breastfeeding to the baby and the lack of evidence of harm for most drugs. Sertraline is a suitable antidepressant for women who plan to breastfeed.

Explanation
As many as 81% of women in the United Kingdom breastfeed their infants [11]. It is usually advisable to continue the antidepressant prescribed during pregnancy or to restart the previously effective medication. Switching drugs post-partum for breastfeeding is usually not advisable.

In Karen's case, sertraline was previously effective, and sertraline is also known to have undetectable or low infant plasma concentration levels, making it a suitable antidepressant in treating post-natal depression. Maternal use of sertraline is not associated with adverse effects in breastfeeding infants [12]. Sertraline is in Dr Hale's lactation risk category L2.

Antidepressants are excreted in varying degrees in breast milk. For instance, fluoxetine's long half-life and potential for accumulation in breast milk have prompted some recommendations to avoid its use in women who are breastfeeding young infants.

The 'pump-and-dump' method (discarding expressed breastmilk close to the time of medication administration) or formula milk feeding are alternatives for breastfeeding mothers concerned about the breastmilk's drug concentration for the baby.

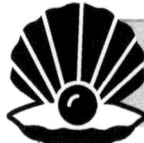

Clinical Pearls

- When initiating an antidepressant post-partum, sertraline or mirtazapine may be considered
- It is usually advisable to continue the drug that has shown effectiveness

Question 6

What are the general guiding principles when prescribing mood-stabilising medications to pregnant women?

Answer

In women who have been stable without relapse, consider switching to a safer medication (e.g., an antipsychotic)

If the risk of relapse is high or symptoms severe, consider continuing the existing mood stabilisers after discussing the fetal risks with close support from a multidisciplinary team

Discontinuing medications should be done gradually to avoid relapse during and after pregnancy

Lithium should be avoided in pregnancy, if possible

Carbamazepine and valproate should almost always be avoided. Valproate should be avoided in females of child-bearing age

Electroconvulsive therapy can be considered if pharmacotherapy is ineffective in acute mania

In bipolar depression in pregnancy, consider using CBT for moderate depression and an SSRI for more severe depression. Lamotrigine is safer than carbamazepine and valproate and can be a treatment option.

Explanation

The United Kingdom's National Institute for Health and Care Excellence (NICE) guidelines [3] recommend the use of mood-stabilising antipsychotics over mood stabilisers due to their safer side-effect profile.

Lithium completely equilibrates across the placenta and has been known to cause the cardiac malformation of Ebstein's anomaly in the fetus, with a 20-fold relative increased risk of this abnormality [13]. While the overall risk of congenital malformations was twice as great in exposure, the increase in absolute risk of congenital abnormalities (7 per 1,000) is considered small. Other fetal side effects include neonatal goitre, hypotonia, lethargy and cardiac arrhythmias.

However, if lithium is the best medication for the patient, she should be advised of the increased risk but supported to continue lithium with regular high-resolution ultrasound and echocardiography performed in liaison with fetal medicine obstetric services.

Both carbamazepine and valproate have a clear causal link with various fetal abnormalities, particularly neural tube defects, including spina bifida. Valproate carries a 10% higher risk of neural tube defects than carbamazepine and causes atrial septal defects, cleft palate, hypospadias, polydactyly, craniosynostosis and motor and neurodevelopmental problems [14–16]. There is also a 40% risk of long-term cognitive difficulties in children exposed to it during pregnancy [5].

Exam Essentials

- Refer to Case 2 on delusional disorder for more information on psychosis and pregnancy and breastfeeding

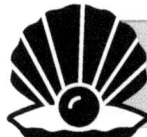

Clinical Pearls

- Lithium has been known to cause cardiac malformation of Ebstein's anomaly in the fetus

Question 7
What are the general guiding principles when prescribing mood-stabilising medications to women who are breastfeeding?

Answer
The effective medication that has been used during pregnancy should be continued during breastfeeding, except lithium. Carbamazepine, lamotrigine and valproate are generally safe to use while breastfeeding.

If initiation of a medication is required, consider a mood-stabilising antipsychotic such as olanzapine or quetiapine.

Explanation
The NICE guidelines [3] recommend that women on lithium should avoid breastfeeding. Breastfeeding while on lithium has been associated with early feeding problems, hypotonia, lethargy and lithium toxicity with raised creatinine.

Quetiapine and olanzapine plasma concentrations in infants are undetectable or minimal despite maternal breastfeeding and they are generally safe.

433

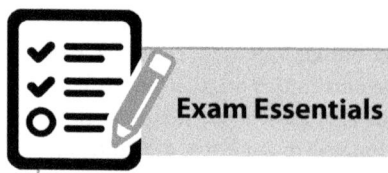

Exam Essentials

- For patients not on psychotropics, consider a mood-stabilising antipsychotic

Question 8
What are the general guiding principles when prescribing antipsychotics to women who are pregnant?

Answer
Pregnant women who are stable on an antipsychotic and are at risk of relapse without it should be advised to continue the antipsychotic under close monitoring. Switching antipsychotics risks a relapse and is generally not advised.

First-generation antipsychotics (FGAs) and second-generation antipsychotics (SGAs) are unlikely to be major teratogens. Antipsychotics, as a class, carry a 15% risk of anti-psychotic discontinuation symptoms in neonates when used in the third trimester [17]. Antipsychotics increase the risk of maternal weight gain and SGA use in pregnancy is associated with gestational diabetes. FGAs carry a higher risk of pre-term birth and low birth weight compared to SGAs or no antipsychotic exposure. FGAs have also been associated with neonatal dyskinesia and neonatal jaundice. SGA use in pregnancy was associated with increased birth weight and a modestly increased risk of cardiac septal defects (although the study mentioned screening bias or co-exposure to SSRIs).

Clozapine appears to present no increased risk of malformation, although there is a higher risk of gestational diabetes and neonatal seizures.

Explanation
The following antipsychotics have the most reproductive safety data available: quetia-pine, olanzapine, risperidone and haloperidol, with more limited data for clozapine, aripiprazole and ziprasidone. Women on antipsychotics should give birth in a unit that has access to paediatric intensive care facilities for closer monitoring if required. Psychiatric stability is crucial as, during a relapse, the fetus may ultimately be exposed to greater concentrations of antipsychotics if multiple drugs and higher doses are required to reach stability.

Symptoms of discontinuation syndrome include, for example, crying, agitation and increased suckling. Mixed (breast/bottle) feeding can be carried out to minimise with-drawal symptoms. Pregnant women on antipsychotics should be monitored for gesta-tional diabetes with an oral glucose tolerance test.

Olanzapine is widely considered to be a safer option and most reproductive data exist for it; however, it has also been associated with both lower birth weight and increased risk of intensive care admission, a large head circumference and macrosomia.

Exam Essentials

- FGAs and SGAs are unlikely to be major teratogens

Question 9
How would you advise Renée on the use of antipsychotics while breastfeeding?

Answer
There is limited evidence, but reassuring data which indicate that Renée may continue to breastfeed while on olanzapine based on the risks and benefits ratio.

Explanation
Maternal doses of olanzapine up to 20 mg daily produce low levels in milk and undetectable levels in the serum of breastfed infants [18]. In most cases, short-term side effects have not been reported, but sedation has occurred. Most antipsychotics are in Dr Hale's lactation risk category L3, while olanzapine is in category L2. Generally, patients on clozapine are advised not to breastfeed due to the risks of agranulocytosis in infants.

The pump-and-dump method or formula milk feeding are alternatives for breastfeeding mothers who are concerned about the drug concentration in the breastmilk for the baby.

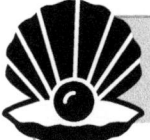

Clinical Pearls

- When initiating a drug post-partum:
    - Consider the previous response to treatment
    - Avoid psychotropic drugs with high reported infant plasma levels
    - Consider the half-lives of the drugs: drugs with a long half-life can accumulate in breast milk and infant serum

Diving Deep ...

The FDA pregnancy risk categories [19] indicate the potential of a drug to cause birth defects if used during pregnancy. The categories were determined by assessing the reliability of documentation and the risk–benefit ratio. The categories are:

435

- A. adequate and well-controlled studies have failed to demonstrate a risk to the fetus in the first trimester of pregnancy (and there is no evidence of risk in later trimesters)

- B. animal reproduction studies have failed to demonstrate a risk to the fetus and there are no adequate and well-controlled studies in pregnant women

- C. animal reproduction studies have shown an adverse effect on the fetus and there are no adequate and well-controlled studies in humans, but potential benefits may warrant the use of the drug in pregnant women despite potential risks

- D. there is positive evidence of human fetal risk based on adverse reaction data from investigational or marketing experience or studies in humans, but potential benefits may warrant the use of the drug in pregnant women despite potential risks

- X: studies in animals or humans have demonstrated fetal abnormalities and/or there is positive evidence of human fetal risk based on adverse reaction data from investigational or marketing experience, and the **risks involved in the use of the drug in pregnant women outweigh potential benefits**

Dr Hale's lactation risk categories are as follows [20]:

- L1: drug without any observed increase in adverse effects in infants in a large number of mothers, controlled studies fail to demonstrate a risk to the infant and the possibility of harm to the infant is remote

- L2: drug without an increase in adverse effects in infants in a limited number of mothers, and evidence of demonstrated risk which is likely following the use of the medication is remote

- L3: drug with no controlled studies in mothers, but the risk of untoward effects to an infant is possible, or controlled studies show only minimal non-threatening adverse effects

- L4: drug with positive evidence of risk to the infant, but benefits from use in mothers may be acceptable despite risks to the infant (i.e., if the drug is needed in a life-threatening situation)

- L5: drug with significant and documented risk to the infant from studies in mothers, or has a high risk of causing significant damage to the infant; the risk of using the drug clearly outweighs any possible benefit from breastfeeding

Post-natal blues occurs in about 50–75% of women, it typically develops within two to three days post-partum, peaks on the third to fifth day and resolves within two weeks of onset [9]. It is a brief psychological disturbance characterised by mild depressive symptoms such as insomnia, exhaustion, decreased concentration, tearfulness, emotional lability and confusion in mothers. Post-natal blues usually resolves spontaneously with support and reassurance, pharmacological treatment is not necessary. In this case, the later onset (two weeks post-partum) and prolonged duration of symptoms make a diagnosis of post-natal blues less likely.

In post-partum psychosis, peak occurrence is at two weeks post-partum. Up to 80% of patients present with prominent affective symptoms [9]. Common features include lability of symptoms, insomnia, perplexity, bewilderment and disorientation. Thoughts of suicide or infanticide are also present at times, and are important to screen for.

Infanticide is most often associated with post-partum psychotic episodes that are characterised by command hallucinations to kill the infant or delusions that the infant is possessed, but psychotic symptoms can also occur in severe post-partum mood episodes without such specific delusions of hallucinations.

The data on rapid tranquillisation use in pregnant women are limited. However, if chemical restraints are required, the use of short-acting benzodiazepines (e.g., lorazepam) and sedative antihistamines (e.g., promethazine) is preferable. The United Kingdom's NICE guidelines [3] also recommend the use of an antipsychotic.

References

1. Ban L, Gibson J, West J, Fiaschi L, Sokal R, Smeeth L, et al. Maternal depression, antidepressant prescriptions, and congenital anomaly risk in offspring: a population-based cohort study. *BJOG*. 2014 Nov;121(12):1471–81.

2. Ter Horst PGJ, Jansman FGA, van Lingen RA, Smit JP, de Jong-van den Berg LTW, Brouwers JRBJ. Pharmacological aspects of neonatal antidepressant withdrawal. *Obstet Gynecol Surv*. 2008 Apr;63(4):267–79.

3. National Institute for Health and Care Excellence (NICE). Antenatal and postnatal mental health: clinical management and service guidance. Clinical guideline [CG192]. NICE; 2014. Available from: www.nice.org.uk/guidance/cg192

4. Cohen LS, Altshuler LL, Harlow BL, Nonacs R, Newport DJ, Viguera AC, et al. Relapse of major depression during pregnancy in women who maintain or discontinue antidepressant treatment. *JAMA*. 2006 Feb 1;295(5):499–507.

5. Taylor DM, Barnes TRE, Young A. *The Maudsley prescribing guidelines in psychiatry*, 14th edition. Chichester Hoboken, NJ: Wiley Blackwell; 2021.

6. Davis RL, Rubanowice D, McPhillips H, Raebel MA, Andrade SE, Smith D, et al. Risks of congenital malformations and perinatal events among infants exposed to antidepressant medications during pregnancy. *Pharmacoepidemiol Drug Saf*. 2007 Oct;16(10):1086–94.

7. Cuijpers P, Weitz E, Karyotaki E, Garber J, Andersson G. The effects of psychological treatment of maternal depression on children and parental functioning: a meta-analysis. *Eur Child Adolesc Psychiatry*. 2015 Feb;24(2):237–45.

437

8. Paulzen M, Goecke TW, Stickeler E, Gründer G, Schoretsanitis G. Sertraline in pregnancy: therapeutic drug monitoring in maternal blood, amniotic fluid and cord blood. *J Affect Disord*. 2017 Apr 1;212:1–6.

9. Semple D, Smyth R. *Oxford handbook of psychiatry*, 4th edition. Oxford: Oxford University Press; 2019.

10. Cox JL, Holden JM, Sagovsky R. Detection of postnatal depression. Development of the 10-item Edinburgh Postnatal Depression Scale. *Br J Psychiatry*. 1987 Jun;150:782–6.

11. McAndrew F, Thompson J, Fellows L, Large A, Speed M, Renfrew MJ. Infant feeding survey 2010. Health and Social Care Information Centre; 2010. Available from: https://doc.ukdataservice.ac.uk/doc/7281/mrdoc/pdf/7281_ifs-uk-2010_report.pdf

12. Pinheiro E, Bogen DL, Hoxha D, Ciolino JD, Wisner KL. Sertraline and breastfeeding: review and meta-analysis. *Arch Womens Ment Health*. 2015 Apr;18(2):139–46.

13. Boland RJ, Verduin ML, Ruiz P, Shah A, Sadock BJ, editors. *Kaplan & Sadock's synopsis of psychiatry*, 12th edition. Philadelphia: Wolters Kluwer; 2022.

14. Wide K, Winbladh B, Källén B. Major malformations in infants exposed to antiepileptic drugs *in utero*, with emphasis on carbamazepine and valproic acid: a nation-wide, population-based register study. *Acta Paediatr*. 2004 Feb;93(2):174–6.

15. Wyszynski DF, Nambisan M, Surve T, Alsdorf RM, Smith CR, Holmes LB, et al. Increased rate of major malformations in offspring exposed to valproate during pregnancy. *Neurology*. 2005 Mar 22;64(6):961–5.

16. Weston J, Bromley R, Jackson CF, Adab N, Clayton-Smith J, Greenhalgh J, et al. Monotherapy treatment of epilepsy in pregnancy: congenital malformation outcomes in the child. *Cochrane Database Syst Rev*. 2016 Nov 7;11(11):CD010224.

17. Gentile S. Antipsychotic therapy during early and late pregnancy. A systematic review. *Schizophr Bull*. 2010 May;36(3):518–44.

18. Olanzapine. In Drugs and Lactation Database (LactMed®). Bethesda, MD: National Institute of Child Health and Human Development; 2006. Available from: www.ncbi.nlm.nih.gov/books/NBK501056

19. Boothby LA, Doering PL. FDA labeling system for drugs in pregnancy. *Ann Pharmacother*. 2001 Nov;35(11):1485–9.

20. Hale TW, Krutsch K. *Hale's medications & mothers' milk 2023: a manual of lactational pharmacology*, 20th edition. Springer Publishing Company; 2022.

Case 53: Hepatic Impairment

Is my liver alright?

Our patients often present with co-morbid medical conditions which may affect their hepatic and renal functioning. The liver is responsible for the metabolism of certain medications and the synthesis of plasma proteins and clotting factors. Therefore, several clinical considerations are important when prescribing psychotropics to patients with hepatic impairment.

- **Question 1: What are the general principles of prescribing in patients with hepatic impairment?**

Clifford is a 48-year-old gentleman with advanced liver cirrhosis secondary to hepatitis B. He recently developed auditory hallucinations and delusions of persecution and was diagnosed with schizophrenia.

- **Question 2: Given his background of impaired hepatic function, what antipsychotics would you consider starting him on?**

Clifford was started on amisulpride and his symptoms of schizophrenia went into remission. A year later, he presents with symptoms of low mood, poor appetite, poor sleep, poor concentration and thoughts of suicide. You plan to start him on an antidepressant.

- **Question 3: Given his background of impaired hepatic function, what antidepressant would you consider starting him on?**

Clifford was started on sertraline and his depressive symptoms went into remission. Sertraline was subsequently discontinued and amisulpride continued for the treatment of his schizophrenia. Unfortunately, Clifford returned two years later with one week of irritability, reduced need for sleep, increased energy, flight of ideas and increased talkativeness. Despite increasing his amisulpride dose, he remains symptomatic.

- **Question 4: Given his background of impaired hepatic function, what mood stabiliser would you prescribe to him?**

During his inpatient admission, Clifford continues to display symptoms of agitation and your consultant is keen to prescribe a sedative.

- **Question 5: Given his background of impaired hepatic function, if required, which benzodiazepine would you consider?**

Answers to Case 53

Question 1
What are the general principles of prescribing in patients with hepatic impairment?

Answer
Avoid polypharmacy where possible
Initiate medications at a lower starting dose
Exercise caution when prescribing medications that are extensively hepatically metabolised, and avoid hepatotoxic medications
Consider longer intervals between dosage increases
Patients with hepatic encephalopathy are often sensitive to sedating medications (e.g., benzodiazepines)

Explanation
A lower starting dose is required, especially for highly protein-bound medications, such as tricyclic antidepressants, selective serotonin reuptake inhibitors (SSRIs) (except citalopram), trazodone and antipsychotic drugs. Most psychotropics are extensively hepatically metabolised except sulpiride, amisulpride, lithium pregabalin and gabapentin.

Consider closely monitoring liver function (as frequently as weekly, initially) if hepatically metabolised drugs are used. The half-life of medications may be prolonged in hepatic impairment and require more time to reach a steady state.

Ascites and reduced albumin may be present in patients with hepatic impairment. Dosing has to be adjusted for highly protein-bound medications, given the increased volume of distribution for water-soluble drugs.

Avoid using medication with a long half-life or prodrugs that require hepatic metabolism to become active.

Aside from sedating medications, drugs that may cause constipation should be used cautiously because of the risk of precipitating hepatic encephalopathy.

Exam Essentials

- The liver extensively metabolises most psychotropics except sulpiride, amisulpride, lithium, pregabalin and gabapentin

Question 2

Given his background of impaired hepatic function, what antipsychotics would you consider starting him on?

Answer

Amisulpride, sulpiride or paliperidone

Explanation

Most antipsychotics, except for amisulpride and sulpiride, are extensively hepatically metabolised.

Amisulpride and sulpiride are predominantly renally excreted; hence, dose adjustments are not required. Amisulpride is also unlikely to cause transaminitis and hepatocellular injury. Sulpiride has a low potential to cause sedation or constipation; however, elevations in liver enzymes are more common. Isolated case reports of cholestatic jaundice and primary biliary cirrhosis have been associated with sulpiride use.

If an intramuscular depot preparation is required, paliperidone is the medication of choice as it is mainly excreted unchanged by the kidneys. While clozapine is contraindicated in active liver disease, it can be used with caution in patients with hepatic disease in consultation with a hepatologist.

Exam Essentials

- Non-alcoholic fatty liver disease can occur as a result of metabolic syndrome arising from chronic antipsychotic use

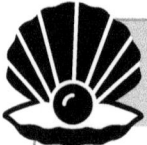

Clinical Pearls

- Antipsychotic medications can cause abnormal liver function tests (LFTs) in one-third of patients that occur within one to six weeks of initiation [1]. However, only rarely do they cause clinically significant hepatic damage

- In liver-impaired patients presenting with psychosis, always exclude delirium and encephalopathy before attributing the condition to psychiatric causes

Question 3
Given his background of impaired hepatic function, what antidepressant would you consider starting him on?

Answer
Paroxetine, sertraline, citalopram, vortioxetine or mirtazapine

Explanation
Paroxetine, sertraline and citalopram belong to the SSRI class of antidepressants which are hepatically metabolised but have a relatively lower effect on hepatic enzymes. While vortioxetine undergoes significant hepatic metabolism, pharmacokinetic studies suggest no dose reduction is required and it does not seem to be associated with hepatotoxicity. Mirtazapine may be used with caution and at a reduced starting dose with careful titration.

Antidepressants that should not be used in patients with hepatic impairment include agomelatine, which has been associated with liver failure, with a dose-related increase in transaminases reported, requiring frequent LFT monitoring during initiation. Duloxetine is also contraindicated in hepatic impairment with significantly reduced clearance even in mild liver impairment. Non-selective monoamine oxidase inhibitors have also been associated with hepatotoxicity and hepatitis and are best avoided. Tricyclic antidepressants are hepatically metabolised and highly protein bound with additional side effects of constipation and sedation, leaving them as an undesirable treatment option. Antidepressants with long half-lives (e.g., fluoxetine) are hard to dose as it may take many days to weeks to reach a steady state.

Exam Essentials

- Agomelatine should not be used in liver impairment

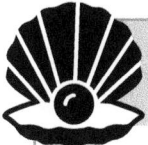

Clinical Pearls

- Melatonin may be used for insomnia in those with liver impairment. Hydroxyzine may be used with caution. Avoid long-acting benzodiazepines (diazepam, clonazepam)

Question 4
Given his background of impaired hepatic function, what mood stabiliser would you prescribe to him?

Answer
Lithium

Explanation
Amongst the mood stabilisers available, lithium is the only medication that is not hepatically metabolised, therefore dose adjustments are not required. However, if ascites develops as a complication of liver cirrhosis, a note should be made of the change in volume of distribution. Serum lithium levels are useful in guiding the titration of the dose required.

While lamotrigine can still be used with caution and with a 50–75% reduction in initial dose (based on the degree of hepatic impairment) it is more commonly used in the treatment of bipolar depression as opposed to acute mania [2].

Carbamazepine is extensively hepatically metabolised and a potent inducer of cytochrome P450 enzymes and should be avoided in acute liver disease. It has been associated with hepatitis, cholangitis, cholestatic and hepatocellular jaundice and hepatic failure, all of which occur most commonly in the first two months of treatment. If prescribed, it should be started at 50% of the usual starting dose and guided with regular carbamazepine serum levels [2].

Valproate is similarly extensively hepatically metabolised and is contraindicated in severe and/or active hepatic impairment, or a family history of severe impairment. If prescribed, it should be started at 50% of the usual starting dose and guided with regular valproate serum levels [2]. It is associated with elevated LFTs and serious hepatotoxicity including hepatic failure.

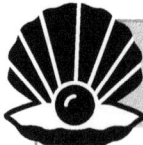

Clinical Pearls

- Monitor fluid status and degree of ascites/oedema when starting lithium – as the dose may need to be adjusted

Question 5
Given his background of impaired hepatic function, if required, which benzodiazepine would you consider?

Answer
Benzodiazepine with a short half-life, such as lorazepam

Explanation
Benzodiazepines are extensively hepatically metabolised and therefore medications without active metabolites and with a short half-life are preferred. Lorazepam is well tolerated in advanced liver disease and is commonly used in alcohol withdrawal. Other preferred benzodiazepines include oxazepam and temazepam. Diazepam, midazolam and clonazepam have active metabolites and a prolonged duration of effect.

Promethazine is commonly used as a sedative agent but is extensively hepatically metabolised and should be used with caution. Z-drugs (e.g., zopiclone) are hepatically metabolised but have a short half-life (one to seven hours) and may be used at a low dose and with caution.

Exam Essentials

- Benzodiazepines with a short half-life are preferred in hepatic impairment

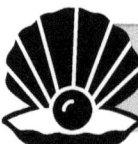

Clinical Pearls

- Normal aspartate transaminase (AST) and alanine transaminase (ALT) in LFTs may not necessarily indicate normal liver function. Always check:

- ○ Albumin level
- ○ Prothrombin time/partial thromboplastin time
- ○ Clotting factors
- ○ Consider ultrasound liver if needed

Diving Deep …

While many cases of antipsychotic- and antidepressant-induced mild transaminitis are not clinically significant, close monitoring of LFTs should be performed to monitor for the progression of drug-induced hepatitis. If the serum ALT or AST is more than three times the upper limit of normal (ULN), and the serum total bilirubin is elevated to more than twice the ULN, discontinuation of treatment should be considered. If the ALT is increased more than five times the ULN, treatment should be immediately discontinued [3].

References

1. Marwick KFM, Taylor M, Walker SW. Antipsychotics and abnormal liver function tests: systematic review. *Clin Neuropharmacol.* 2012;35(5):244–53.

2. Taylor DM, Barnes TRE, Young A. *The Maudsley prescribing guidelines in psychiatry,* 14th edition. Chichester Hoboken, NJ: Wiley Blackwell; 2021.

3. Chalasani NP, Hayashi PH, Bonkovsky HL, Navarro VJ, Lee WM, Fontana RJ, et al. ACG clinical guideline: the diagnosis and management of idiosyncratic drug-induced liver injury. *Am J Gastroenterol.* 2014 Jul;109(7):950–66; quiz 967.

Case 54: Renal Impairment

Are my kidneys ok?

In renal impairment, the pharmacokinetics (absorption, distribution, metabolism, excretion) of medications are altered, and there is a reduced capacity to excrete drugs and their metabolites.

- **Question 1: What are the general principles of prescribing in patients with renal impairment?**

Michelle is a 24-year-old lady who has a history of systemic lupus erythematosus complicated by impaired renal function due to lupus nephritis. She presents to your clinic with symptoms of hallucinations and delusions.

- **Question 2: Which antipsychotics would you avoid in patients with renal impairment?**

You started Michelle on olanzapine and her symptoms entered remission. Unfortunately, Michelle later developed symptoms of depression.

- **Question 3: Which antidepressants are suitable first-line treatment options in the treatment of patients with depression and renal impairment?**

You prescribed escitalopram for the treatment of her depression. Three years later, Michelle presents with symptoms of mania. Despite discontinuing her escitalopram, she continues to display delusions of grandeur and irritability.

- **Question 4: Which mood stabilisers are best avoided in patients with renal impairment?**

Michelle displays symptoms of agitation, and your consultant is keen to prescribe a sedative.

- **Question 5: Given her history of renal impairment, if required, which benzodiazepine would you consider?**

Unfortunately, with time, Michelle's lupus nephritis progresses, and she develops end-stage renal failure. She was started on regular haemodialysis treatment.

- **Question 6: How does renal replacement therapy affect the clearance of psychotropics?**

Answers to Case 54

Question 1
What are the general principles of prescribing in patients with renal impairment?

Answer
The stage of renal impairment should be assessed by calculating the estimated glomerular filtration rate (eGFR)/creatinine clearance and checking for proteinuria

As individuals age, renal function naturally decreases and in elderly patients (age > 65 years) closer attention should be paid to the assessment of their renal function

Avoid medications that are nephrotoxic and exercise caution when using medications that are extensively renally cleared

Renally excreted medications should be initiated at a low dose and increased slowly as the half-life of medications may take a longer time to reach a steady state

Avoid polypharmacy to reduce the risk of drug–drug interactions

Avoid long-acting medications (e.g., depot preparations)

Avoid medications known to prolong the QTc interval. Electrolyte derangements are common in chronic kidney disease and therefore the risk of QTc prolongation is further increased

Exercise caution when using medications with anticholinergic effects

Exercise caution when prescribing medications that can cause neuroleptic malignant syndrome (NMS) and serotonin syndrome (SS)

Monitor weight gain caused by psychotropics

Explanation
An assessment of the degree of renal impairment helps one to adjust the dose of medications which are renally excreted. Additionally, one should monitor for any progression in declining renal function and risk of progression to renal replacement therapy.

NMS and SS can result in rhabdomyolysis, which further worsens kidney functioning. Medications with anticholinergic effects can cause urinary retention, further impairing renal function. Weight gain increases the risk of developing metabolic syndrome, contributing to renal impairment.

447

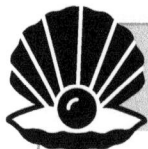

Clinical Pearls

- **Uraemia** in kidney impairment can directly inhibit the activity of the cytochrome P450s and drug transporters, impairing the hepatic metabolism of medications [1]

Question 2
Which antipsychotics would you avoid in patients with renal impairment?

Answer
Amisulpride and sulpiride

Explanation
Both amisulpride and sulpiride are predominantly renally excreted and best avoided in renal impairment.

Fifty per cent of amisulpride is excreted unchanged in the urine and 95% of sulpiride is excreted in the urine and faeces as unchanged sulpiride [2]. If either is prescribed, they require a dose reduction depending on the degree of renal impairment. There is a case report of renal failure associated with sulpiride use due to diabetic coma and rhabdomyolysis [3].

If an antipsychotic must be prescribed, one should avoid highly anticholinergic agents, which can cause urinary retention. A suitable first-generation antipsychotic is haloperidol, which is less than 1% excreted unchanged in the urine. A suitable second-generation antipsychotic is olanzapine, which is well tolerated.

Question 3
Which antidepressants are suitable first-line treatment options in the treatment of patients with depression and renal impairment?

Answer
Most antidepressants can be prescribed in renal impairment, with dose adjustments made. In advanced renal impairment, it is generally recommended that antidepressants be initiated at a low dose and increased slowly with caution.

Explanation
If cognitive behavioural therapy (CBT) is not available or is insufficient, selective serotonin reuptake inhibitors (SSRIs) should be considered.

Fluoxetine has conflicting evidence for the treatment of depression in renal disease and requires a lower dose in GFR < 20 mL/min. While no dose adjustments are required for sertraline, its efficacy in treating depression in chronic kidney disease is limited. The

Maudsley guidelines [2] have suggested that citalopram and escitalopram are effective in treating depression in chronic renal failure and improving quality of life. However, when prescribed to patients on haemodialysis, both are associated with a higher risk of sudden cardiac death (due to prolonged QTc) versus other SSRIs [4].

Only 0.5% of bupropion is excreted unchanged in the urine and it has been used to treat sexual dysfunction in mild to moderately depressed patients with chronic kidney disease [2]. Mirtazapine can be used but requires dose adjustments in patients with GFR < 10 mL/min.

Medications such as desvenlafaxine and tricyclic antidepressants can be given in renal impairment but have anticholinergic effects, increasing the risk of urinary retention, and hence are less preferable. Duloxetine is contraindicated in patients with a GFR < 30 mL/min as it can accumulate in chronic kidney disease.

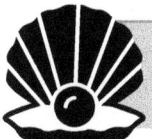

Clinical Pearls

- Vortioxetine does not require dose adjustments in renal impairment and end-stage renal failure and is also safe for use in hepatic impairment

Question 4
Which mood stabilisers are best avoided in patients with renal impairment?

Answer
Lithium

Explanation
Ninety-five per cent of lithium is excreted unchanged in the urine and it is nephrotoxic and contraindicated in severe renal impairment [2]. Long-term treatment may result in progressive irreversible impaired renal function, changes in kidney histology, nephrogenic diabetes insipidus, nephrotic syndrome and collecting duct renal carcinoma. Lithium causes chronic kidney disease through chronic interstitial nephritis, glomerulonephritis and the formation of renal cysts. However, the risk can be mitigated through regular lithium serum level monitoring to reach target maintenance serum levels, avoiding chronic lithium toxicity and active monitoring of kidney function by both psychiatrist and nephrologist. Major risk factors for lithium-induced nephrotoxicity include the duration of lithium exposure and its cumulative dose. Other risk factors include episodes of acute intoxication, increased age, lower initial eGFR, female gender, concomitant nephrotoxic drugs and medical co-morbidities (e.g., hypertension and diabetes) and concomitant use of other antipsychotic medications. If lithium is still required, significant dose reductions are required. If the GFR is 10–50 mL/min, avoid, or reduce

449

the dose to 50–75% of the normal dose. At GFR < 10 mL/min, avoid, or reduce the dose to 25–50% of the normal dose. There are case reports of lithium used successfully in patients on haemodialysis [5].

Topiramate is primarily renally excreted, and chronic kidney disease can affect the clearance of topiramate. If prescribed for moderate to severe renal impairment, topiramate should be initiated at half of the usual dose. As topiramate is removed by dialysis, a supplemental dose may be required during haemodialysis. Additionally, caution should be exercised as topiramate use is associated with urolithiasis formation in < 3% of patients.

Only 2–3% of carbamazepine is excreted unchanged in the urine, and dose reduction is not necessary. While there are case reports of renal failure, tubular necrosis and tubulointerstitial nephritis, it is less likely than lithium to cause chronic kidney disease. Stevens–Johnson syndrome and toxic epidermal necrolysis are known complications of carbamazepine, which can cause renal impairment.

Only 2% of valproate is excreted unchanged, and dose adjustment is not required. While there are case reports of valproate causing renal impairment [6], interstitial nephritis [7], Fanconi syndrome [8], renal tubular acidosis [9] and renal failure, it is less likely than lithium to cause chronic kidney disease.

While < 10% of lamotrigine is excreted unchanged in the urine, inactive metabolites can accumulate, and it should be started at a low dose and increased slowly.

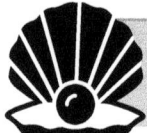

Clinical Pearls

- Lithium may cause chronic kidney disease with long-term treatment

Question 5
Given her history of renal impairment, if required, which benzodiazepine would you consider?

Answer
Lorazepam

Explanation
While all benzodiazepines can be prescribed for renal impairment, active metabolites may accumulate in renal impairment causing excessive sedation, therefore short-acting benzodiazepines, such as lorazepam, are preferred.

Amongst the Z-drugs, both zolpidem and zopiclone do not require dose adjustments, although the clearance of zolpidem is moderately reduced in renal impairment. Therefore, zopiclone is a reasonable choice.

Both pregabalin and gabapentin should used with caution and at a reduced dose as both are predominantly renally excreted unchanged in the urine, with clearance reduced in renal impairment. While gabapentin and pregabalin have been used to treat pruritus, neuropathic pain, muscle cramps and restless leg syndrome in patients on haemodialysis, there is a risk of toxicity and it has been associated with acute renal failure, myoclonus, altered mental state and falls.

Question 6
How does renal replacement therapy affect the clearance of psychotropics?

Answer
While haemodialysis affects the volume of distribution, plasma albumin/globulin ratio and body weight, most drugs with high protein binding (> 90%) are less likely to be dialysed, and most antipsychotics are not dialysed due to the larger size of the antipsychotic–protein complex [10, 11].

Most antidepressants are hepatically metabolised and highly protein bound, therefore they are not significantly removed during dialysis. However, albumin can be low in chronic kidney disease, which affects the serum level of some antidepressants (e.g., fluvoxamine and amitriptyline).

Amongst the mood stabilisers, only the use of lithium requires specific dose adjustments in patients on haemodialysis.

Amongst anxiolytics and sedatives, pregabalin and gabapentin are removed during haemodialysis. Both benzodiazepines and Z-drugs are not removed during haemodialysis.

Explanation
The caution regarding prescribing amisulpride and sulpiride in renal impairment holds for patients on renal replacement therapy. Given the changes in haemodynamics perihaemodialysis, there is modest evidence favouring multiple dosing regimens of oral aripiprazole, ziprasidone, risperidone and quetiapine, which are less likely to be affected by haemodialysis. Long-acting injections of olanzapine risk significant sedation, and those of haloperidol risk extrapyramidal symptoms. If a long-acting injection is required, two case reports have shown successful use of a long-acting risperidone injection.

Bupropion has been used in haemodialysis patients at a low dose of 150 mg every three days. Escitalopram and citalopram have been used in patients on haemodialysis; however, there is a higher risk of sudden cardiac death compared to other SSRIs. Fluoxetine has been used in patients on haemodialysis at a reduced once-weekly dosing regimen. Paroxetine has been used in patients on haemodialysis at a reduced dose of 10 mg/day. Sertraline is safe but lacks efficacy in the treatment of depression in patients on haemodialysis. Venlafaxine can be used to treat peripheral diabetic neuropathy in patients on haemodialysis. Mirtazapine can be used to treat pruritus caused by renal failure and appetite loss.

Lithium requires a single supplementary dose given post dialysis to maintain steady-state plasma levels. As lithium is removed during haemodialysis, haemodialysis is often emergently required during severe acute lithium toxicity.

451

Haemodialysis extracts 35% of gabapentin and 50%–60% of pregabalin from the blood [12] and therefore a supplementary dose should be considered after each session while monitoring for toxicity. Both gabapentin and pregabalin are predominantly renally excreted, and therefore if required by patients on haemodialysis, they should be prescribed judiciously.

Exam Essentials

- The only antipsychotic with well-researched plasma levels for monitoring is clozapine

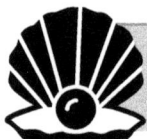

Clinical Pearls

- CBT is efficacious in the management of depression in patients on dialysis [13]

Diving Deep …

The interaction between psychiatric and physical medical co-morbidities poses a challenge to any physician and multidisciplinary management is always preferred. For patients on regular haemodialysis treatment, fluctuations in mental states may affect compliance to the haemodialysis regimen and any missed haemodialysis sessions may cause electrolyte imbalances and fluid overload, which contribute to delirium, further affecting compliance and the patient's mental state.

For patients who have received a renal or hepatic transplant, special consideration should be given to potential drug–drug interactions between immunosuppressants and psychiatric medications. Cytochrome P450 (CYP) 3A4 inducers (e.g., carbamazepine or valproate) can reduce serum concentrations of immunosuppressants, which may unwittingly lead to subtherapeutic concentrations of immunosuppressants and subsequent transplant rejection; whereas CYP 3A4 inhibitors (e.g., fluoxetine, paroxetine and fluvoxamine) can increase the plasma level of immunosuppressants.

References

1. Yeung CK, Shen DD, Thummel KE, Himmelfarb J. Effects of chronic kidney disease and uremia on hepatic drug metabolism and transport. *Kidney Int*. 2014 Mar;85(3):522–8.

2. Taylor DM, Barnes TRE, Young A. *The Maudsley prescribing guidelines in psychiatry*, 14th edition. Chichester Hoboken, NJ: Wiley Blackwell; 2021.

3. Toprak O, Cirit M, Ersoy R, Uzüm A, Ozümer O, Cobanoğlu A, et al. New-onset type II diabetes mellitus, hyperosmolar non-ketotic coma, rhabdomyolysis and acute renal failure in a patient treated with sulpiride. *Nephrol Dial Transplant*. 2005 Mar;20(3):662–3.

4. US Food & Drug Administration (FDA). Clarification of dosing and warning recommendations for Celexa. FDA; 2016. Available from: www.fda.gov/Drugs/ResourcesForYou/SpecialFeatures/ucm297764.htm

5. Chang CWL, Ho CSH. Lithium use in a patient with bipolar disorder and end-stage kidney disease on hemodialysis: a case report. *Front Psychiatry*. 2020 Feb 3;11:6.

6. Zaki EL, Springate JE. Renal injury from valproic acid: case report and literature review. *Pediatr Neurol*. 2002 Oct;27(4):318–9.

7. Fukuda Y, Watanabe H, Ohtomo Y, Yabuta K. Immunologically mediated chronic tubulo-interstitial nephritis caused by valproate therapy. *Nephron*. 1996;72(2):328–9.

8. Smith GC, Balfe JW, Kooh SW. Anticonvulsants as a cause of Fanconi syndrome. *Nephrol Dial Transplant*. 1995;10(4):543–5.

9. Tanaka H, Onodera N, Ito R, Monma N, Waga S, Yokoyama M. Distal type of renal tubular acidosis after anti-epileptic therapy in a girl with infantile spasms. *Clin Exp Nephrol*. 1999 Dec 20;3(4):311–3.

10. Sutar R, Atlani MK, Chaudhary P. Antipsychotics and hemodialysis: a systematic review. *Asian J Psychiatr*. 2021 Jan;55:102484.

11. Hashimoto M, Maeda H, Oniki K, Yasui-Furukori N, Watanabe H, Saruwatari J, et al. New insight concerning therapeutic drug monitoring: the importance of the concept of psychonephrology. *Biol Pharm Bull*. 2022 Jul 1;45(7):834–42.

12. Raouf M, Atkinson TJ, Crumb MW, Fudin J. Rational dosing of gabapentin and pregabalin in chronic kidney disease. *J Pain Res*. 2017;10:275–8.

13. Zegarow P, Manczak M, Rysz J, Olszewski R. The influence of cognitive–behavioral therapy on depression in dialysis patients: meta-analysis. *Arch Med Sci*. 2020;16(6):1271–8.

Case 55: Forensic Psychiatry

Minds on trial

Forensic psychiatry is defined by the American Academy of Psychiatry and the Law as 'a subspecialty of psychiatry in which scientific and clinical expertise is applied in legal contexts involving civil, criminal correctional regulatory or legislative matters, and in specialised clinical consultations in areas such as risk assessment or employment'[1]. Forensic psychiatry has evolved since its inception and now covers a range of issues from civil matters (e.g., psychiatric disabilities and child custody), regulatory issues (e.g., the right to refuse treatment and informed consent) and clinical topics with legal implications (e.g., assessment of dangerousness and risk management).

- **Question 1: What is the difference in the roles of a forensic psychiatrist and a general psychiatrist when interacting with a patient?**

- **Question 2: Before a forensic psychiatric consult, what is a typical warning that should be given to the examinee by the forensic psychiatrist?**

- **Question 3: Can a forensic psychiatrist who has been treating a patient act as an expert witness for the same patient?**

- **Question 4: How does one assess a defendant's fitness to plead?**

- **Question 5: How does one determine if the examinee is criminally responsible for a crime committed?**

- **Question 6: Based on the 2002 MacArthur study of mental disorder and violence, what is the prevalence of crime among individuals with mental disorders?**

- **Question 7: Medical malpractice is a civil wrong resulting from a physician's negligence. How does one prove that malpractice has occurred?**

Answers to Case 55

Question 1
What is the difference in the roles of a forensic psychiatrist and a general psychiatrist when interacting with a patient?

Answer
A forensic psychiatrist may not necessarily have a collaborative clinical relationship that advocates for the patient, which is typical between a general psychiatrist and a patient.

Explanation
The altered relationship is the consequence of the law and medicine intersecting. The general psychiatrist's primary duty is to the patient and adheres to the ethical pillars of non-maleficence. However, the forensic psychiatrist is often retained by the court to provide psychiatric expertise to inform the court of psychiatric disorders and their relationship to the examined crime; in turn, their testimony may harm the examinee, for example when the defendant is found guilty and criminally responsible.

Question 2
Before a forensic psychiatric consult, what is a typical warning that should be given to the examinee by the forensic psychiatrist?

Answer
1. There is an emphasis on the lack/absence of confidentiality in the entire interaction, and of the physician's overriding duty to the court. The content and results of the examination may be transmitted to attorneys and judges and may be revealed in open court

2. The examination does not entail therapy; the examiner is not the treating doctor

3. While the examinee need not answer questions, any refusal may be noted

4. The examinee should be informed about who has retained the forensic psychiatrist: the prosecution/plaintiff, the defence or the court. The forensic psychiatrist should also explain that for the testimony to be useful, it must be objective. What is reported might help, hurt, or make no difference to the examinee's case, and this will not be known until after the case has been concluded.

Explanation
As there are multiple agencies at play during court proceedings, care should be taken by the forensic psychiatrist to avoid any deceptions that may inadvertently arise. The

455

examinee may have certain societal expectations of a doctor and assume that any disclosure will be kept confidential by the forensic psychiatrist and used only for their benefit. Therefore, informed consent should be obtained before the interview and examinees made aware of their vulnerability and different contextual circumstances of the forensic interview they are about to undergo. A transparent approach allows the forensic psychiatrist to uphold their responsibilities to the examinee, to the court and to the medical community and profession.

Exam Essentials

- Examinees must be made aware of their vulnerability and different contextual circumstances of the forensic interview they are about to undergo as compared to a normal psychiatric consult

Question 3
Can a forensic psychiatrist who has been treating a patient act as an expert witness for the same patient?

Answer
The forensic psychiatrist should avoid holding the dual role of therapist and forensic evaluator, which will inevitably lead to a conflict of interest and affect the credibility of the physician

Explanation
While is it common for attorneys to call upon treating clinicians to testify as expert witnesses for their patients, this should be avoided for many reasons. First, treating clinicians may be affected by personal bias resulting from the therapeutic alliance with their patients and may lack objectivity in their attempts to be their patients' advocates. The therapeutic relationship may also be strained by the process of the forensic evaluation, which requires corroborative history and exposure of information to public scrutiny and the patient themselves to possible cross-examinations. Moreover, issues of confidentiality arise when the treating clinician is no longer able to honour their patient's confidentiality to the same extent during their ongoing consultations.

Exam Essentials

- The forensic psychiatrist should avoid holding the dual role of therapist and forensic evaluator

Question 4
How does one assess a defendant's fitness to plead?

Answer
Taking reference to the Pritchard criteria [2], a defendant is fit to plead if they fulfil the following:

- Capacity to understand the charge(s)

- Capacity to enter a plea

- Ability to understand and question the evidence involved

- Ability to follow the proceedings to make a proper defence

- Know their right to challenge a juror

- Ability to instruct their legal representatives

Explanation
Fitness to plead relates to the mental abilities of the defendant to comply with trial proceedings. The Pritchard criteria arise from the 1836 British case of R v Pritchard, whereby the defendant, accused of bestiality, was deaf and mute. People are assumed to have the capacity to plead unless found otherwise. If the defendant's fitness to plead comes under question, a forensic psychiatrist is often called to assess the defendant. If one or more of the Pritchard criteria are not satisfied, the judge may decide to divert the defendant(s) to psychiatric services for treatment first as a conventional trial cannot proceed.

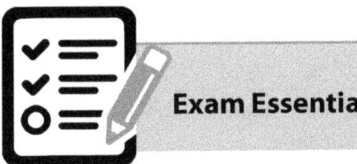

Exam Essentials

- The Pritchard criteria [2] are often referenced in assessing fitness to plead

Question 5
How does one determine if the examinee is criminally responsible for a crime committed?

Answer
The forensic psychiatrist must determine if the examinee had *actus reus* and *mens rea*

Explanation
The term *actus reus* refers to voluntary conduct and *mens rea* refers to evil intent. The latter cannot exist if the patient does not have soundness of mind due to a deficient or abnormal mental status. Such a diseased mental state would have deprived the offender

of the capacity for rational evil intent, as they would not have been able to appreciate the wrongfulness of their act or to conform their conduct to the requirement of the law.

Therefore, to be found not guilty by reason of insanity, it must be proved that the defendant had committed the act at a time in which there was a disease of the mind resulting in an inability to know the nature and quality of the act they were doing. Or if they did understand their actions, they must not have recognised that what they were doing was wrong.

Exam Essentials

- The M'Naghten rule established in 1843 in the British courts was the precedent for determining legal responsibility

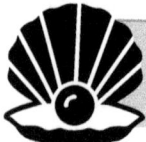

Clinical Pearls

- The age of criminal responsibility in England and Wales is 10 years old

Question 6
Based on the 2002 MacArthur study of mental disorder and violence [3], what is the prevalence of crime among individuals with mental disorders?

Answer
Twenty-seven and a half per cent of patients committed violent acts post-discharge during a one-year follow-up study period. However, Monahan and colleagues also showed that there was no higher propensity for violence among psychiatric patients without concomitant substance abuse than among other residents in the same neighbourhood [3].

Explanation
While violence may be more common in individuals with mental disorders, they are also much more likely to be victimised than the general population. Risk is multifactorial and risk assessments are notoriously challenging. However, there are tools to aid the psychiatrist in evaluation with various approaches to risk assessments.

The actuarial approach uses formal, algorithmic and objective procedures for quantifying risks in numerical terms of a future outcome. The actuarial approach is useful in predicting the risk of violence and sexual offending and typically uses group data obtained from high-risk individuals to calculate the risk for the patient in question. The cons of the actuarial approach include a heavier weightage on historical risk factors and does not guide how risk can be mitigated. Examples of actuarial instruments include the Violence Risk Appraisal Guide and the Violence Risk Appraisal Guide – Revised [4], Violence Risk Scale [5] and Psychopathy Checklist-Revised [6] to diagnose psychopathy and inform risk assessment.

The structured risk tools approach uses structured clinical assessments to systematise the exercise of discretion for risk assessments. The cons of the structured approach include reduced reliability due to human bias. Examples include the Historical Clinical Risk Management-20 [7] to predict inpatient violence and community violence in discharged patients, the Spousal Assault Risk Assessment guide [8] to gauge the risk of future violence in men arrested for spousal assault and the Sexual Violence Risk-20 [9] scale for assessing violence risk in sex offenders.

Question 7

Medical malpractice is a civil wrong resulting from a physician's negligence. How does one prove that malpractice has occurred?

Answer

The following factors must be established:

1. A doctor–patient relationship existed that created a duty of care

2. There was a deviation from the standard of care

3. The patient was damaged

4. The aforementioned deviation directly caused the damage sustained by the patient

Explanation

Two common tests employed to determine if malpractice occurred are the Bolam test and the Montgomery test.

The Bolam test was derived from the 1957 British case of Bolam v Friern Hospital Management Committee [10], which stated that the standard of care expected of a professional practising a special skill is that of an 'ordinary skilled man exercising and professing to have that special skill'. Therefore, the court has to determine if the doctor in question had acted in accordance with a practice accepted as proper by a responsible body of medical men skilled in that particular discipline. Hence, even if a minority body holds a contrary view on the practice undertaken, the doctor will not be liable. The Bolitho addendum is a logical corollary to the Bolam test, which states that the body of opinion relied upon must meet a satisfactory threshold test of logic, failing which the court could choose to disregard that body of opinion.

However, in 2015, in matters of informed consent, the Supreme Court rejected the Bolam test in favour of the Montgomery test. This arose from the Scottish case of Montgomery v Lanarkshire Health Board in 2015 [11], where a woman was not informed of the increased risk of shoulder dystocia (she was of short stature and diabetic) during vaginal delivery, with her child ultimately suffering from cerebral palsy due to the birth complication. The Montgomery test now states that doctors are under a duty to take reasonable care to ensure that the patients are provided information about all material risks involved in any recommended treatment and of any reasonable alternative or variant treatments; they must disclose any risk to which a reasonable person in the patient's position would attach significance. When discussing risks and harms, clinicians should recognise and highlight risks of harm that they believe anyone in the patient's position would want to know. The Supreme Court ruled that information can be withheld in rare situations where being given this information would be seriously detrimental to the patient's health.

Exam Essentials

- The elements of malpractice claims can be recalled through the four Ds:
  - Duty
  - Deviation
  - Damage
  - Direct causation

Diving Deep ...

While the retention of individuals in prisons takes away their liberty as part of the justice system, it does not reduce the individual's right to access healthcare. Taking reference to the European Convention on Human Rights and United Nations International Resolutions concerning standard minimum rules for the treatment of prisoners, there is a principle of equivalence in the setting of prison healthcare. Therefore, health services should not be treated as an arm of the legal system used to punish or repress prisoners.

References

1. American Academy of Psychiatry and the Law. Ethics guidelines for the practice of forensic psychiatry. American Academy of Psychiatry and the Law; 2005. Available from: www.aapl.org/docs/pdf/ETHICSGDLNS.pdf
2. R v Pritchard [1836] 7 C&P 303. 1836.
3. Monahan J, Steadman HJ, Silver E, Appelbaum PS, Robbins PC, Edward P. Mulvey EP et al. *Rethinking risk assessment: the MacArthur study of mental disorder and violence.* New York: Oxford University Press; 2001.

4. Morgan RD. *The SAGE encyclopedia of criminal psychology.* Thousand Oaks, CA: SAGE Publications, Inc.; 2019. Available from: https://sk.sagepub.com/reference/the-sage-encyclopedia-of-criminal-psychology-1e

5. Wong SCP, Gordon A. Violence Risk Scale. American Psychological Association; 2013. Available from: http://doi.apa.org/getdoi.cfm?doi=10.1037/t22640-000

6. Hart SD, Hare RD, Harpur TJ. The Psychopathy Checklist – Revised (PCL-R). In Rosen JC, McReynolds P, editors. *Advances in psychological assessment.* Boston, MA: Springer; 1992, 103–30. Available from: http://link.springer.com/10.1007/978-1-4757-9101-3_4

7. Douglas KS, Hart SD, Webster CD, Belfrage H, Guy LS, Wilson CM. Historical–Clinical–Risk Management-20, Version 3 (HCR-20 V3): development and overview. *Int J Forensic Ment Health.* 2014 Apr 3;13(2):93–108.

8. Kropp PR, Hart SD. The Spousal Assault Risk Assessment (SARA) guide: reliability and validity in adult male offenders. *Law Hum Behav.* 2000 Feb;24(1):101–18.

9. Otto RK, Douglas KS, editors. *Handbook of violence risk assessment,* 2nd edition. Taylor and Francis Group; 2015.

10. Bolam v Friern Hospital Management Committee [1957] 1 WLR 582. 1957.

11. Montgomery v Lanarkshire Health Board [2015] UKSC 11. 2015.

Part II: Topical MCQs

Case 1: Schizophrenia

Question 1: Which of the following is NOT a Schneiderian first-rank symptom of schizophrenia?

A. Auditory hallucinations
B. Delusion of control
C. Delusional perception
D. Thought broadcasting
E. Visual hallucinations

Question 2: A 34-year-old patient is experiencing an acute relapse of schizophrenia. During your consultation, he tells you, 'I know they are out to get me, and if they threaten me again, I will throw a *momotoo* at them'. What psychopathology in speech is demonstrated here?

A. Derailment
B. Logoclonia
C. Mutism
D. Neologism
E. Word salad

Question 3: What is the efficacy of neuroleptic agents in the treatment of schizophrenia?

A. < 5% of patients with schizophrenia are unresponsive to conventional neuroleptics
B. 5–25% of patients with schizophrenia are unresponsive to conventional neuroleptics
C. 25–50% of patients with schizophrenia are unresponsive to conventional neuroleptics
D. 50–75% of patients with schizophrenia are unresponsive to conventional neuroleptics
E. 75–90% of patients with schizophrenia are unresponsive to conventional neuroleptics

Question 4: Which of the following is NOT a component of expressed emotions?

A. Criticism
B. Emotional over-involvement
C. Hostility
D. Positive comments and warmth
E. Social isolation

Question 5: A 28-year-old man is being treated for treatment-resistant schizophrenia with clozapine and haloperidol. The patient's recent white blood cell count is below 3,000/mm³. The most appropriate immediate intervention is?

A. Discontinue the clozapine
B. Discontinue the haloperidol
C. Reduce the dose of both haloperidol and clozapine
D. Reduce the dose of clozapine
E. Reduce the dose of haloperidol

Case 2: Delusional Disorder

Question 1: Which of the following types of delusional disorder does de Clérambault's syndrome refer to?

A. Erotomania
B. Grandiose
C. Jealous
D. Persecutory
E. Somatic

Question 2: A male patient is treated with clozapine, and his psychotic symptoms are well controlled. Despite lifestyle changes to control weight gain, he has gained 12 kg in three months. What is the next immediate step of management?

A. Reduce the dose of clozapine
B. Start metformin
C. Stop clozapine
D. Switch clozapine to olanzapine
E. Switch clozapine to high dose haloperidol

Question 3: Which of the following antipsychotics is the least likely to cause QTc prolongation?

A. Aripiprazole
B. Clozapine
C. Haloperidol
D. Risperidone
E. Ziprasidone

Question 4: In which delusional misidentification syndromes does the patient believe others have been replaced by identical or near identical imposters?

A. Autoscopic syndrome
B. Capgras syndrome
C. Frégoli syndrome
D. Intermetamorphosis delusion
E. Subjective doubles delusion

Question 5: Which of the following is TRUE concerning depot antipsychotics?

A. Depot preparation reaches peak plasma concentration on the same day
B. Dose for dose, the efficacy of depot preparations is the same as oral medication
C. It is given as a subcutaneous injection
D. Only typical antipsychotics are available in depot formulations
E. The risk of neuroleptic malignant syndrome is higher compared to oral drugs

Case 3: Major Depressive Disorder

Question 1: Which part of the history is MOST concerning for post-partum depression?

A. Increased anxiety
B. Labile mood
C. Loss of appetite
D. Poor quality of sleep
E. Suicidal ideations

Question 2: During a consultation, a lady diagnosed with major depressive disorder tells you, 'It's been 10 minutes, and my friend Rachel hasn't texted me back. She probably hates me ... What if my other friends hate me too ... '?

What type of cognitive error is demonstrated here?

A. Blaming
B. Catastrophising
C. Magnification
D. Overgeneralisation
E. Splitting

Question 3: Which of the following is the most common endocrine abnormality seen in patients with depression?

A. Decreased prolactin serum levels
B. Decreased thyroxine (T4) serum levels
C. Decreased vasopressin serum levels
D. Increased cortisol serum levels
E. Increased ghrelin serum levels

Question 4: How does a patient's history of a major depressive disorder affect her child's risk of developing a depressive episode in the future?

A. No relationship
B. 2 times less likely
C. 3–10 times more likely
D. 10–20 times more likely
E. > 20 times more likely

Question 5: Which of the following antidepressants is LEAST likely to cause hyponatraemia?

A. Amitriptyline
B. Escitalopram
C. Fluoxetine
D. Mirtazapine
E. Venlafaxine

Case 4: Dysthymic Disorder and Premenstrual Dysphoric Disorder

Question 1: Which of the following personality disorders, when present, carries the highest risk of persistent depressive disorder?

A. Antisocial personality disorder
B. Schizoid personality disorder
C. Obsessive–compulsive personality disorder
D. Borderline personality disorder
E. Avoidant personality disorder

Question 2: In the treatment of depression, which antidepressant carries the highest risk if overdosed?

A. Amitriptyline
B. Fluvoxamine
C. Venlafaxine
D. Mirtazapine
E. Agomelatine

Question 3: Response in clinical trials is generally defined as a 50% reduction in depression rating scale scores. It is reported that 20% will recover with no treatment at all, 30% will respond to placebo and 50% will respond to antidepressant drug treatment. What is the number needed to treat for antidepressant response in the treatment of depression?

A. 1
B. 3–5
C. 10–12
D. 15–20
E. > 20

Question 4: Which of the following is NOT a poor prognostic factor for depression?

A. Co-morbid personality disorder
B. Acute onset
C. Incomplete symptomatic remission
D. Co-morbid substance misuse
E. Lack of social support

Question 5: Which of the following is the most suitable first-line treatment for depressive illness with psychotic features?

A. Olanzapine and fluoxetine
B. Mirtazapine and fluoxetine
C. Mirtazapine and venlafaxine
D. Lithium and sertraline
E. Lithium and valproate

Case 5: Grief

Question 1: Which of the following features is NOT seen in grief?

A. Dysphoria is likely to decrease in intensity over days to weeks and occurs in waves
B. The pain of grief may be accompanied by positive emotions and humour
C. The predominant effect is feelings of emptiness and loss
D. The thought content associated with grief generally features a preoccupation with thoughts and memories of the deceased
E. Thoughts of death are because of low self-esteem and feelings of worthlessness

Question 2: Which of the following is NOT part of the five stages of grief as described by Elisabeth Kübler-Ross?

A. Anger
B. Bargaining
C. Denial
D. Depression
E. Emptiness

Question 3: The following are risk factors for prolonged grief disorder, EXCEPT?

A. Death of a spouse/partner or child
B. Increased dependency on the deceased before the death
C. Lack of dependent children
D. Previous history of depression
E. Violent or unexpected deaths

Case 6: Bipolar Disorder

Question 1: When asked about her thoughts on being an excellent tennis player, Jane says, 'I am the undisputed best tennis player of all time. I need to train daily. I hope there won't be a traffic jam to the gym later. I often get hungry while playing tennis. The Japanese food down the corner is authentic and nice. Oh, the weather in Japan is lovely. You know any Japanese anime?' What psychopathology in thought is demonstrated?

A. Circumstantiality
B. Flight of ideas
C. Loosening of associations
D. Tangentiality
E. Thought insertion

Question 2: Dylan is a 24-year-old gentleman brought in by the police after he was found trespassing at a soccer stadium. He was recently fired from his job, and according to his employer, he was 'talking really fast and scaring customers away'. Dylan claims to no longer need a job as he is a billionaire from all the 'championship money' he won from various soccer competitions. He proclaims, 'Money is no issue. I will have a new Rolls Royce delivered to all my friends and family'.

What kind of delusion is demonstrated?

A. Grandiosity
B. Jealousy
C. Nihilistic
D. Reference
E. Persecutory

Question 3: The following are side effects of lithium, EXCEPT?

A. Hepatotoxicity
B. Hypothyroidism
C. Hypercalcaemia
D. Nephrotoxicity
E. Polyuria

Question 4: James is being treated for bipolar disorder with lithium. During a follow-up appointment three months later, he reports worsening low mood in the past four weeks. There is an accompanying loss of appetite and lack of energy. James finds himself tearful at times and no longer finds pleasure in things he formally found pleasure in (e.g., watching his favourite television shows). He has neither recent illness nor new medications initiated. What is the next immediate step in the management of his current episode of bipolar depression?

A. Add imipramine
B. Add omega-3 fatty acids
C. Add quetiapine
D. Switch lithium to fluoxetine monotherapy
E. Check compliance with lithium and lithium serum levels

Question 5: What does rapid cycling bipolar disorder refer to?

A. Patients who experience at least three episodes during a 12-month period
B. Patients who experience at least four episodes during a 12-month period
C. Patients who experience at least five episodes during a 12-month period
D. Patients who experience at least two episodes during a 6-month period
E. Patients who experience at least three episodes during a 6-month period

Case 7: Generalised Anxiety Disorder

Question 1: Jenna is a 39-year-old woman brought in by her husband for excessive worrying. These symptoms started around two years ago. She worries about not paying her bills on time, being stuck in the lift, missing her medical appointments, and even the whereabouts of her five-year-old daughter. Her family describes her as a 'worrier' since young, but her anxiety seems to have worsened over the past two years. She has been feeling restless and having difficulties with sleep and concentration. Her work performance has suffered, and she was recently fired. What is your diagnosis?

A. Panic disorder
B. Social phobia
C. Paranoid personality disorder
D. Generalised anxiety disorder
E. Agoraphobia

Question 2: Which of the following is FALSE regarding generalised anxiety disorder?

A. Genes contribute 30–50% to the development of an anxiety disorder
B. There is anticipatory anxiety described by patients in between episodes
C. Generalised anxiety disorder is associated with disrupted coordination between the amygdala and prefrontal cortex
D. Patients with generalised anxiety disorder are in a state of physiological dysregulation
E. Non-genetic factors contribute 50–70% in the development of anxiety disorders

Question 3: Which of the following statements about generalised anxiety disorder and its management is FALSE?

A. Concurrent psychotherapy has synergistic effects with pharmacotherapy in the treatment of generalised anxiety disorder
B. The first-line pharmacological treatment option for generalised anxiety disorder management is selective serotonin reuptake inhibitors (SSRIs)
C. Tricyclic antidepressants can be considered in patients who do not respond well to trials of SSRIs and serotonin–noradrenaline reuptake inhibitors
D. A primary treatment goal of generalised anxiety disorder management is to achieve early treatment response and remission
E. Benzodiazepines should be used for at least 12 months to alleviate the symptoms of generalised anxiety disorder

Case 8: Panic Disorder and Agoraphobia

Question 1: Which of the following is the first-line pharmacotherapy in the treatment of panic disorder?

A. Agomelatine
B. Alprazolam
C. Bupropion
D. Clomipramine
E. Sertraline

Question 2: In patients with panic disorder, the following are poor prognostic factors for treatment response, EXCEPT?

A. Divorce
B. Female sex
C. Low socioeconomic status
D. Marked agoraphobia
E. Severe initial symptoms

Question 3: Two years after having started paroxetine for panic disorder, Georgina found a reduction in the number of panic attacks over the past six months and decided to stop her medications on her own accord. She comes for her follow-up clinic three days later and complains of giddiness. She also experiences an increase in anxiety, low mood, poor sleep, headache, diarrhoea, reduced appetite, nausea and vomiting.

On examination, her blood pressure is 132/78 mmHg, and her pulse is 72 beats per minute. General physical examination and preliminary blood investigations are also unremarkable. What is the most likely diagnosis for her presentation?

A. Gastroenteritis
B. Generalised anxiety disorder
C. Major depression disorder
D. Mania
E. SSRI discontinuation syndrome

Question 4: Which of the following conditions is the most common co-morbidity in patients with panic disorder?

A. Agoraphobia
B. Alcohol use disorder
C. Bipolar disorder
D. Depression
E. Social phobia

Case 9: Social Anxiety Disorder

Question 1: Which of the following is TRUE about the pharmacological management of social anxiety disorder?

A. Antidepressants must be given at a higher dose than for depression
B. Benzodiazepines should be used regularly as a chronic medication
C. Beta-blockers like atenolol are useful in generalised social anxiety
D. Pharmacotherapy is recommended over CBT as the first-line treatment for social anxiety
E. The risk of relapse is high if antidepressants are discontinued soon after an acute response to treatment is seen

Question 2: Which of the following features is most associated with social phobia?

A. Avoidance to reduce anxiety
B. Compulsion to reduce anxiety
C. Generalisation to other phobias
D. Obsessions
E. Paranoia

Question 3: Which of the following is the most common form of specific phobia?

A. Animals
B. Death
C. Heights
D. Illness
E. Storms

Question 4: Which of the following specific phobias has the highest familial tendency?

A. Animals
B. Blood–injection–injury
C. Height
D. Illness
E. Flying

Case 10: Separation Anxiety and Selective Mutism

Question 1: Liam is an eight-year-old boy who was diagnosed with selective mutism in your clinic after he was referred for an inability to speak in school despite being able to converse in a home setting. Which of the following is TRUE regarding selective mutism?

A. Ten per cent of children develop selective mutism
B. The majority resolve after six months
C. Many children with selective mutism have pre-morbid speech and language problems
D. More common in boys than girls
E. The onset of selective mutism is usually after 12 years of age

Question 2: For the past month, a 10-year-old boy has been having episodes of severe anxiety and has difficulty sleeping without his mother present. He complains about having nightmares of his parents passing away from a mysterious illness. He has been refusing to go to school and complains of nausea and vomiting each morning. What is the likely diagnosis?

A. Generalised anxiety disorder
B. Panic disorder
C. Selective mutism
D. Separation anxiety disorder
E. Social anxiety disorder

Question 3: Which of the following psychotherapies is a suitable first-line treatment for separation anxiety disorder?

A. Cognitive behavioural therapy (CBT)
B. Eye movement desensitisation and reprocessing
C. Interpersonal therapy
D. Mindfulness-based cognitive therapy
E. Psychodynamic therapy

Case 11: Obsessive–Compulsive Disorder

Question 1: Which of the following about obsessive–compulsive disorder (OCD) is FALSE?

A. Rituals may be personal and private or they may involve the participation of others
B. Compulsions are repetitive behaviours or mental acts in response to an obsession
C. Rituals compensate for egosyntonic feelings of the obsessional thoughts
D. Most common obsessions include fear of contamination, fear of aggression and harm
E. Compensatory compulsions include repeating, ordering and arranging

Question 2: What is the first-line pharmacotherapy option for patients with OCD?

A. Sertraline
B. Melatonin
C. Milnacipran
D. Clomipramine
E. Clozapine

Question 3: Joseph is a five-year-old boy who is brought in for behavioural changes. In the past two weeks, Joseph kept changing his shirt multiple times until 'it felt right'. He was never this particular before, as reported by his mother. If prematurely stopped, Joesph would cry as he fears something bad will happen to him as he is not wearing the 'right shirt'. He was often fretful, waking up in the middle of the night due to nightmares in the past two weeks. On further questioning, Joseph was ill with recurrent fevers and sore throat for around two months before the onset of behavioural symptoms. His birth history and developmental history were otherwise unremarkable. What is the likely diagnosis?

A. Pediatric autoimmune neuropsychiatric disorders associated with streptococcal infections (PANDAS)
B. Obsessive–compulsive disorder (OCD)
C. Obsessive–compulsive personality disorder
D. Temper tantrums, child is normal
E. Autism spectrum disorder

Case 12: Body Dysmorphic Disorder

Question 1: A 26-year-old model presents to your clinic with concerns that her nose has grown bigger and become unsightly. This concern began after she was involved in an accident and was hit on the nose three months ago. Despite consulting multiple doctors and being told that her nose is normal, she is only reassured temporarily before the concerns return. It distresses her and leads her to wear a mask to cover her face, affecting her work as a model. What is the diagnosis?

A. Anorexia nervosa
B. Body dysmorphic disorder
C. Bulimia nervosa
D. Delusional disorder, somatic type
E. Obsessive–compulsive disorder (OCD)

Question 2: Which of the following is an appropriate first-line treatment option for body dysmorphic disorder?

A. Clomipramine
B. Fluoxetine
C. Lithium
D. Mirtazapine
E. Risperidone

Question 3: Which of the following psychiatric disorders is most associated with body dysmorphic disorder?

A. Alcohol use disorder
B. Depression
C. OCD
D. Panic disorder
E. Schizophrenia

Case 13: Trichotillomania and Excoriation Disorder

Question 1: Amongst the following listed sites, which area is most commonly affected in trichotillomania?

A. Axillary
B. Eyebrows
C. Facial
D. Perirectal
E. Pubic

Question 2: Which of the following forms of psychotherapy has the best evidence in treating excoriation disorder?

A. Dialectical behavioural therapy
B. Habit reversal therapy
C. Mindfulness therapy
D. Motivational interviewing
E. Psychodynamic therapy

Question 3: What is the usual age of onset for trichotillomania?

A. Elderly
B. Infancy
C. Middle-aged
D. Prepubescent
E. Puberty

Question 4: With which of the following syndromes is excoriation disorder associated?

A. Beckwith–Wiedemann syndrome
B. Down syndrome
C. Klinefelter syndrome
D. Noonan syndrome
E. Prader–Willi syndrome

Case 14: Hoarding Disorder

Question 1: Which of the following is NOT a common co-morbidity associated with hoarding disorder?

A. Generalised anxiety disorder
B. Major depressive disorder
C. Obsessive–compulsive disorder (OCD)
D. Schizophrenia
E. Social phobia

Question 2: Which of the following is TRUE about hoarding disorder?

A. Persistent difficulty in parting with objects of spiritual significance
B. Persistent difficulty in parting with possessions regardless of their actual value
C. They are usually able to keep their living area tidy
D. The items should not be discarded as they were expensive
E. The hoarding does not cause significant distress

Question 3: Which of the following factors predict poor treatment response to hoarding disorder?

A. Biological abnormalities on imaging in the occipital cortex
B. Late onset of hoarding disorder
C. Having a belief that hoarding is not a significant problem
D. Female sex
E. Lower baseline levels of clutter

Case 15: Anorexia Nervosa

Question 1: What is the most common cardiac complication you would expect to find in a 16-year-old person with anorexia nervosa?

A. Aortic stenosis
B. Atrial fibrillation
C. Bradycardia
E. Hypertension
E. Hypertrophic cardiomyopathy

Question 2: 24-year-old Bernice has a relapse in anorexia nervosa; she has not had her period for more than three months. Menarche occurred at 11 years old, and she denies any previous sexual intercourse. You explain that this secondary amenorrhoea is an adverse effect of anorexia nervosa. Which of the following regarding anorexia nervosa-associated secondary amenorrhoea is TRUE?

A. Amenorrhoea may precede weight loss in up to 20% of women with anorexia nervosa
B. Early use of sex hormones leads to better outcomes
C. Fertility rates in women with a lifetime history of anorexia nervosa are lower than in women in the general population
D. Patients with secondary amenorrhoea due to anorexia nervosa cannot become pregnant
E. Rigorous exercise can aid in recovery from secondary amenorrhoea

Question 3: Which of the following features in a patient with anorexia nervosa would warrant consideration for inpatient admission?

A. Age less than 18 years old
B. Asymptomatic sinus bradycardia of 45 beats per minute
C. BMI 15.2
D. Orthostatic hypotension with giddiness
E. Secondary amenorrhoea

Question 4: 22-year-old Nikki was admitted to the hospital for a low BMI of 14 on a background of anorexia nervosa. Three days after the initiation of a new feeding regimen, she complained of left upper abdominal discomfort associated with a sensation of 'bloating' after each meal. After just a few bites of her prescribed meal, this was associated with a sense of nausea and occasional 'burning' sensation in her chest. She last had bowel movements two days ago and is still able to pass flatus. On examination, her abdomen is not distended. On palpation of her abdomen, there is mild generalised discomfort, but the abdomen is soft with no guarding or signs of peritonism. Bowel sounds are reduced. Preliminary blood investigations are unremarkable.

What is the most likely diagnosis?

A. Acute cholecystitis
B. Acute pancreatitis
C. Gastroenteritis
D. Gastroparesis
E. Superior mesenteric artery syndrome

Question 5: What electrolyte derangement would you expect to see in refeeding syndrome?

A. Hyperphosphataemia and hyperkalaemia, hypomagnesaemia
B. Hypophosphataemia, hypokalaemia, hypomagnesaemia
C. Hyperphosphataemia and hypokalaemia, hypermagnesaemia
D. Hypophosphataemia, hypokalaemia, hypomagnesaemia
E. Hypophosphataemia, hypokalaemia, hypermagnesaemia

Case 16: Bulimia Nervosa

Question 1: Which of the following physical signs is suggestive of possible purging?

A. Brittle nails
B. Dry skin
C. Gottron papules
D. Raynaud's phenomenon
E. Russell's sign

Question 2: Cassandra is a 29-year-old woman who presented with binge eating followed by self-induced vomiting and was diagnosed with bulimia nervosa. Which of the following forms of psychotherapy would be offered as the first line of treatment?

A. Bulimia-nervosa-focused family therapy
B. Eating-disorder-focused focal psychodynamic therapy
C. Individual eating-disorder-focused cognitive behavioural therapy (CBT)
D. Interpersonal therapy
E. Supportive counselling

Question 3: Which of the following pharmacological treatments are typically used in the treatment of bulimia nervosa?

A. Amitriptyline
B. Fluoxetine
C. Haloperidol
D. Mirtazapine
E. Lithium

Question 4: Which of the following questions is NOT part of the SCOFF questionnaire?

A. Do you believe yourself to be fat when others say you are too thin?
B. Do you make yourself sick because you feel uncomfortably full?
C. Do you worry that you have lost control over how much you eat?
D. Have you recently lost more than one stone (14 lb/ 6.35 kg) in a three-month period?
E. Would you say that friendships are lost because of your eating habits?

Case 17: Pica and Rumination Disorder

Question 1: Which of the following medical conditions is pica associated with?

A. Asthma
B. Episcleritis
C. Iron deficiency anaemia
D. Psoriasis
E. Rheumatoid arthritis

Question 2: The following are known complications of pica, EXCEPT?

A. Atopic dermatitis
B. Intestinal obstruction
C. Lead poisoning
D. Nutritional deficiency
E. Parasitosis

Question 3: Which of the following is TRUE of rumination disorder?

A. Failure to thrive is necessary for the diagnosis of rumination disorder
B. It is more common in female infants
C. Rumination disorder is associated with hiatal hernia
D. Rumination is caused by low intragastric pressure
E. Rumination occurs only in adults

Case 18: Acute Stress Disorder, Post-Traumatic Stress Disorder and Adjustment Disorder

Question 1: Martin recently got into a car accident three weeks back. He comes into the psychiatric clinic for difficulties in sleeping and recurrent nightmares, with themes surrounding the car accident. He gets frequent flashbacks of the car accident when getting into the driver's seat. This results in difficulties in driving, and he has avoided driving since. What is the most likely diagnosis?

A. Adjustment disorder
B. Post-traumatic stress disorder (PTSD)
C. Acute stress disorder
D. Anxiety disorder
E. Traumatic brain injury

Question 2: Which of the following neurotransmitters is NOT responsible for the development of PTSD?

A. Noradrenaline
B. Serotonin
C. Dopamine
D. Brain-derived neurotropic factor
E. Testosterone

Question 3: Which of the following statements is FALSE regarding the management of PTSD?

A. First-line pharmacological options include selective serotonin reuptake inhibitors (SSRIs), serotonin–noradrenaline reuptake inhibitors and tricyclic antidepressants
B. Prazosin may be prescribed to patients with PTSD who are experiencing distressing nightmares
C. Psychological debriefing after a mass casualty event has no benefit in preventing the development of PTSD
D. Eye movement desensitisation and reprocessing (EMDR) therapy is not an approved treatment for PTSD
E. Antipsychotics may be used in the augmentation of SSRIs in the treatment of PTSD

Case 19: Illness Anxiety Disorder and Somatic Symptom Disorder

Question 1: A 55-year-old man presents with complaints of chest pain, shortness of breath, headaches and abdominal pain. These symptoms have been present for the past six months and have led to multiple emergency department visits and consultations with various specialists. Repeated medical investigations have been unremarkable; nonetheless, he remains concerned and anxious about the symptoms he experiences. When reassured by the cardiologist that his chest pain is unlikely to be due to a sinister cause, he expresses frustration that his symptoms are not being taken seriously. These various symptoms have affected his ability to carry on work as a car mechanic.

What is the most likely diagnosis?

A. Conversion disorder
B. Factitious disorder
C. Illness anxiety disorder
D. Malingering
E. Somatic symptom disorder

Question 2: Which of the following personality traits are associated with somatic symptom disorder?

A. High in neuroticism
B. Low in agreeableness
C. Low in conscientiousness
D. Low in extraversion
E. Low in openness

Question 3: Which of the following psychiatric disorders is the most associated with illness anxiety disorder?

A. Dysthymia
B. Generalised anxiety disorder
C. Panic disorder
D. Phobias
E. Substance use disorder

Case 20: Conversion Disorder and Factitious Disorder

Question 1: In a patient presenting with unilateral right lower limb weakness, which of the following physical findings suggest a functional weakness?

A. Babinski reflex
B. Hoover's sign
C. Hyperflexia
D. Numbness
E. Romberg's sign

Question 2: A 25-year-old man was admitted to the medical ward for repeated episodes of fainting. During the night, one of the staff nurses observes him injecting an unknown substance into his abdomen and then hiding the needle in his bag. On confrontation, it was noted that he had insulin and needles in his possession. He denies any financial motivation or other external pressures behind his actions.

Which of the following is the most likely diagnosis?

A. Borderline personality disorder
B. Conversion disorder
C. Factitious disorder (previously known as Munchausen syndrome)
D. Illness anxiety disorder
E. Somatic symptom disorder

Question 3: Patients with conversion disorder may unconsciously model their symptoms on those of someone important to them. What is this phenomenon known as?

A. Identification
B. La belle indifference
C. Factitious disorder, imposed by another
D. Primary gain
E. Secondary gain

Case 21: Delirium and Neurocognitive Disorders

Question 1: Which of the following are risk factors for Alzheimer's disease?

A. Asthma, hyperlipidaemia, cerebrovascular disease, type 2 diabetes, obesity, brain trauma

B. Hypertension, cerebrovascular disease, type 2 diabetes, obesity, osteoporosis

C. Hypertension, hyperlipidaemia, cerebrovascular disease, type 2 diabetes, obesity, brain trauma

D. Hypertension, hyperlipidaemia, type 2 diabetes, brain trauma, high level of pre-morbid education

E. Hypertension, hyperlipidaemia, cerebrovascular disease, brain trauma, chronic non-steroidal anti-inflammatory drug (NSAID) use

Question 2: What changes would you most expect to see on the MRI brain scan of an individual with Alzheimer's disease?

A. Atrophy of the putamen and dorsal mesopontine grey matter

B. Focal frontal or temporal atrophy manifests

C. Hyperintense signal on diffusion-weighted, fluid-attenuated inversion recovery (FLAIR), and T2-weighted images involving the cerebral cortex and corpus striatum caudate head and putamen

D. Reduced hippocampal volume or medial temporal lobe atrophy

E. Small lacunar infarcts in the subcortical brain regions

Question 3: Which of the following statements regarding apolipoprotein E (APOE) genotyping is most accurate?

A. APOE genotyping in presymptomatic individuals is generally encouraged because of the high sensitivity and specificity of testing, which adds to the predictive value of clinical criteria for Alzheimer's disease

B. APOE genotyping in presymptomatic individuals is generally encouraged because early detection allows for early intervention and prevention of Alzheimer's disease

C. APOE genotyping in presymptomatic individuals is generally discouraged because of the high costs involved in testing despite its high sensitivity and specificity

D. APOE genotyping in presymptomatic individuals is generally discouraged because patients who are APOE epsilon 4 (APOE4)-positive suffer undue psychological harm in the short term after results are released

E. APOE genotyping in presymptomatic individuals is generally discouraged because of the low sensitivity and specificity of testing and the lack of preventive options

Question 4: Which of the following is a reasonable treatment option for Alzheimer's disease?

A. Oestrogen replacement in post-menopausal women to improve cognitive outcomes
B. Formal exercise programmes to improve physical functioning to slow the progression of functional decline
C. Ginkgo biloba to improve cognitive outcomes
D. Omega-3 fatty acid supplementation to improve cognitive outcomes
E: Vitamin B supplements to improve cognitive outcomes

Question 5: Elizabeth is a 72-year-old lady who is on follow-up for mild cognitive impairment secondary to Alzheimer's disease. Her daughter reports that her mother's memory loss has progressed, and repeat Mini-Mental State Examination scores show a further decline to 18/30. She was started on donepezil.

How does donepezil aid in the treatment of mild to moderate Alzheimer's disease?

A. Cholinesterase inhibitors are neuroprotective and reverse the decline in cognition
B. Cholinesterase inhibitors delay institutionalisation by 12 months
C. Cholinesterase inhibitors provide a modest improvement in ADLs
D. Cholinesterase inhibitors show an increase in efficacy with an increase in the duration of use
E. Cholinesterase inhibitors work by decreasing the concentration of acetylcholine at sites of neurotransmission

Question 6: Lidia is 88 years old with advanced Alzheimer's disease. The Global Deterioration Scale screen shows a score of 7 out of 7 (severe dementia). Lidia is unable to carry out activities of daily living (ADLs), bedbound, uncommunicative and urinary incontinent. Her daughter is concerned about Lidia's food refusal. Over the past few months, Lidia has been more selective with her food, and her appetite has been steadily decreasing with a loss of weight. Lidia takes several spoonfuls of porridge for each meal and occasionally refuses food entirely. Lidia's daughter enquires about the role of inserting a nasogastric or percutaneous endoscopic gastrostomy (PEG) tube to aid in feeding, as the thought of her mother 'starving to death' terrifies her.

How would you advise her on the role of a nasogastric or PEG tube concerning feeding?

A. Do not insert a long-term feeding tube. Hand feeding improves survival outcomes over long-term feeding tube
B. Do not insert a long-term feeding tube. Tube feeding in advanced dementia does not prolong survival
C. Insert a long-term feeding tube. It allows the delivery of prescribed daily caloric intake and improves nutritional status
D. Insert a long-term feeding tube. It decreases discomfort from hunger or thirst
E. Insert a long-term feeding tube. It reduces the risk of aspiration

Case 22: Mental Capacity Assessment

Question 1: Which of the following scenarios suggests that the patient lacks the mental capacity to give consent to a colonoscopy procedure?

A. The patient is unable to perform the serial sevens test
B. The patient is unable to speak
C. The patient is unable to hear
D. The patient is unable to understand the benefits and risks of the procedure
E. The patient has just recovered from delirium

Question 2: John is a 45-year-old male who has a significant medical history of diabetes mellitus, hypertension and end-stage renal failure. Which of the following statements suggest that John may not have decision-making capacity and should be evaluated further?

A. His decision not to go for dialysis was communicated via an inpatient translator
B. He can retain the information relayed to him by the translator
C. His family claims that he is 'not in the right mind' and his decision should not be trusted
D. John does not want to go for dialysis, knowing that he will die within two weeks if he doesn't go for it
E. Laboratory tests show significant uraemia and John appears to be confused and agitated, with an inability to engage with the clinician meaningfully

Question 3: In the Mental Capacity Act, what does it mean that 'a person must be assumed to have capacity unless it is established that he lacks capacity'?

A. If there is no disease of the mind or evidence of impaired thinking, a person is assumed to have mental capacity
B. It is a default position that doctors assume the patient has mental capacity until they make an unwise decision
C. There is no need to assess a patient's capacity if they refuse medical treatment thrice
D. There is no need to assess a patient's capacity unless it is a complex operation
E. There is no need to assess a patient's capacity when they can maintain eye contact throughout your interview with them

Case 23: Attention Deficit Hyperactivity Disorder

Question 1: James is a three-year-old boy brought to the clinic for concerns over his behaviour. James appears 'always on the go' and does not interact with his younger brother. He has difficulties waiting his turn, which leads to conflicts with his peers. He does not appear to pay attention despite being spoken to directly. On examination in the clinic, you notice it is very difficult to sit James down in a chair. Physical examination is normal and developmentally appropriate for his age. What is the most likely diagnosis?

A. Global developmental delay
B. Autism spectrum disorder
C. Attention deficit hyperactivity disorder (ADHD)
D. Intellectual disability
E. Reassure that child is normal

Question 2: Tim has been recently diagnosed with ADHD. He has a background history of epilepsy. Which of the following management plans is NOT suitable for Tim?

A. Atomoxetine
B. Behavioural therapy
C. Bupropion
D. Clonidine
E. Methylphenidate

Question 3: Moses is a six-year-old boy who was recently diagnosed with ADHD and started on methylphenidate. He has developed short, sudden, repetitive and purposeless hand movements over the past month. What is your diagnosis?

A. Transient tic disorder
B. Chronic motor/vocal tic disorder
C. Tourette's syndrome
D. Methylphenidate-related tics
E. Epilepsy

Question 4: Mary is concerned about her 10-year-old son Joseph, who was recently diagnosed with ADHD. She comes into the clinic with concerns over the upcoming school examinations. How would you advise her?

A. Joseph is inevitably going to have poor academic performance due to his fluctuating attention
B. A request can be made on medical grounds for Joseph to have access arrangements for his upcoming school examinations

C. Joseph should take a medication break during the upcoming examinations
D. Joseph should double the medication dosing in preparation for the upcoming examinations
E. Mary should withhold all co-curricular activities to allow John to have more time to revise

Question 5: All the following are conditions associated with ADHD, EXCEPT?

A. Anxiety disorders
B. Depression
C. Oppositional defiant disorder
D. Post-traumatic stress disorder (PTSD)
E. Substance use disorder

Case 24: Autism Spectrum Disorder and Intellectual Developmental Disorder

Question 1: Ryan is a six-year-old boy who was brought to the clinic after his teachers were concerned he had features of autism. He was noted to have poor eye contact, poor social interactions with his peers and repetition of phrases, such as 'bang bang bang'. On physical examination, you note the following features:

- Relative macrocephaly, a long narrow face with a prominent forehead and chin, and large ears
- Midface hypoplasia with sunken eyes and pale blue irises
- Arched palate
- Heart – S1 S2, apical mid systolic click

Apart from autism spectrum disorder (ASD), what co-morbid condition does Ryan likely have?

A. Down's syndrome
B. Fragile X syndrome
C. Klinefelter syndrome
D. Marfan syndrome
E. Tuberous sclerosis complex

Question 2: The following are risk factors for ASD, EXCEPT?

A. Advanced parental age
B. Exposure to sodium valproate *in utero*
C. Male sex
D. Measles, mumps and rubella (MMR) vaccination
E. Preterm birth

Question 3: Which of the following statements regarding the non-pharmacological management of ASD is FALSE?

A. Cognitive behavioural therapy can be used if the child has the cognitive and verbal ability to engage and stay motivated
B. Children with a diagnosis of ASD should have ongoing follow-ups with a specialist (e.g., developmental and behavioural paediatrician, neurologist, psychologist, psychiatrist)
C. Early diagnosis and intensive behavioural and educational treatment programmes have limited benefits on the natural course of autism and subsequent outcomes
D. Families and carers should be offered personal, social and emotional support through local support groups

E. In each area, a specialist community-based multidisciplinary team for adults with autism (the specialist autism team) should be established

Question 4: Caleb is a 16-year-old boy with ASD. He has been having trouble with sleep onset. He has no other significant symptoms of note. Non-pharmacological methods have not been successful. Which of the following would be the most appropriate initial pharmacological treatment for him?

A. Diazepam
B. Melatonin
C. Mirtazapine
D. Quetiapine
E. Zolpidem

Case 25: Alcohol Use Disorder

Question 1: Janish has been admitted for alcoholic pancreatitis. It has been four days since admission, and he has been complaining of little humans walking towards him from the nurse counter. The nurse calls you as she noted him to be uprolling his eyes and his limbs jerking. He was also noted to have tachycardia and labile blood pressure. What is your diagnosis?

A. Acute alcohol withdrawal
B. Alcohol intoxication
C. Delirium tremens
D. Hypocalcaemia-induced seizures
E. Provoked seizure by sepsis

Question 2: Cherie presents with auditory hallucinations. She hears aliens whisper into her ear about how they will take her to Jupiter. She is orientated to time, place and person. She has been diagnosed with alcohol use disorder and is currently in the process of reducing her alcohol intake. Which of the below diagnoses explain her presentation?

A. Delirium tremens
B. Korsakoff syndrome
C. Wernicke's encephalopathy
D. Acute alcohol withdrawal
E. Alcoholic hallucinosis

Question 3: Kenneth was diagnosed with alcohol use disorder and has since been abstinent from alcohol use. However, he is keen on medications to help with the maintenance of abstinence. Which of the following medications listed below would be most suitable for him?

A. Naloxone
B. Disulfiram
C. Haloperidol
D. Diazepam
E. Sertraline

Question 4: Marcus is referred by his general practitioner for concerns of alcohol use disorder. Which of the following is NOT part of the CAGE screening questionnaire?

A. Have you felt the need to cut down on your drinking?
B. Do you feel annoyed by people complaining about your drinking?
C. Do you ever feel guilty about your drinking?

D. Do you require a drink to go to sleep?
E. All of the questions are part of the CAGE questionnaire

Question 5: Which of the following individuals should be evaluated for complications of alcohol use?

A. A 36-year-old female who takes one shot of vodka a day for the past six months
B. A 25-year-old male who consumes four shots of vodka (350 mL) before clubbing once a month for the past three years
C. A 30-year-old male who goes for a post-work drink daily with his colleagues at a wine bar, drinking two standard pours each time for the past five years
D. A 27-year-old male who drinks four cans of beer daily over the past three years while watching movies on his couch
E. A 37-year-old female who drinks a cocktail fortnightly with her friends for the past three years

Case 26: Cannabis Use Disorder

Question 1: Sharon presents with complaints of recurrent vomiting occurring every few months, which is relieved with hot showers. These symptoms have been ongoing for the past year. She is known to have a psychiatric history of an alcohol use disorder, major depressive disorder in remission and ongoing multiple substance abuse – methamphetamines and cannabis. What is the most likely diagnosis?

A. Acute alcohol withdrawal
B. Cannabinoid hyperemesis syndrome
C. Cyclical vomiting syndrome
D. Gastroenteritis
E. Pancreatitis

Question 2: Jesse is on follow-up for bipolar disorder, which was diagnosed three years ago. During the consult, you find out that she has been self-medicating with cannabis. What would you advise her?

A. Continue taking the cannabis as it has been helping her control her symptoms
B. Continue taking the cannabis as it will not affect her condition
C. Discontinue the cannabis as it may worsen the severity of her symptoms
D. Discontinue the cannabis as it is expensive
E. Leave it to Jesse as you respect her autonomy

Question 3: Which of the following signs and symptoms are NOT characteristic of cannabis intoxication?

A. Bradycardia
B. Conjunctival injection
C. Dry mouth
D. Euphoria
E. Increased appetite

Case 27: Stimulant Use Disorder

Question 1: Donovan, a 24-year-old male, presents to the emergency department with an altered mental state. On physical examination, he is noted to have clonus of his eyes, patellar clonus and hypertonia. His vitals are heart rate 92 beats per minute, respiratory rate 13 breaths per minute, pulse oximetry 99% on room air and a temperature of 38.6 °C. He has no significant past medical history. Which substance is likely the reason for his presentation?

A. Alcohol
B. Caffeine
C. Amoxicillin/clavulanic acid
D. Gingko extract
E. 3, 4-Methylenedioxymethamphetamine (MDMA)

Question 2: Rachel is brought in by her friends for an altered mental state. Her friends reported that they were clubbing together when she suddenly became confused. They admitted that they took the illicit drug ecstasy (MDMA). Which of the following physical findings do you NOT expect to find on physical examination?

A. Decreased respiratory rate
B. Nausea
C. Psychomotor agitation
D. Pupillary constriction
E. Sweating

Question 3: Which of the following medical co-morbidities is highly suggestive of cocaine use?

A. Allergic rhinitis
B. Hepatitis B/C
C. HIV
D. Infective endocarditis
E. Nasal septum perforation

Case 28: Opioid Use Disorder

Question 1: David is a 60-year-old gentleman who has repeatedly visited your clinic for a chronic productive cough for the past two years. He is a smoker of 40 pack years. He reports having a persistent cough for the past two years, and only cough syrups containing codeine are effective for him. He requests to have more prescribed to him as his last prescription from a month ago has since run out. His medical record shows that he has visited the clinic multiple times with similar prescriptions filled. Which of the following actions would NOT be appropriate?

A. Refer to a respiratory physician for further evaluation
B. Evaluate for symptoms of opioid dependence
C. Evaluate for possible underlying lung malignancy with further imaging
D. Prescribe the same cough medication to him
E. Screen for other substance use disorders

Question 2: Which of the following statements regarding opioid use is FALSE?

A. The onset of withdrawal symptoms typically occurs after two to three times the half-life of the withdrawn opioid
B. Pharmacological management of withdrawals includes clonidine and methadone
C. The severity of opioid withdrawal is correlated to the total daily amount of use
D. The severity of opioid withdrawal is variable based on the individual's physical health, and stress coping mechanism
E. Withdrawal symptoms of opioid use include having pinpoint pupils

Question 3: Which of the following is the best predictor of opioid toxicity?

A. Altered mental state
B. Euphoria
C. Pinpoint pupils
D. Reduced appetite
E. Respiratory rate < 12 breaths per minute

Case 29: Hallucinogen Use Disorder

Question 1: The following are signs and symptoms of acute phencyclidine intoxication, EXCEPT?

A. Ataxia
B. Numbness
C. Psychomotor retardation
D. Tachycardia
E. Vertical or horizontal nystagmus

Question 2: Which of the following statements about hallucinogen-persisting perception disorder is FALSE?

A. Duration of visual disturbances may be episodic or nearly continuous
B. It can be triggered by the use of other substances (e.g. cannabis or alcohol)
C. It is most commonly associated with previous lysergic acid diethylamide (LSD) use
D. It is not strongly correlated with the number of occasions of hallucinogen use
E. Reality testing is lost in hallucinogen-persisting perception disorder

Question 3: Which of the following statements about ketamine is FALSE?

A. Ketamine can induce a dissociated state
B. Ketamine causes cardiovascular stimulation
C. Ketamine can cause cystitis
D. Ketamine causes respiratory depression
E. Ketamine causes salivation

Question 4: Which of the following is TRUE about LSD withdrawal?

A. Benzodiazepines are the first line of management for LSD withdrawal
B. There are no withdrawal symptoms in LSD use
C. Withdrawal may last up to 6–12 hours
D. Withdrawal occurs within 72 hours of intoxication
E. Withdrawal symptoms include perceptual changes such as illusions, hallucinations and body distortions

Question 5: Brandon is a 30-year-old male who comes in with a three-year history of lower urinary tract symptoms – increased frequency and incontinence. He has no other significant urological medical history. He reported using ketamine for seven years. What is your main diagnosis?

A. Benign prostatic hypertrophy
B. Ketamine bladder syndrome
C. Pupillary dilatation
D. Type I diabetes mellitus
E. Urinary tract infection

Case 30: Gambling Disorder

Question 1: The following disorders are significantly co-morbid with gambling disorder, EXCEPT?

A. Attention deficit hyperactivity disorder (ADHD)
B. Bipolar disorder
C. Depression
D. Obsessive–compulsive disorder (OCD)
E. Substance use disorder

Question 2: Which of the following is NOT part of the four phases typically described in gambling disorder?

A. Bargaining phase
B. Desperate phase
C. Hopeless phase
D. Progressive-loss phase
E. Winning phase

Question 3: The following is true of gambling disorder, EXCEPT?

A. Early expression of gambling disorder is more common among young women
B. Gambling can increase during periods of stress, depression and substance use
C. Gambling patterns may be regular or episodic
D. Gambling that begins in childhood or early adolescence is associated with increased rates of gambling disorder
E. Most gambling disorder develops over years

Case 31: Borderline Personality Disorder

Question 1: Which of the following statements regarding recurrent suicidal and self-harm behaviour in borderline personality disorder is FALSE?

A. Approximately 6% of patients with borderline personality disorder complete suicide
B. Self-harm acts are usually precipitated by threats of separation or rejection by others
C. Self-harm acts may bring relief by reaffirming the individual's ability to feel
D. Self-harm acts may occur during periods in which the individual is experiencing dissociative symptoms
E. Rates of suicide attempts remain stable throughout the course of borderline personality disorder

Question 2: Which defence mechanism is commonly seen in patients with borderline personality disorder?

A. Denial
B. Sublimation
C. Projective identification
D. Rationalisation
E. Suppression

Question 3: Which of the following sleep architectural changes is NOT seen in borderline personality disorder?

A. Increased total sleep time
B. Increased N2
C. Increased rapid eye movement (REM) density
D. Reduced N3
E. Reduced REM latency

Case 32: Antisocial Personality Disorder

Question 1: Which of the following is NOT characteristic of antisocial personality disorder?

A. Aggression towards people and animals
B. Deceitfulness or theft
C. Destruction of property
D. Odd beliefs or magical thinking that is inconsistent in the given cultural context
E. Serious violation of rules

Question 2: What is FALSE about antisocial personality disorder?

A. Diagnosis cannot be made in individuals younger than 18 years old
B. Diagnosis is more common in males than in females
C. Diagnosis is synonymous with criminality
D. Diagnosis should adjust for the distorting effects of socioeconomic status, cultural background and sex
E. Patients with antisocial personality disorder can be amenable to psychotherapy

Question 3: Bryant is a 19-year-old male, who is brought in by his parents for challenging behaviour. As an adolescent, he was caught shoplifting multiple times, scammed others at betting games and abused cats. He had trouble maintaining friendships and was sent to a juvenile reformatory at 17. During his stay, he picked up fights with the juvenile inmates. He was recently picked up by the police again after robbing a convenience store. What is his diagnosis?

A. Antisocial personality disorder
B. Attention deficit hyperactivity disorder
C. Criminal behaviour
D. Conduct disorder
E. Histrionic personality disorder

Case 33: Schizoid, Schizotypal and Paranoid Personality Disorder

Question 1: The following are symptoms of schizoid personality disorder, EXCEPT?

A. Appears emotionally detached
B. Lack of desire for close relationships
C. Little interest in sexual experiences with another person
D. Paranoia
E. Prefers solitary activities

Question 2: The following disorders are significantly co-morbid with schizoid personality disorder, EXCEPT?

A. Avoidant personality disorder
B. Major depressive disorder
C. Panic disorder
D. Paranoid personality disorder
E. Schizotypal personality disorder

Question 3: Which of the following defence mechanisms is seen commonly in paranoid personality disorder?
A. Dissociation
B. Fantasy
C. Isolation
D. Projection
E. Splitting

Case 34: Dependent Personality Disorder

Question 1: John is a 22-year-old male who is overly reliant on his mother – asking her to make the majority of decisions for him, ranging from clothes to wear to jobs to apply for. He has difficulty expressing his opinions to others and often follows what has been suggested to him. He is often anxious when his mother goes on long overseas trips and worries about being unable to care for himself. What is his diagnosis?

A. Borderline personality disorder
B. Dependent personality disorder
C. Normal, no psychiatric disorder
D. Panic disorder
E. Separation anxiety disorder

Question 2: What is FALSE about dependent personality disorder?

A. An essential feature of dependent personality disorder is the pervasive and excessive need to be taken care of
B. Dependent personality disorder occurs more commonly in women than men
C. Patients frequently experience dissociative episodes
D. The degree to which dependent behaviours are considered appropriate varies with age and sociocultural groups
E. There is a fear of becoming or appearing more competent in fear of losing support

Question 3: Which of the following is NOT a known treatment for dependent personality disorder?

A. Antipsychotics
B. Assertiveness training
C. Behavioural therapy
D. Family therapy
E. Group therapy

Case 35: Suicide Risk Assessment

Question 1: In which period is the risk of suicide greatest in patients with a previous suicide attempt?

A. Within six months from the last suicide attempt
B. Within nine months from the last suicide attempt
C. Within 12 months from the last suicide attempt
D. Within 18 months from the last suicide attempt
E. Within 24 months from the last suicide attempt

Question 2: Which of the described methods of suicide poses the highest rate of fatality?

A. Cutting
B. Drowning
C. Fall from height – four storeys
D. Gas poisoning
E. Hanging

Question 3: Which of the following is NOT a warning sign for suicide?

A. Chronic pain
B. Impulsive and reckless behaviour
C. Significant mood changes
D. Sudden increase in alcohol use
E. Talking or writing about suicide

Case 36: Catatonia and Electroconvulsive Therapy

Question 1: How would you counsel a patient on the safety of electroconvulsive therapy (ECT)?

A. Antegrade and retrograde memory loss is an expected adverse effect of ECT
B. ECT increases the risk of dementia slightly
C. Mortality from ECT is higher than that of minor procedures involving general anaesthesia
D. There is a higher risk of adverse effects from concurrent use of ECT and antidepressants and antipsychotics
E. There is a small risk of structural brain damage from ECT

Question 2: The following are indications for ECT, EXCEPT?

A. Bipolar mania
B. Catatonia
C. Depression with food refusal complicated by dehydration
D. Depression with high suicidal risk
E. Severe generalised anxiety disorder

Question 3: Which of the following is the most common psychiatric cause of catatonia?

A. Bipolar disorder
B. Delusional disorder
C. Brief psychotic disorder
D. Generalised anxiety disorder
E. Schizophrenia

Case 37: Neuroleptic Malignant Syndrome and Serotonin Syndrome

Question 1: What is the most common cause of death in neuroleptic malignant syndrome (NMS)?

A. Disseminated intravascular coagulation
B. Heart failure
C. Liver failure
D. Renal failure
E. Respiratory failure

Question 2: Which of the following is NOT a symptom of serotonin syndrome (SS)?

A. Agitation
B. Bradycardia
C. Hyperreflexia
D. Hyperthermia
E. Mydriasis

Question 3: Which of the following factors increases the risk of developing NMS?

A. Dehydration
B. Hypothyroidism
C. Long-term use of antipsychotics
D. Low-potency antipsychotics
E. Younger age

Question 4: Which of the following medications, when added to fluoxetine, carries the greatest risk of developing SS?

A. Agomelatine
B. Bupropion
C. Mirtazapine
D. Olanzapine
E. St John's wort

Case 38: Insomnia Disorder

Question 1: Which of the following regarding Klein–Levin syndrome is FALSE?

A. Associated with hypnagogic hallucinations
B. Hyperphagia
C. Hyposexuality
D. Largely affects male adolescents
E. Recurrent episodes of severe hypersomnia

Question 2: Which of the following symptoms is less indicative of depression in patients who are medically ill?

A. Anhedonia
B. Depressed mood
C. Insomnia
D. Suicidal thoughts
E. Worthlessness

Question 3: How do benzodiazepines affect sleep?

A. Decrease in rapid eye movement (REM) sleep duration
B. Decrease in N2 of non-REM (NREM) sleep
C. Increase in N1 of NREM sleep
D. Increase in N3 of NREM sleep
E. Increase in sleep latency

Case 39: Narcolepsy Disorder

Question 1: Which of the following statements about nocturnal sleep polysomnography in patients with narcolepsy is FALSE?

A. Antidepressants should be stopped for at least one week before testing
B. Multiple Sleep Latency Test (MSLT) shows a mean sleep latency of less than or equal to eight minutes
C. MSLT shows two or more sleep-onset rapid eye movement (REM) periods
D. Stimulants and other psychoactive medications should be stopped one week before the tests
E. There is an REM sleep latency of less than or equal to 15 minutes

Question 2: Which of the following statements regarding cataplexy is FALSE?

A. Cataplexy occurs in type 1 narcolepsy
B. Cataplexy typically develops within three to five years of the onset of sleepiness in 60% of people with narcolepsy
C. Consciousness remains intact during cataplexy
D. Deep tendon reflexes are preserved during cataplexy
E. The majority of cataplexy attacks begin in the face

Question 3: Which of the following medications treats cataplexy in narcolepsy but has no effect on sleepiness?

A. Armodafinil
B. Modafinil
C. Prazosin
D. Solriamfetol
E. Venlafaxine

Case 40: Breathing-Related Sleep Disorders

Question 1: Which of the following can worsen the symptoms of obstructive sleep apnoea (OSA)?

A. Alcohol
B. Melatonin
C. Opioid use
D. Simvastatin
E. Telmisartan

Question 2: The following are risk factors for OSA, EXCEPT?

A. Age > 50 years
B. Female
C. Increased neck circumference
D. Obesity
E. Tonsillar and adenoid hypertrophy

Question 3: Which of the following is the gold-standard diagnostic test for OSA?

A. Actigraphy
B. History of snoring from the bed partner
C. Polysomnography
D. Sleep diary
E. Video recording

Case 41: Non-Rapid Eye Movement Sleep Arousal Disorder

Question 1: How does melatonin help in the treatment of insomnia?

A. Decreases sleep apnoea
B. Decreases sleep-onset latency
C. Improves sleep maintenance
D. Increases rapid eye movement (REM) onset latency
E. Reduces sleep duration

Question 2: A five-year-old boy was brought into the clinic by his mother over concerns of sleepwalking. Which of the following statements is FALSE regarding sleepwalking?

A. Injury may occur during sleepwalking
B. It is familial
C. It typically peaks between the ages of 8 and 12
D. Sleepwalking is more common in children
E. The child usually wakes up during sleepwalking

Question 3: At any given time, what is the proportion of the general population that reports insomnia symptoms?

A. 5%
B. 10%
C. 30%
D. 50%
E. 70%

Question 4: A boy, aged 11, has been diagnosed with a non-REM (NREM) sleep disorder. The most likely diagnosis is?

A. Nocturnal panic attacks
B. Sleepwalking
C. Sleep paralysis
D. Sleep talking
E. Sleep terrors

Case 42: Rapid Eye Movement Sleep Behaviour Disorder

Question 1: Which of the following statements is TRUE about rapid eye movement (REM) sleep disorder?

A. Avoid treatment with clonazepam
B. It is not associated with Parkinson's disease
C. It is seen more commonly in elderly females
D. It occurs during the early part of the night
E. In REM sleep disorder, there is no loss of muscle tone

Question 2: Which among the following is the best evidence-based non-pharmacological treatment for insomnia?

A. Interpersonal psychotherapy
B. Mindfulness psychotherapy
C. Psychodynamic psychotherapy
D. Acceptance and commitment therapy
E. Stimulus control therapy

Question 3: The following medications are approved for the treatment of chronic insomnia, EXCEPT?

A. Diazepam
B. Doxepin
C. Lemborexant
D. Ramelteon
E. Zolpidem

Case 43: Dissociative Amnesia and Dissociative Identity Disorder

Question 1: When a 38-year-old prisoner was asked, 'What is the colour of a lemon?', he answered 'blue'. What is the most appropriate diagnosis?

A. Derealisation
B. Dissociative identity disorder
C. Fugue
D. Dissociative amnesia
E. Ganser's syndrome

Question 2: Dissociative identity disorder is linked to severe experiences of early childhood trauma, usually maltreatment. What is the rate of reported severe childhood trauma for patients with dissociative identity disorder?

A. 10–20%
B. 30–40%
C. 50–60%
D. 70–80%
E. > 85%

Question 3: In which of the following psychiatric disorders is depersonalisation/derealisation a known diagnostic symptom?

A. Autism spectrum disorder
B. Major depressive disorder
C. Obsessive–compulsive disorder
D. Panic disorder
E. Schizophrenia

Question 4: A 14-year-old girl was noted by her mother to be more quiet and reserved in the past three days. Recently, her uncle was charged with an allegation of sexual abuse against one of his nieces. Today, she was found to be mute and unresponsive by her mother at home. She did not move nor accept any food or drink despite her mother's offer. She did not respond to anything that anyone else did or said. She was admitted to the hospital, but investigations did not reveal any significant abnormalities. What is the most appropriate diagnosis?

A. Depression
B. Depersonalisation
C. Dissociative amnesia
D. Dissociative stupor
E. Fugue

Case 44: Voyeuristic, Exhibitionistic, Frotteuristic and Sexual Masochism and Sadism Disorders

Question 1: Which of the following paraphilic disorders is characterised by the touching and rubbing of genitals against a non-consenting person?

A. Exhibitionistic disorder
B. Fetishistic transvestism
C. Frotteuristic disorder
D. Coercive sexual sadism disorder
E. Voyeuristic disorder

Question 2: Which of the following is NOT classified as a disruptive impulse-control and conduct-related disorder?

A. Exhibitionistic disorder
B. Intermittent explosive disorder
C. Kleptomania
D. Oppositional defiant disorder
E. Pyromania

Question 3: Which of the following is TRUE of voyeuristic disorder?

A. It involves the use of physical force or coercion to obtain sexual gratification
B. It is a paraphilic disorder which involves the patient exposing their genitals to a non-consenting person
C. Masturbation to orgasm usually accompanies or follows the act
D. The first voyeuristic act usually occurs after the age of 50
E. Voyeuristic disorder only occurs in men

Case 45: Paedophilic Disorder

Question 1: Which of the following statements about paedophilia is FALSE?

A. A significant number of paedophiles have concomitantly or previously been involved in exhibitionism, voyeurism or rape
B. The majority of offenders are strangers, unknown to the victims
C. One-third of the offenders are adolescents
D. The offender is usually a male
E. The presence of antisocial traits portends a poorer prognosis in paedophilic disorder

Question 2: Which of the following factors in paedophilic disorder is most likely to increase the risk of sexual reoffending?

A. Antisocial personality traits
B. High motivation for treatment
C. History of depression
D. Lack of emotional congruence with children
E. Lack of victim empathy

Question 3: Which of the following is TRUE of paraphilic disorders?

A. The majority of paraphilic disorders have their onset after 18 years old
B. Paedophilic disorder is the most common paraphilic disorder which presents to the legal system
C. Paraphilic disorders can be diagnosed if the patient has experienced intense and recurrent arousal from their deviant fantasy for at least one month and has acted on the paraphilic impulse
D. Paraphilic disorders have an equal prevalence in males and females
E. Persons with fetishistic disorder are often involved in criminal proceedings

Case 46: Transvestic and Fetishistic Disorders

Question 1: Kennedy is a 37-year-old married male whose sexual preferences include cross-dressing and a sexual interest in feet. He is in a heterosexual relationship and has no other sexual partners apart from his wife. He can achieve sexual stimulation without cross-dressing and involving the feet. What is his diagnosis?

A. Fetishistic disorder
B. Normal paraphilia
C. Sexual sadism disorder
D. Sexual masochism disorder
E. Transvestic disorder

Question 2: Which of the following is a poor prognostic feature of paraphilic disorder patients?

A. Late age of onset
B. Normal intelligence
C. Singular paraphilic disorder
D. Successful adult attachments
E. Substance abuse

Question 3: A 45-year-old gentleman was caught by the police for stealing women's undergarments. He later admitted to using these for masturbation. Which of the following specifiers would be appropriate if he was diagnosed with fetishistic disorder?

A. Body part(s)
B. Combined
C. Non-living object(s)
D. Transvestic fetishism
E. Other

Case 47: Gender Dysphoria

Question 1: Which of the following conditions is the most common significant co-morbid disorder in adult patients with gender dysphoria?

A. Autism spectrum disorder
B. Depression
C. Personality disorders
D. Post-traumatic stress disorder
E. Substance misuse

Question 2: The presentation of gender dysphoria manifests differently between children and adults. The following are symptoms of gender dysphoria in children, EXCEPT?

A. A strong preference for cross-gender roles in make-believe play or fantasy play
B. A strong preference for playmates of the same gender
C. A strong preference for the toys, games or activities stereotypically used or engaged in by the other gender
D. In boys, a strong preference for cross-dressing or simulating female attire
E. In girls, a strong rejection of typically feminine toys, games and activities

Question 3: Which of the following statements regarding gender dysphoria is FALSE?

A. A diagnosis of gender dysphoria requires marked incongruence between one's experienced/expressed gender and assigned gender of at least six months' duration
B. An older age at presentation makes the persistence of gender dysphoria into adolescence and adulthood more likely
C. Biological males with gender dysphoria more commonly have older brothers when compared with cisgender males
D. More biological females than males with gender dysphoria seek gender-affirming treatment
E. More than half of children diagnosed with gender dysphoria later identify with their birth-assigned gender once they reach adulthood

Case 48: Pyromania

Question 1: Which of the following signs and symptoms is NOT characteristic of pyromania?

A. There is deliberate and purposeful fire setting on more than one occasion
B. There is fascination and attraction to fire
C. There is gratification when setting fires
D. There is tension or affective arousal just before the act
E. The act of fire setting can be done for monetary gain

Question 2: The following psychiatric disorders are common co-morbid conditions of pyromania, EXCEPT?

A. Bipolar disorder
B. Depression
C. Gambling disorder
D. Schizophrenia
E. Substance use disorder

Question 3: What is the common age of onset for pyromania?

A. Adulthood
B. Early childhood
C. Geriatric
D. Late adolescence
E. Middle age

Case 49: Kleptomania

Question 1: Which of the following signs and symptoms is NOT characteristic of kleptomania?

A. There is a recurrent failure to resist impulses to steal objects that are needed for personal use
B. There is gratification at the time of committing the theft
C. There is tension built up before committing the theft
D. Theft committed is not done in response to a delusion or a hallucination
E. Theft is not better explained by antisocial personality disorder

Question 2: What is the common age of onset for kleptomania?

A. Adolescence
B. Adulthood
C. Early childhood
D. Geriatric
E. Middle age

Case 50: Child and Adolescent Mental Health Services

Question 1: Paediatric autoimmune neuropsychiatry disorder associated with strepto-coccal infections (PANDAS) occurs between three years and the onset of puberty. Which of the following manifestations is commonly seen in PANDAS?

A. Binge eating
B. Intellectual disability
C. Obsessive–compulsive disorder
D. Panic disorder
E. Psychosis

Question 2: Which of the following signs and symptoms are suspicious for child abuse?

A. Frenulum tears
B. Injury to genitalia
C. Multiple fractures in various stages of healing
D. Retinal or subconjunctival haemorrhage
E. All of the above

Question 3: Which of the following would be an appropriate first-line medical treatment for an adolescent with depression?

A. Clomipramine
B. Mirtazapine
C. Olanzapine
D. Escitalopram
E. Venlafaxine

Case 51: Old Age Psychiatry

Question 1: An 82-year-old gentleman was hospitalised following a hip fracture for which he has undergone hip surgery. He was referred to the psychiatry team as he presents with agitation and confusion. Which of the following is NOT a risk factor for the development of delirium?

A. Acute retention of urine
B. Constipation
C. Family history of delirium
D. Pain
E. Post-operative infection

Question 2: A 74-year-old gentleman is receiving chemotherapy for lymphoma. He experiences low mood, anhedonia, hopelessness, lethargy, poor appetite and chemotherapy-induced nausea. Given the constellation of symptoms, which of the following antidepressants would be most appropriate for the treatment of his depression?

A. Clomipramine
B. Mirtazapine
C. Sertraline
D. Trazodone
E. Venlafaxine

Question 3: A 77-year-old woman with a history of dense cataracts presents to the clinic complaining about seeing colourful tigers walking around the house. They last for a few minutes each time. She is aware that it is impossible for these tigers to be physically in her home and finds it amusing. She does not have any auditory or visual hallucinations or other complaints. Which of the following conditions best fit her descriptions?

A. Balint syndrome
B. Charles Bonnet syndrome (CBS)
C. Delusional disorder
D. Lewy body dementia (LBD)
E. Late-onset schizophrenia

Question 4: Over the past year, an 80-year-old woman has been having visual hallucinations of little kids running around. Her daughter reports fluctuating memory difficulties during this period, accompanied by hand tremors. Which of the following medications would be most appropriate?

A. Melatonin
B. Vortioxetine
C. Quetiapine
D. Risperidone
E. Rivastigmine

Case 52: Pregnancy and Breastfeeding

Question 1: Which of the following antidepressants should be avoided in patients who are in their first trimester of pregnancy?

A. Escitalopram
B. Fluoxetine
C. Mirtazapine
D. Paroxetine
E. Sertraline

Question 2: Which of the following antipsychotics taken by pregnant women has the lowest relative rate of placental passage?

A. Aripiprazole
B. Clozapine
C. Haloperidol
D. Quetiapine
E. Risperidone

Question 3: What of the following complications is associated with lithium use during pregnancy?

A. Cleft palate
B. Ebstein's anomaly
C. Hypospadias
D. Polydactyly
E. Spina bifida

Question 4: Which of the following antipsychotics should NOT be taken while breastfeeding?
A. Amisulpride
B. Clozapine
C. Haloperidol
D. Olanzapine
E. Quetiapine

Question 5: Breastfeeding by mothers on lithium can lead to the following adverse effects on infants, EXCEPT?

A. Hypotonia
B. Increased infections
C. Lethargy
D. Lithium toxicity
E. Raised serum creatinine

Case 53: Hepatic Impairment

Question 1: A 52-year-old gentleman was admitted following a fall. He has a history of Child–Pugh class C liver cirrhosis secondary to alcohol use disorder. During his inpatient stay, he started to experience signs and symptoms of alcohol withdrawal. Which of the following medications would be most suitable for the management of his alcohol withdrawals?

A. Chlordiazepoxide
B. Clobazam
C. Clonazepam
D. Diazepam
E. Lorazepam

Question 2: Which of the following antipsychotics is NOT affected in patients with hepatic impairment?

A. Amisulpride
B. Aripiprazole
C. Asenapine
D. Clozapine
E. Risperidone

Question 3: Which of the following antidepressants is most likely to cause hepatic impairment?

A. Agomelatine
B. Brexanolone
C. Sertraline
D. Vilazodone
E. Vortioxetine

Question 4: Which of the following mood stabilisers is preferred in the treatment of patients with bipolar disorder with known advanced liver cirrhosis?

A. Carbamazepine
B. Lamotrigine
C. Lithium
D. Topiramate
E. Valproate

Question 5: Hy's rule is used in assessing the hepatotoxicity of new drugs; what is the rule defined as?

ALT = alanine transaminase, AST = aspartate transaminase

A. ALT > three times the upper limit of normal and serum bilirubin > two times the upper limit of normal

B. ALT > four times the upper limit of normal and serum bilirubin > two times the upper limit of normal

C. ALT > three times the upper limit of normal and serum bilirubin > four times the upper limit of normal

D. AST > three times the upper limit of normal and serum bilirubin > two times the upper limit of normal

E. AST > four times the upper limit of normal and serum bilirubin > two times the upper limit of normal

Case 54: Renal Impairment

Question 1: A 68-year-old gentleman with bipolar disorder has elevated serum creatinine levels suggestive of kidney injury. Which of the following medications is the most likely cause of kidney injury?

A. Carbamazepine
B. Diazepam
C. Lithium
D. Olanzapine
E. Valproate

Question 2: Which of the following antipsychotics should be avoided in renal impairment?

A. Clozapine
B. Haloperidol
C. Olanzapine
D. Sulpiride
E. Ziprasidone

Question 3: Which of the following psychotropics is significantly removed by haemodialysis?

A. Aripiprazole
B. Fluoxetine
C. Pregabalin
D. Risperidone
E. Valproate

Question 4: Which of the following selective serotonin reuptake inhibitors (SSRIs) is less preferable in patients on haemodialysis?

A. Citalopram
B. Fluoxetine
E. Fluvoxamine
D. Paroxetine
A. Sertraline

Case 55: Forensic Psychiatry

Question 1: There are special scenarios where the physician must breach confidentiality to ensure the safety of threatened third parties. This duty to warn a potential victim of a patient is also known as?

A. ALI test
B. Durham rule
C. M'Naughten rule
D. Tarasoff I
E. Tarasoff II

Question 2: In criminal law, what does *mens rea* mean?

A. Guilty act
B. Guilty intent
C. Innocent intent
D. Innocent act
E. Suspected culprit

Question 3: Which of the following tests is commonly employed to determine if medical malpractice has occurred?

A. Bernard's test
B. Drummond's test
C. Edward's test
D. Montgomery test
E. Simmon's test

Answers to Topical MCQs

Answers to Case 1

Q1: E

Explanation
Options A–D are part of Schneiderian first-rank symptoms. Visual hallucinations are present in schizophrenia (up to 27% of patients with schizophrenia) [1] but are NOT part of Schneiderian first-rank symptoms of schizophrenia.

Q2: D

Explanation
Neologism refers to the creation of new, idiosyncratic words that hold special meaning for the speaker and are not found in the English language.

Q3: B

Explanation
Only 5–25% of patients with schizophrenia are unresponsive to conventional antipsychotics [2]. The efficacy of antipsychotics for acute symptoms has been clearly proven. Patients with 'positive' schizophrenic symptoms respond better than 'negative' symptoms. Of the patients who stop medication, 60–70% relapse within a year and 85% within two years, compared to 10–30% of those who are continued on medications. Adequacy of a medication trial requires optimum dosage for four to six weeks.

Q4: E

Explanation
High expressed emotion (EE) occurs in an adverse family environment, reflected in the quality of interaction patterns and the nature of family relationships among the family caregivers and patients. The five components of EE are: critical comments, hostility, emotional over-involvement, positive remarks and warmth. Emotional over-involvement, critical comments and hostility are the most predictive measures for relapse of schizophrenia.

Q5: A

Explanation
Clozapine should be discontinued immediately in the presence of agranulocytosis. Agranulocytosis occurs in 1% of people taking clozapine in the first few months of

treatment. The risk is greatest at around three months but decreases significantly thereafter to 0.01% at one year [3]. A low baseline white cell count has been associated with future neutropenia but NOT agranulocytosis. The risk of agranulocytosis increases with age, while that of neutropenia decreases with age.

References

1. Waters F, Collerton D, Ffytche DH, Jardri R, Pins D, Dudley R, et al. Visual hallucinations in the psychosis spectrum and comparative information from neurodegenerative disorders and eye disease. *Schizophr Bull.* 2014 Jul;40(Suppl_4):S233–45.

2. Puri BK, Hall AD, Ho R. *Revision notes in psychiatry*, 3rd edition. Boca Raton, FL: CRC Press/Taylor & Francis Group; 2014.

3. Alvir JM, Lieberman JA, Safferman AZ, Schwimmer JL, Schaaf JA. Clozapine-induced agranulocytosis. Incidence and risk factors in the United States. *N Engl J Med.* 1993 Jul 15;329(3):162–7.

Answers to Case 2

Q1: A

Explanation
De Clérambault's syndrome refers to erotomaniac delusional disorder. Patients with erotomania present with the belief that some important person is secretly in love with them. The person of whom this conviction is held is usually of higher status.

Q2: B

Explanation
Lifestyle modifications are helpful in most early cases and are the first line of intervention in treating antipsychotic-associated weight gain. Metformin is commonly used as an adjunct in the treatment of antipsychotic-induced weight gain in adults with psychosis. Stopping or reducing the dose of clozapine is not advised as the next immediate intervention, as the patient is likely to experience a relapse in psychotic symptoms. Clozapine is used in treatment-resistant psychosis; therefore, switching to another antipsychotic is likely to cause a relapse in symptoms and is not advised as an initial intervention.

Q3: A

Explanation
QTc prolongation is important to note as it is a risk factor for ventricular arrhythmia torsades de pointes, which is often fatal. Among the listed antipsychotics, the risk of QTc prolongation is lowest in aripiprazole. Risperidone and clozapine have similar low effects, and haloperidol has a moderate effect on QTc prolongation. Ziprasidone has a high effect on QTc prolongation.

Q4: B

Explanation

In Capgras syndrome, the patient believes others have been replaced by identical or near identical imposters. In Frégoli syndrome, an individual, most often unknown to the patient, is someone they know 'in disguise'. In other words, the stranger is thought to be a 'friend'. In autoscopic syndrome, the patient sees a double of themselves projected onto other people or objects nearby. In intermetamorphosis delusion, the patient believes they can see others change (usually temporarily) into someone else (both external appearance and internal personality). In subjective doubles delusion, the patient believes there is a double ('doppelgänger') who exists and functions independently.

Q5: B

Explanation

Depot antipsychotics are given intramuscularly. Both typical and atypical antipsychotics are available in depot formulation. Dose for dose, the efficacy of depot preparations is the same as oral medication, but depot antipsychotics can be more successful than oral medication in preventing relapse in patients with previously poor compliance. Depot preparations have long half-lives and may take several weeks for peak plasma concentrations to be reached. The risk of neuroleptic malignant syndrome is the same as for oral drugs, though reversibility may be poorer given the long half-life.

Answers to Case 3

Q1: E

Explanation

Options A–D are not specific to post-partum depression and can be seen in the acute puerperium period as part of post-partum blues. The presence of suicidal ideations and symptoms of post-partum blues worsening or persisting beyond two weeks is concerning for post-partum depression.

Q2: B

Explanation

'Catastrophising' is the process of giving greater weight to the worst possible outcome, however unlikely. 'Overgeneralisation' is the hasty generalisation of failure in one area of life to other areas of life with insufficient evidence. 'Magnification' is the tendency to give greater weight to a perceived failure, with dismissal of all previous successes. In 'blaming', other people are held responsible for the harm caused by the individual, especially for their intentional or negligent infliction of emotional distress. 'Splitting' is commonly seen as a defence mechanism in borderline patients and happens when patients adopt a polarised view of the world where people are either idealised as all 'good' or devalued as all 'bad'. There is a failure to see that each person has positive and negative aspects to their being.

Q3: D

Explanation

Hypercortisolaemia is commonly seen in those with major depression. This is evident by measuring the excretion of urinary free cortisol or salivary cortisol. Dexamethasone administration fails to stimulate the feedback loop and, in turn, fails to suppress the cortisol level. This is one of the most consistent and robust findings in depression. However, it is not specific to depression – it is also seen in mania, schizophrenia, dementia and other psychiatric disorders. Lower plasma ghrelin serum levels are expected instead. Serum T4 levels in the upper range of normal or slightly higher have been reported in depressed patients as compared to healthy or psychiatric controls. These levels have been found to regress after successful treatment of depression. There is no evidence for decreased vasopressin serum levels or decreased prolactin serum levels in depression.

Q4: C

Explanation

People with a first-degree family member who has experienced depression are 2.8–10 times more likely to develop depression [1].

Q5: D

Explanation

Selective serotonin reuptake inhibitors and serotonin–noradrenaline reuptake inhibitors have a higher risk of causing hyponatraemia. Tricyclic antidepressants have a moderate risk, while mirtazapine, bupropion, agomelatine and monoamine oxidase inhibitors have a lower risk.

References

1. Wallace J, Schnieder T, McGuffin P. *Handbook of depression*. The Guilford Press; 2002.

Answers to Case 4

Q1: D

Explanation

Having borderline personality disorder is a particularly robust risk factor for persistent depressive disorder. Early onset persistent depressive disorder (i.e., before age 21 years) is associated with a higher likelihood of co-morbid personality disorders and substance use disorder.

Q2: A

Explanation

Amitriptyline is a tricyclic antidepressant, which is toxic in overdoses. All tricyclic antidepressants may slow cardiac conduction and lower seizure threshold, leading to fatal arrhythmias in overdoses.

Q3: B

Explanation

The number needed to treat (NNT) is the number of patients you need to treat to prevent one additional bad outcome (death, stroke, etc.).

To find the NNT, it is important to first find the absolute risk reduction (ARR) due to the intervention. The NNT is the inverse of the ARR (i.e., NNT = 1/ARR). The ARR is calculated as (control event rate) − (experimental event rate).

Therefore, in the above example, to arrive at the NNT of 3 and 5, the calculations are as below. The control event in this case refers to antidepressant treatment in patients, of which the control event rate is 50% (i.e., 0.5).

Experimental event	No treatment	Placebo
ARR	0.5 − 0.2 = 0.3	0.5 − 0.3 = 0.2
NNT	1/0.3 = approximately 3	1/ 0.2 = 5

Hence, the NNT of 3 for antidepressant over true no treatment control and NNT of 5 for antidepressant over placebo.

Q4: B

Explanation
Acute onset of depression carries a better prognosis.

Q5: A

Explanation
The Maudsley [1] and NICE [2] guidelines suggest a combination of an antipsychotic and an antidepressant in the treatment of psychotic depression. A combination of an antipsychotic and antidepressant is superior to either medication alone, and treatment with antidepressant medication alone is unlikely to be successful.

References

1. Taylor DM, Barnes TRE, Young A. *The Maudsley prescribing guidelines in psychiatry*, 14th edition. Chichester Hoboken, NJ: Wiley Blackwell; 2021.
2. National Institute for Health and Care Excellence (NICE). Depression in adults: treatment and management. NICE guideline [NG222]. NICE; 2022. Available from: www.nice.org.uk/guidance/ng222

Answers to Case 5

Q1: E

Explanation

In grief, the predominant affect is feelings of emptiness and loss, while in major depressive disorder, it is a persistent depressed mood and anhedonia. Unlike major depressive disorder, where there is pervasive unhappiness and misery, grief comes in waves. Self-critical or pessimistic ruminations associated with low self-esteem are more commonly seen in major depressive disorder than in grief. If a bereaved individual thinks about death and dying, such thoughts are generally focused on the deceased and possibly about 'joining' them.

Q2: E

Explanation

The five stages of grief by Elisabeth Kübler-Ross are denial, anger, bargaining, depression and acceptance.

Q3: C

Explanation

It is thought that if the survivor has to care for dependent children and is unable to show their grief easily, they are at risk of abnormal grief.

Answers to Case 6

Q1: B

Explanation

Flight of ideas is characterised by a continuous stream of speech where topics jump rapidly from one to another, but there is a logical link between topics.

Q2: A

Explanation

Delusion of grandiosity is characterised by exaggerated power or importance.

Q3: A

Explanation

Lithium is not hepatotoxic. Adverse renal effects may be functional and reversible but may eventually progress to structural, permanent changes. Lithium is known to cause polyuria, polydipsia, goitre, hypothyroidism, chronic autoimmune thyroiditis, hyperthyroidism, hypercalcaemia, elevated serum parathyroid hormone and hyperparathyroidism.

Q4: E

Explanation

Checking compliance and lithium serum levels is the first step in the management of bipolar depression in patients already on an anti-manic drug. The use of monotherapy antidepressants to treat bipolar depression is concerning due to the risk of treatment-induced mania and rapid cycling. If prescribed, antidepressants are usually given with mood stabilisers such as lithium, valproate, carbamazepine or a second-generation antipsychotic. The evidence for omega-3 fatty acids as monotherapy is limited; however, they can be added at any point during treatment because they are well tolerated. Mood switching occurs in more patients who receive tricyclic antidepressants than other antidepressants.

Q5: B

Explanation

Patients who experience at least four episodes during a 12-month period are deemed to have rapid cycling bipolar disorder. The risk factors of rapid cycling include usage of tricyclic antidepressants, low thyroxine level, being a female patient, bipolar II pattern of illness and the presence of neurological disease. 'Ultra-rapid cycling' refers to rapid shifts between mood states alternating between periods of mania/hypomania, depression and euthymia, with each mood state lasting approximately 24 hours.

Answers to Case 7

Q1: D

Explanation

She fulfils the criteria for generalised anxiety disorder as evidenced by her pervasive excessive anxiety, difficulties controlling it and three of the following symptoms (restlessness, sleep disturbance, poor concentration) lasting more than six months.

Q2: B

Explanation

The symptoms described are more typical of panic disorder symptoms rather than generalised anxiety disorder [1, 2].

Q3: E

Explanation

Multiple guidelines suggest that benzodiazepine therapy for adults should be limited to a short course, varying from two weeks up to six months, due to concerns about possible misuse and dependence.

References

1. Cackovic C, Nazir S, Marwaha R. Panic disorder. *StatPearls*. Treasure Island, FL: StatPearls Publishing; 2023. Available from: www.ncbi.nlm.nih.gov/books/NBK430973
2. Patriquin MA, Mathew SJ. The neurobiological mechanisms of generalized anxiety disorder and chronic stress. *Chronic Stress*. 2017 Feb;1:247054701770399.

Answers to Case 8

Q1: E

Explanation

Most guidelines suggest a selective serotonin reuptake inhibitor as the first-line treatment option for panic disorder. Venlafaxine is an alternative first-line treatment option as well. Benzodiazepines should be limited to two weeks until the effects of a co-administered antidepressant are seen. Tricyclic antidepressants are effective but are not a first-line option. There is limited evidence on the efficacy of bupropion and agomelatine in panic disorder.

Q2: B

Explanation

Female sex is a good prognostic factor for treatment response.

Q3: E

Explanation

Discontinuation syndrome results from the abrupt cessation/rapid tapering of anti-depressants. These symptoms occur within a few days (typically one to four days) of abruptly stopping antidepressants or tapering them rapidly (typically one to seven days). Antidepressants with a short half-life are particularly prone to discontinuation syndrome, with paroxetine carrying one of the highest risks. The most common discontinuation symptoms include giddiness, fatigue, headache and nausea. It can also cause agitation, anxiety, diaphoresis, dysphoria, insomnia and diarrhoea. The history of abrupt cessation of her SSRI and normal blood test results make the diagnosis of discontinuation syndrome most likely.

Q4: D

Explanation

Depressive disorders appear to be the most common co-morbid condition, occurring in up to 68% of patients with panic disorder. Agoraphobia occurs in 30–50% of patients in community surveys [1].

References

1. Semple D, Smyth R. *Oxford handbook of psychiatry*, 4th edition. Oxford: Oxford University Press; 2019.

Answers to Case 9

Q1: E

Explanation

Some benefit of antidepressant use is usually seen within eight weeks, and treatment should be continued for at least a year and probably longer. Long-term use of benzodiazepines carries the risks of dependence and should not be used as monotherapy for social anxiety disorder. Beta-blockers (atenolol and propranolol) are indicated in specific social phobias (e.g., performance anxiety) and given one hour before the performance.

The United Kingdom's NICE guidelines recommend CBT as the first-line treatment for social anxiety disorder.

Q2: A

Explanation
The marked fear or anxiety about one or more social situations in which the individual is exposed to possible scrutiny by others leads to avoidance of the social situations.

Q3: A

Explanation
The following specific phobias are listed in descending frequency of appearance: animals, storms, heights, illness, injury and death [1].

Q4: B

Explanation
Specific phobia tends to run in families. The blood–injection–injury type has the highest familial tendency [2].

References

1. Boland RJ, Verduin ML, Ruiz P, Shah A, Sadock BJ, editors. *Kaplan & Sadock's synopsis of psychiatry*, 12th edition. Philadelphia: Wolters Kluwer; 2022.
2. Samra CK, Abdijadid S. Specific phobia. *StatPearls*. Treasure Island, FL: StatPearls Publishing; 2023. Available from: www.ncbi.nlm.nih.gov/books/NBK499923

Answers to Case 10

Q1: C

Explanation
Many children with selective mutism have pre-morbid speech and language problems. Common co-morbidities include developmental delay/disorder, communication disorder, elimination disorders and anxiety disorders [1]. Onset is usually between three and five years of age after normal speech has been acquired. It is slightly more common in girls. Selective mutism is chronic, with a remission rate of only 58% 13 years after the first referral [2].

Q2: D

Explanation
The increased and disproportionate anxiety around separation from attachment figures is characteristic of separation anxiety disorder. This is supported by the other features of sleep disturbances and nightmares surrounding themes of separation, somatisation and school refusal.

Q3: A

Explanation

CBT is a suitable first-line treatment option for separation anxiety disorder. CBT replaces negative beliefs with realistic, neutral thoughts. Patients are encouraged to face their fears, and this reduces the element of avoidance. This can be achieved through graded exposure to the feared situation.

References

1. Semple D, Smyth R. *Oxford handbook of psychiatry*, 4th edition. Oxford: Oxford University Press; 2019.

2. Harrison PJ, Cowen P, Burns T, Fazel M. *Shorter Oxford textbook of psychiatry*, 7th edition. Oxford: Oxford University Press; 2018.

Answers to Case 11

Q1: C

Explanation

OCD is an egodystonic condition as opposed to obsessive–compulsive personality disorder, which is egosyntonic. Egodystonic experience is defined by an individual's negative assessment of their thoughts and emotions on a background of preserved consciousness. OCD patients are often distressed by their obsessions, and the compulsions are performed in an attempt to relieve the distress.

Q2: A

Explanation

Selective serotonin reuptake inhibitors (SSRIs) are generally the first-line option for OCD due to good response rates and positive long-term results. There are no significant differences among the SSRI drug class. Melatonin is used in the treatment of OCD to restore circadian rhythm. Serotonin–noradrenaline reuptake inhibitors (SNRIs) are usually combined with SSRIs to synergise noradrenaline reuptake. Milnacipran is an SNRI that has received attention for the possibility of OCD treatment; however, its effectiveness requires further examination. Clomipramine is reported to be equivalent to or slightly better than SSRIs; however, its side-effect profile is less favourable, making it a second-line treatment option. Clozapine is not recommended for OCD due to poor evidence for efficacy.

Q3: A

Explanation

PANDAS usually occurs in children who develop streptococcal autoimmunity. Such children usually suddenly present with childhood-onset OCD and tic disorders, including Tourette's syndrome. Diagnosis is through the fulfilment of the DSM-5-TR for obsessive–compulsive and related disorder due to another medical condition. Other supportive investigations include antistreptococcal antibody titres, throat cultures, EEG, ECG and brain MRI. Possible management options for PANDAS include intravenous immunoglobulins, therapeutic plasmapheresis and early administration of corticosteroids.

Answers to Case 12

Q1: B

Explanation

There is an overvalued idea that can be challenged concerning her belief that her nose is abnormal, making body dysmorphic disorder the best option here.

Q2: B

Explanation

Selective serotonin reuptake inhibitors (SSRIs) are the first-line treatment option for body dysmorphic disorder. Clomipramine is a suitable second-line treatment option. Antipsychotics are used to augment SSRIs for treatment-resistant body dysmorphic disorder. Lithium is not used for body dysmorphic disorder.

Q3: B

Explanation

The lifetime rate of co-morbid depression in patients with body dysmorphic disorder is 75%. Approximately one-third of patients have a lifetime history of OCD, and 30% experience panic attacks [1].

References

1. Boland RJ, Verduin ML, Ruiz P, Shah A, Sadock BJ, editors. *Kaplan & Sadock's synopsis of psychiatry*, 12th edition. Philadelphia: Wolters Kluwer; 2022.

Answers to Case 13

Q1: B

Explanation

The most commonly affected sites are the eyebrows, eyelids and scalp. Less commonly affected sites are the axillary, facial, pubic and perirectal regions.

Q2: B

Explanation

Habit reversal therapy, together with cognitive behavioural therapy and acceptance-enhanced behaviour/acceptance and commitment therapy, have the most evidence in the treatment of excoriation disorder.

Q3: E

Explanation
Trichotillomania most commonly begins following the onset of puberty.

Q4: E

Explanation
Excoriation disorder is a form of impulse-control disorder which is a common feature seen in Prader–Willi syndrome.

Answers to Case 14

Q1: D

Explanation
Generalised anxiety disorder is most commonly associated with hoarding disorder. The others described – major depressive disorder, OCD and social phobia – are other commonly reported co-morbidities. The relationship between schizophrenia and hoarding is not well studied.

Q2: B

Explanation
In hoarding disorder, there is a persistent difficulty in discarding or parting with possessions, regardless of their actual value. The other options are incorrect.

Q3: C

Explanation
Early onset, strong attachment to possessions, poor insight, co-morbid depression/anxiety, cognitive impairment and biological abnormality in the ventral prefrontal cortex could lead to poor treatment response of hoarding disorder. A study [1] found that the female sex predicted larger reductions in overall hoarding severity.

References

1.   Tolin DF, Frost RO, Steketee G, Muroff J. Cognitive behavioral therapy for hoarding disorder: a meta-analysis. *Depress Anxiety*. 2015 Mar;32(3):158–66.

Answers to Case 15

Q1: C

Explanation
Bradycardia commonly occurs in anorexia nervosa due to increased parasympathetic (vagal) activity with an unchanged sympathetic tone.

Q2: A

Explanation

Amenorrhoea may precede weight loss in up to 20% of women with anorexia nervosa [1]. While rare, patients with secondary amenorrhoea may still be able to ovulate. There is no evidence for the early use of sex hormones. Fertility rates in women with a lifetime history of anorexia nervosa do not differ from women in the general population. Rigorous exercise contributes to secondary amenorrhoea.

Q3: D

Explanation

As a general guide, any signs of medical instability warrant inpatient admission for closer monitoring.

Q4: D

Explanation

Gastroparesis frequently develops with food restriction and significant weight loss. The main symptom is bloating (gas and distension), often after eating. Other symptoms include early satiety, fullness, nausea and vomiting.

While acute pancreatitis has been associated with anorexia nervosa, the diagnosis is less likely due to the lack of epigastric tenderness and the rise in amylase. Superior mesenteric artery syndrome is a rare complication that may occur in severe cases of anorexia nervosa. Weight loss reduces the fat pad covering the superior mesenteric artery, which narrows the angle between the two vessels, entrapping the duodenum and causing a small bowel obstruction. While the patient has not had bowel movements for the past two days, she is still able to pass flatus and, clinically, she is not in intestinal obstruction, a prominent feature of superior mesenteric artery syndrome. Gastroenteritis is less likely given the lack of diarrhoea, significant vomiting, sick contact or food consumption history. Acute cholecystitis is less likely given normal investigation findings, the subacute clinical course and the lack of right upper quadrant tenderness on palpation (absent Murphy's sign), nausea and vomiting.

Q5: D

Explanation

In response to carbohydrates, the rise in glucose causes insulin release, triggering cellular uptake of phosphate (and potassium and magnesium) and a decrease in serum phosphorus levels.

References

1. Dalle Grave R, Calugi S, Marchesini G. Is amenorrhea a clinically useful criterion for the diagnosis of anorexia nervosa? *Behav Res Ther.* 2008 Dec;46(12):1290–4.

Answers to Case 16

Q1: E

Explanation

Russell's sign refers to calloused skin over interphalangeal joints from repeated self-induced vomiting. Other signs of repeated self-induced vomiting include erosion of tooth enamel, dental caries and parotid gland enlargement.

Q2: C

Explanation

An evidence-based self-help programme or specialised course of CBT is recommended for bulimia nervosa in adults. CBT has the best evidence.

Q3: B

Explanation

Most evidence exists for high-dose selective serotonin reuptake inhibitors (SSRIs), with fluoxetine being well studied.

Q4: E

Explanation

The five SCOFF questions [1]:

- Do you make yourself **S**ick because you feel uncomfortably full?

- Do you worry that you have lost **C**ontrol over how much you eat?

- Have you recently lost more than **O**ne stone (14 lb/6.35 kg) in a three-month period?

- Do you believe yourself to be **F**at when others say you are too thin?

- Would you say that **F**ood dominates your life?

References

1. Morgan JF, Reid F, Lacey JH. The SCOFF questionnaire: a new screening tool for eating disorders. *West J Med.* 2000 Mar;172(3):164–5.

Answers to Case 17

Q1: C

Explanation

Iron studies should be considered in patients with pica as iron deficiency anaemia has been implicated.

Q2: A

Explanation

Pica can lead to medical or surgical emergencies due to poisoning, obstruction, nutritional deficiencies or parasitosis.

Q3: C

Explanation

Rumination disorder may be associated with medical conditions such as hiatal hernia that results in oesophageal reflux. Developmentally normal infants may have acts of rumination that are not pathological. Rumination syndromes can also be found in children and adolescents. Rumination varies in severity and can cause malnutrition, but failure to thrive is not a necessary criterion for this disorder. It is more common in male infants and emerges between three months and one year of age. Rumination results from high intragastric pressure, causing retrograde movement of the gastric contents into the oesophagus.

Answers to Case 18

Q1: C

Explanation

Acute stress disorder should be considered in patients who develop symptoms similar to post-traumatic stress disorder (PTSD) within three days to one month following exposure to the traumatic event.

Q2: E

Explanation

Testosterone was noted to have a protective effect in the development of PTSD, as there are studies to suggest that higher serum levels of testosterone correlate with a lower risk of PTSD development. The other four options are known to be neurochemical factors in the development of PTSD.

Q3: D

Explanation

EMDR is a trauma-focused psychotherapy which is approved for the treatment of PTSD.

Answers to Case 19

Q1: E

Explanation

The lack of preoccupation with acquiring a specific serious illness makes illness anxiety disorder less likely than somatic symptom disorder.

Q2: A

Explanation

Neuroticism, one of the Big Five personality traits, has been identified as an independent risk factor for many somatic symptoms.

Q3: B

Explanation

Seventy-one per cent of patients with illness anxiety disorder have generalised anxiety disorder, making it the most common co-morbid psychiatric disorder [1].

References

1. Barsky AJ, Wyshak G, Klerman GL. Psychiatric comorbidity in DSM-III-R hypochondriasis. *Arch Gen Psychiatry*. 1992 Feb;49(2):101–8.

Answers to Case 20

Q1: B

Explanation

Hoover's sign is useful to identify patients with conversion disorder who have paralysis in one or more limbs or one side of the face or body.

Q2: C

Explanation

In this case, there is clear evidence of the falsification of physical symptoms (syncope likely secondary to hypoglycaemia) with deception behind it. The patient had also presented himself as ill, leading to his current hospitalisation. There are no obvious external rewards for his actions, and there is no other evidence of another mental disorder (e.g., psychosis).

Q3: A

Explanation

Identification refers to the process where patients with conversion disorder may unconsciously model their symptoms on those of someone important to them. For example, a patient whose father recently had a stroke may serve as a model for conversion disorder, and they may have a weakness which mimics that of their father.

Answers to Case 21

Q1: C

Explanation

A high level of pre-morbid education is protective. Chronic NSAID use, osteoporosis and asthma are not risk factors for Alzheimer's disease

Q2: D

Explanation

Structural MRI findings in Alzheimer's disease include both generalised and focal atrophy, as well as white matter lesions. The most characteristic focal finding in Alzheimer's disease is reduced hippocampal volume or medial temporal lobe atrophy.

Q3: E

Explanation

The APOE4 allele is neither necessary nor sufficient to cause Alzheimer's disease and has a low sensitivity and specificity. There is a lack of evidence-based preventives, and even homozygotes for the APOE4 allele may not develop Alzheimer's disease in the future.

Q4: B

Explanation

Formal exercise programmes may improve physical functioning and the ability to perform ADLs, which slows the progression of functional decline in Alzheimer's disease.

Q5: C

Explanation

A Cochrane review [1] of 13 trials showed evidence of benefits for ADLs. The AD2000 study [2] found no significant benefit of donepezil compared with placebo for institutionalisation. NICE guidelines [3] concluded that although it was clinically plausible that treatment with an acetylcholinesterase inhibitor may delay the time to institutionalisation, limited direct evidence was available to assess the size of this effect. Cholinesterase inhibitors may show modest improvement in cognitive symptoms but do not prevent a decline in cognition. The Cochrane review and meta-analysis of the three studies reporting conversion to dementia gives no strong evidence of a beneficial effect of cholinesterase inhibitors on the progression to dementia at one, two or three years. Cholinesterase inhibitors work by increasing the acetylcholine concentration at the neurotransmission sites. There is no evidence that the efficacy of cholinesterase inhibitors increases with the duration of use.

Q6: B

Explanation

There is no evidence that tube feeding in advanced dementia prolongs survival; these procedures carry antecedent risks, such as agitation, use of physical and chemical restraints, tube-related complications and new pressure ulcers. There is no evidence that hand feeding improves survival outcomes over long-term feeding tubes. Feeding tubes will not prevent aspiration in severely demented patients as they aspirate oral secretions and regurgitated gastric contents. Tube feeding does not improve nutritional status or pressure ulcers. No measurable increase in discomfort following a decision to withhold artificial nutrition or hydration has been seen among patients with advanced dementia.

References

1. Birks J. Cholinesterase inhibitors for Alzheimer's disease. *Cochrane Database Syst Rev.* 2006 Jan 25;2006(1):CD005593.

2. Courtney C, Farrell D, Gray R, Hills R, Lynch L, Sellwood E, et al. Long-term donepezil treatment in 565 patients with Alzheimer's disease (AD2000): randomised double-blind trial. *Lancet.* 2004 Jun 26;363(9427):2105–15.

3. National Institute for Health and Care Excellence (NICE). Donepezil, galantamine, rivastigmine and memantine for the treatment of Alzheimer's disease. Technology appraisal guidance [TA217]. National Institute for Health and Care Excellence; 2011. Available from: www.nice.org.uk/guidance/ta217

Answers to Case 22

Q1: D

Explanation
A lack of mental capacity is considered when one is unable to decide for oneself if one is unable to (1) understand, (2) retain, (3) weigh information relevant to that decision or (4) communicate one's decision by any means.

Q2: E

Explanation
The use of a translator is acceptable when assessing a patient for mental capacity. Patients may make unwise decisions but still retain mental capacity. Mental capacity should not be decided solely based on information given by family members. Co-morbid medical conditions causing delirium (e.g., uraemia) should prompt a closer evaluation by the clinician.

Q3: A

Explanation
A person should not be regarded as unable to make a decision merely because they make an unwise decision. Repeated refusal of medical treatment does not mean that a patient has mental capacity if the physician suspects the presence of a disease of the mind. The degree of complexity of treatment offered does not determine if a mental capacity assessment should be done. The ability to maintain eye contact is not a criterion when assessing mental capacity.

Answers to Case 23

Q1: C

Explanation
James displays hallmarks of ADHD, such as hyperactivity and inattention, which are present in two or more settings.

Q2: C

Explanation
Bupropion is known to lower the seizure threshold and is not recommended in patients with epilepsy.

Q3: D

Explanation

In patients on methylphenidate, look out for tics as a potential side effect. Methylphenidate tics should prompt a change of ADHD management to non-stimulant options such as atomoxetine and alpha agonists. Tic disorders should not be due to underlying substance usage or medical condition.

Q4: B

Explanation

Following a comprehensive assessment by qualified professionals before the examinations, John can be evaluated for his eligibility for a spectrum of access arrangements (e.g., additional time) depending on local school policies.

Q5: D

Explanation

PTSD is not a known co-morbidity of ADHD.

Answers to Case 24

Q1: B

Explanation

Fragile X syndrome is a common co-morbidity of autism spectrum disorder. Various physical features suggestive of fragile X syndrome include the apical mid-systolic click suggestive of a mitral valve prolapse, large testicles and ears, smooth skin, hyperextensible fingers, flat feet, inguinal and hiatus hernia and facial features (long, narrow face with underdevelopment of the mid-face, pale blue irises, macrocephaly).

Q2: D

Explanation

There is no association between MMR vaccinations and the development of autism. The initial controversy arose from a 1998 paper by Andrew Wakefield and his colleagues, who published a case series in the *Lancet* that suggested an association between the MMR vaccine and autism. Subsequent papers refuted this posited link, and Wakefield et al. were held guilty of ethical violations and deliberate fraud (they had selected data that supported their case and falsified data).

Q3: C

Explanation

There is evidence that intervention is more effective when initiated as early as possible, with improvements concerning behaviour, functional skills and communication. Although there is no cure, symptoms can decrease over time and, in a small minority, be minimised to the extent that they no longer cause disability.

Q4: B

Explanation

Sleep disturbance is relatively common in people with ASD. This is thought to be due to an abnormality in circadian rhythm and is best treated with melatonin.

Answers to Case 25

Q1: C

Explanation

Delirium tremens is characterised by autonomic instability and profound confusion, alongside other signs and symptoms of alcohol withdrawal. It often occurs 72 hours from the last drink; this is in line with the fact Janish has already been admitted for four days.

Q2: E

Explanation

Alcoholic hallucinosis occurs in a patient with preserved sensorium and typically involves auditory hallucinations, usually involving voices uttering insults or threats. The hallucinations are not due to acute alcohol withdrawal and can persist after several months of abstinence.

Q3: B

Explanation

Disulfiram works by blocking alcohol oxidation so that acetaldehyde accumulates. This accumulation of acetaldehyde leads to unpleasant effects, such as facial flushing, throbbing headache, hypotension, palpitations, tachycardia and nausea and vomiting. Therefore, it acts as a deterrent to impulsive drinking when a person is abstinent. It should not be initiated in patients still consuming alcohol as it could lead to a fatal disulfiram reaction (hypotension and tachycardia). Other commonly used medications in the maintenance phase (but not listed above) include naltrexone and acamprosate. Benzodiazepines are helpful in the treatment of withdrawal symptoms. Naloxone is used in the treatment of opioid overdose. Sertraline is not used to curb cravings for alcohol during the period of abstinence.

Q4: D

Explanation

The CAGE [1] consists of four questions:

- Have you felt the need to Cut down on your drinking?

- Do you feel Annoyed by people complaining about your drinking?

- Do you ever feel Guilty about your drinking?

- Do you ever drink an Eye-opener in the morning to relieve the shakes?

It is often used as a screening tool to assess whether the individual has an alcohol use disorder.

Q5: D

Explanation

A standard drink is 30 mL of hard liquor or 300 mL of beer or 120 mL of wine. Risky use of alcohol refers to drinking more than 21 units (males) or 14 units (females) in a week. Option D qualifies for risky use of alcohol and should be evaluated for alcohol use disorder and its accompanying complications.

References

1. Ewing JA. Detecting alcoholism. The CAGE questionnaire. *JAMA*. 1984 Oct 12;252(14):1905–7.

Answers to Case 26

Q1: B

Explanation

Cannabinoid hyperemesis syndrome is likely in Sharon's case due to the chronic use of cannabis alongside symptoms of cyclical nausea, vomiting and abdominal pain. The defining characteristic of cannabinoid hyperemesis syndrome is the relief of symptoms with hot baths/showers.

Q2: C

Explanation

Cannabis use has been found to be associated with earlier onset of bipolar disorder, prolonged or worsened manic episodes and increased likelihood of suicidal attempts. The use of cannabis seems to be associated with decreased long-term remission and poor treatment outcomes.

Q3: A

Explanation

Tachycardia occurs in cannabis intoxication.

Answers to Case 27

Q1: E

Explanation

MDMA is known to increase serotonin release and hence precipitate the syndrome. The risk of serotonin syndrome is proportionally related to the dose of MDMA.

Q2: D

Explanation

Pupillary constriction is unlikely to be found in a patient acutely intoxicated with MDMA. MDMA is a type of stimulant which causes pupillary dilation, tachycardia and raised blood pressure. Dose-dependent effects include cardiac arrhythmias, severe hypertension that can lead to cerebrovascular accidents and, occasionally, circulatory collapse. At high doses, patients are likely to present with seizures, altered mental state and coma.

Q3: E

Explanation
Nasal septum perforation is an uncommon condition but could be a presenting sign of drug addiction. Perforation may occur due to cocaine's vasoconstrictive effects causing tissue necrosis and perforation, direct trauma to mucosa or contaminant-induced irritation.

Answers to Case 28

Q1: D

Explanation
Dependence should be suspected in patients with the use of codeine-containing cough mixtures for longer than a month. Other medical causes of chronic cough should be ruled out. Calling the police at this juncture would be premature and would break rapport with the patient. Where substance misuse is suspected, further evaluation and screening for other co-morbid psychiatric conditions should be done.

Q2: E

Explanation
Opioid withdrawal symptoms are associated with a sympathetic response, with dilation of the pupils. Therefore, a constriction of the pupils would instead be expected in opioid intoxication. Other symptoms include intense craving for the drug, restlessness and insomnia, myalgia and arthralgia, rhinorrhoea and tearing and gastrointestinal symptoms.

Q3: E

Explanation
Respiratory rate < 10–12 breaths per minute is known to be the best clinical predictor of opioid intoxication. Other symptoms of opioid intoxication include an altered mental state (euphoria to coma), miotic pupils, bradycardia, hypotension, decreased bowel sounds and dry skin.

Answers to Case 29

Q1: C

Explanation
Psychomotor agitation is a sign of acute hallucinogen intoxication.

Q2: E

Explanation

Reality testing is typically intact in hallucinogen-persisting perception disorder and, if lost, should prompt the clinician to look for an alternative diagnosis to explain the abnormal perceptions better.

Q3: D

Explanation

Ketamine does not cause respiratory depression, making it a commonly used anaesthetic agent in cases of trauma where respiratory and cardiovascular compromise are of concern. The chronic use of ketamine has been associated with severe ulcerative cystitis.

Q4: B

Explanation

There are no withdrawal symptoms in LSD use; however, in chronic use, LSD flashbacks may occur, which are defined to be symptoms that resemble the 'bad trip' of the prior LSD use, such as panic, psychotic symptoms and anxiety.

Q5: B

Explanation

Ketamine bladder syndrome results from chronic ketamine use and results in a small and painful bladder with symptoms of frequency, incontinence, haematuria and upper tract obstruction.

Answers to Case 30

Q1: D

Explanation

Gambling disorder is highly co-morbid with mood disorders (both depression and bipolar), substance use and addictive disorders (especially alcohol and stimulant abuse and caffeine and tobacco). Other associations include ADHD, other impulse-control disorders and personality disorders (especially antisocial, borderline and narcissistic personality disorders). Although many patients with gambling disorder have obsessive personality traits, full-blown OCD is uncommon in this group.

Q2: A

Explanation

The winning phase occurs with the gambler ending with a big win, which hooks patients. The progressive-loss phase occurs when gamblers structure their lives around gambling and take on considerable risks, such as cash in securities, borrowing money, missing work and losing their jobs. The desperate phase occurs with patients frenziedly gambling larger amounts of money, being unable to pay back debts, involving themselves with loan sharks, possibly embezzling money, etc. The hopeless stage occurs with an acceptance that losses can never be made up, but the gambling continues because of the associated arousal or excitement.

Q3: A

Explanation
Early expression of gambling disorder is more common among young men (ages 18–21 years) than among young women [1].

References

1. Boland RJ, Verduin ML, Ruiz P, Shah A, Sadock BJ, editors. *Kaplan & Sadock's synopsis of psychiatry*, 12th edition. Philadelphia: Wolters Kluwer; 2022.

Answers to Case 31

Q1: E

Explanation
Together with an improvement of impulsive symptoms, recurrent suicidal behaviour declines with time. In one study, suicide attempts in patients with borderline personality disorder declined from 83.1% to 46.6% over 10 years [1].

Q2: C

Explanation
Projective identification is found in borderline personality disorder patients where intolerable aspects of themselves are projected onto another to induce the other person to act in the projected role. This has clinical implications for the therapist – who should act neutrally toward the patient.

Q3: A

Explanation
Sleep architectural changes are similar to those seen in depression – reduced total sleep time, reduced sleep efficiency, reduced N3, increased N2 and increased REM density.

References

Soloff PH, Chiappetta L. 10-Year outcome of suicidal behavior in borderline personality disorder. *J Pers Disord*. 2019 Feb;33(1):82–100.

Answers to Case 32

Q1: D

Explanation
The presence of odd beliefs or magical thinking that influences behaviour is more characteristic of schizotypal personality disorder than antisocial personality disorder.

Q2: C

Explanation

The personality disorder is not synonymous with criminality, as criminality is limited to personal gain and is not accompanied by rigid, maladaptive and persistent personality traits. While some patients with antisocial personality disorder may be amenable to psychotherapy, the prognosis remains guarded.

Q3: A

Explanation

Bryant displays multiple features of a pervasive pattern of disregard for, and violation of, the rights of others that begins in childhood or early adolescence and continues into adulthood, fulfilling the DSM-5-TR diagnostic criteria for antisocial personality disorder.

Answers to Case 33

Q1: D

Explanation

Patients with schizoid personality disorder are aloof and eccentric and lack the paranoid ideation seen in paranoid personality disorder.

Q2: C

Explanation

The 'schizophrenic spectrum' concept includes group disorders like schizophrenia and Cluster A personality disorders, including schizoid personality disorders. In response to stress, individuals with schizoid personality disorder may experience very brief psychotic episodes (lasting minutes to hours). In some, schizoid personality disorder may be a pre-morbid antecedent of delusional disorder or schizophrenia. More common co-morbidities include major depressive disorder, schizotypal, paranoid and avoidant personality disorders.

Q3: D

Explanation

Patients with paranoid personality disorder use the defence mechanism of projection frequently. They tend to externalise their own emotions and attribute to others the impulses and thoughts they cannot accept. This excessive fault-finding and sensitivity to criticism may appear to therapists as prejudiced, hypervigilant injustice collecting and should be met with honesty and formal, concerned distance from the therapist. Fantasy is commonly seen in patients with schizoid personality disorder, who seek solace and satisfaction within themselves by creating imaginary lives, especially imaginary friends. Dissociation is seen in patients with histrionic personality disorder and is often seen as dramatising and emotionally shallow. Isolation is seen in patients with obsessive–compulsive personalities and, in a crisis, they may show intensified self-restraint, overly formal social behaviour and obstinacy. Splitting is seen in patients with borderline personality disorders, with the patient's feelings towards the therapist divided into good and bad with no in-between.

Answers to Case 34

Q1: B

Explanation

With various features centred on the pervasive and excessive need to be taken care of by his mother, leading to submissive and clinging behaviour and fears of separation, John fulfils the DSM-5-TR criteria of dependent personality disorder. In both separation anxiety disorder and dependent personality disorder, there is an element of anxiety when separated from the attachment figure; however, John has an additional component of dependency where he needs others to assume responsibility for most major areas of his life.

Q2: C

Explanation

Dissociative episodes are more commonly seen in borderline personality disorder than dependent personality disorder.

Q3: A

Explanation

Pharmacological therapy used in the treatment of dependent personality disorder includes imipramine, benzodiazepines and serotonergic agents for separation anxiety and psychostimulants for depression or withdrawal symptoms. Antipsychotics are not typically used in the treatment of dependent personality disorder.

Answers to Case 35

Q1: A

Explanation

The greatest risk of death by suicide occurs within the first six months after the suicide attempt. Recurrence of suicidal attempts within the first six months occurs at a rate of 75% amongst patients [1]. It is noted that the risk factor for death by suicide is a history of previous suicidal attempts.

Q2: B

Explanation

In the order of decreasing fatality: firearms (83%), drowning (66%), hanging (61%), gas poisoning (42%), falls/jumps (35%), poison ingestion (1.5%), cutting (1.2%) and other methods (8%) [2].

Q3: A

Explanation

Warning signs are characteristics that risk stratify the individual to be at imminent higher risk of suicide [3]. While chronic pain is a risk factor for suicide, it is not a warning sign for it.

559

References

1. Demesmaeker A, Chazard E, Vaiva G, Amad A. Risk factors for reattempt and suicide within 6 months after an attempt in the French ALGOS cohort: a survival tree analysis. *J Clin Psychiatry*. 2021 Feb 18;82(1). Available from: www.psychiatrist.com/jcp/risk-factors-for-reattempt-and-suicide-within-6-months-after-an-attempt-in-the-french-algos-cohort-a-survival-tree-analysis

2. Bachmann S. Epidemiology of suicide and the psychiatric perspective. *IJERPH*. 2018 Jul 6;15(7):1425.

3. Ryan EP, Oquendo MA. Suicide risk assessment and prevention: challenges and opportunities. *FOC*. 2020 Apr;18(2):88–99.

Answers to Case 36

Q1: A

Explanation

Mortality with ECT is comparable to that of minor procedures involving general anaesthesia. Prospective CT and MRI studies show no evidence of ECT-induced structural changes. Many psychotropic medications may be continued during a course of ECT for their synergistic effect without compromising safety, including antidepressants, antipsychotics and lithium. Anticonvulsants and benzodiazepines often interfere with ECT (e.g., decrease seizure duration) and may need to be tapered and discontinued. It does not appear that ECT is associated with an increased risk of dementia. There are three main types of impairment: (1) acute confusion, (2) anterograde amnesia and (3) retrograde amnesia. Anterograde amnesia occurs during a course of ECT and typically resolves within two weeks after completing the course. The period of retrograde amnesia typically involves the period during ECT and weeks to a few months before that.

Q2: E

Explanation

ECT is not indicated in anxiety disorders.

Q3: A

Explanation

Catatonia is most commonly associated with mania (accounts for up to 50% of cases). It is more common in mood disorders than schizophrenia [1].

References

1. Semple D, Smyth R. *Oxford handbook of psychiatry*, 4th edition. Oxford : Oxford University Press; 2019.

Answers to Case 37

Q1: D

Explanation

The usual cause of death in NMS is renal failure secondary to rhabdomyolysis, leading to a high release of myoglobin, which precipitates renal failure.

Q2: B

Explanation

Serotonin syndrome is associated with tachycardia and not bradycardia.

Q3: A

Explanation

Dehydration and other acute medical illnesses carry an increased risk of developing NMS.

Q4: E

Explanation

Serotonergic agents, such as selective serotonin reuptake inhibitors (SSRIs), serotonin-noradrenaline reuptake inhibitors, selective amphetamines, monoamine oxidase inhibitors, tricyclic antidepressants, lithium, dextromethorphan, meperidine, etc., carry an increased risk of SS. St John's wort acts as an SSRI, thereby increasing the risk of SS when combined with other serotonergic agents.

Answers to Case 38

Q1: C

Explanation

There are increased hypersexual behaviours in approximately half of males and one-third of females [1].

Q2: C

Explanation

With physical illnesses, patients may have insomnia, hypersomnia, anorexia, lethargy and psychomotor retardation due to their medical conditions.

Q3: A

Explanation

Benzodiazepines affect sleep architecture by increasing the duration in N2 of NREM sleep, which leads to a subjective improvement of sleep quality. There is a decrease in time in N3 of NREM sleep. There is also a decrease in the duration of REM sleep, which aids in memory consolidation and learning [2].

References

1. Arnulf I, Lin L, Gadoth N, File J, Lecendreux M, Franco P, et al. Kleine–Levin syndrome: a systematic study of 108 patients. *Ann Neurol.* 2008 Apr;63(4):482–93.

2. De Mendonça FMR, De Mendonça GPRR, Souza LC, Galvão LP, Paiva HS, De Azevedo Marques Périco C, et al. Benzodiazepines and sleep architecture: a systematic review. *CNSNDDT*. 2023 Feb;22(2):172–9.

Answers to Case 39

Q1: A

Explanation

Antidepressants should be stopped for at least three weeks before testing (four weeks for fluoxetine with a longer half-life). Individuals without sleep disorders enter REM sleep 80 to 100 minutes after sleep onset.

Q2: D

Explanation

During whole-body cataplexy, there is a transient loss of deep tendon reflexes, which can help clinicians distinguish cataplexy from a functional neurological symptom disorder.

Q3: E

Explanation

Antidepressants such as venlafaxine and fluoxetine are thought to increase noradrenergic and serotonergic signalling, which suppresses REM sleep and reduces cataplexy. However, it does not improve the sleepiness experienced in narcolepsy. Modafinil, armodafinil and solriamfetol have no effect on cataplexy. Prazosin worsens cataplexy.

Answers to Case 40

Q1: A

Explanation

Alcohol can depress the central nervous system, exacerbate OSA, worsen sleepiness and promote weight gain. Other medications which can exacerbate OSA symptoms include benzodiazepine receptor agonists, barbiturates, other anti-epileptic medications, sedating antidepressants, antihistamines and opiates. Opioid use is established to have an association with central sleep apnoea, but the relationship with OSA is not as clear and still requires further studies and research.

Q2: B

Explanation

The prevalence of OSA increases with age, rising from young adulthood through the sixth to seventh decade, then plateauing after. OSA is more common in males than females. The risk of OSA correlates well with the body mass index and obesity, a well-established risk factor for OSA. Craniofacial or upper airway abnormalities, including tonsillar and adenoid hypertrophy, increase the likelihood of having OSA.

Q3: C

Explanation

Polysomnography is the gold-standard diagnostic test for OSA.

Answers to Case 41

Q1: B

Explanation

Melatonin works best when taken a few hours before bedtime, helping to augment natural circadian alignment. Melatonin appears to shorten the time to sleep onset (reduces latency) by decreasing the typical evening suprachiasmatic nucleus-driven arousal, and it helps to reinforce circadian periodicity.

Q2: E

Explanation

Sleepwalking is an NREM sleep disorder and may not always manifest as actual walking but can present as sitting up and doing repetitive movements. During sleepwalking, their eyes may be open, but they do not respond to questions and are very difficult to wake. If awakened during the episode, they are confused and disorientated. Sleepwalking can start at any age but is more common in young children and becomes less common in older childhood. It is rare in adulthood, usually occurring in the context of sleep deprivation, exacerbated by alcohol or other depressant drugs. Sleepwalking may be familial.

Q3: C

Explanation

Approximately 30% of the general population reports insomnia. It is more common in females than males and greater in the elderly. The prevalence of 'clinically significant insomnia' is lower, at 9–12% [1].

Q4: B

Explanation

Sleepwalking is the most common NREM sleep disorder for children aged 6 to 11.

References

1. Semple D, Smyth R. *Oxford handbook of psychiatry*, 4th edition. Oxford: Oxford University Press; 2019.

Answers to Case 42

Q1: E

Explanation

REM sleep is normally accompanied by muscle atonia, episodic rapid eye movements and dreaming. In REM sleep disorder, there is no loss of muscle tone and the dreams are acted out as complex behaviours. During these episodes, patients have limited awareness of their surroundings. REM sleep predominates during the final one-third of the night, and hence, episodes of REM sleep disorders arise during the middle to the latter third of the night. REM sleep disorders are associated with neurological disorders, usually degenerative (e.g., Parkinson's disease), diffuse Lewy body disease, multiple system atrophy and Guillain–Barré syndrome. It is more common in the elderly, particularly men. If symptoms are chronic and problematic, clonazepam (0.5–1.0 mg at night) can be used to treat symptoms, with good evidence of long-term safety and sustained benefit.

Q2: E

Explanation
Stimulus control therapy is part of cognitive behavioural therapy for insomnia (CBT-I), which is the preferred form of treatment for chronic insomnia in adults and has been endorsed as first-line therapy by multiple societies and guideline panels. Examples of stimulus control include going to bed only when sleepy; using the bed only for sleep and sex; if sleep does not occur, not remaining in bed for more than 10–20 minutes, getting up and going to another room and returning to bed only when sleepy; establish a regular time to get up, with no more than one hour variation.

Q3: A

Explanation
Long-acting benzodiazepines like diazepam are not recommended as there is a higher risk of dependence and habituation, especially when alternatives are readily available. There are four main categories of medications (with regulatory approval) based on their mechanism of action:

- Benzodiazepine receptor agonists, which include the non-benzodiazepine receptor agonists (zolpidem, eszopiclone and zaleplon) and five older benzodiazepine hypnotics (estazolam, flurazepam, temazepam, triazolam and quazepam)

- Dual orexin receptor antagonists (lemborexant, daridorexant and suvorexant)

- Histamine receptor antagonists (low-dose doxepin)

- Melatonin receptor agonists (ramelteon)

Answers to Case 43

Q1: E

Explanation
Ganser's syndrome is a rare dissociative disorder characterised by the production of 'approximate answers', psychogenic physical symptoms, hallucinations and apparent clouding of consciousness. 'Approximate answers' refers to answers given to simple questions that are wrong but reflect an understanding of the question and are clearly related to the correct answer.

Q2: E

Explanation

An estimated 85–97% of patients with dissociative identity disorder report a history of severe childhood trauma [1]. Physical and sexual abuse are the most frequently reported sources of childhood trauma.

Q3: D

Explanation

Depersonalisation/derealisation is one of the symptoms of a panic attack and panic disorder. Therefore, depersonalisation/derealisation disorder should not be diagnosed when the symptoms occur only during panic attacks that are part of panic disorder, social anxiety disorder or a specific phobia.

Q4: D

Explanation

Dissociative stupor is one of three dissociative syndromes which are present in ICD-10 but not in DSM-5-TR. Dissociative stupors are rare and characterised by a reduction or absence of voluntary movements, being mute and a lack of responsiveness to external stimuli, potentially induced by stress. While they do not respond to stimulation, they are aware of their surroundings. It is essential to exclude other conditions, such as schizophrenia, depressive disorder, mania and organic brain diseases.

References

1. Boland RJ, Verduin ML, Ruiz P, Shah A, Sadock BJ, editors. *Kaplan & Sadock's synopsis of psychiatry*, 12th edition. Philadelphia: Wolters Kluwer; 2022.

Answers to Case 44

Q1: C

Explanation

Frotteuristic disorder is typically characterised by a man rubbing his penis against the body parts of a fully clothed woman to achieve orgasm.

Q2: A

Explanation

Exhibitionistic disorder is classified as a paraphilic disorder as opposed to an impulse-control disorder.

Q3: C

Explanation

Voyeurism refers to observing the sexual activity of others repeatedly as a preferred means of sexual arousal. Voyeurism is usually accompanied by or followed by masturbation. The lifetime prevalence of voyeuristic disorder is estimated to be as high as 12% in males and 4% in females [1]. The first voyeuristic act usually occurs during childhood. Physical force or coercion is not part of the sexual gratification process in voyeuristic disorder. Exposure of genitals to a non-consenting person is characteristic of exhibition-istic disorder.

References

1. American Psychiatric Association. *Diagnostic and statistical manual of mental disorders*, 5th edition, text revision (DSM-5-TR). Washington, DC. American Psychiatric Association Publishing; 2022. Available from: www.psychiatry.org/psychiatrists/practice/dsm

Answers to Case 45

Q1: B

Explanation
About 93% of children who are victims of sexual abuse know their abuser [1].

Q2: A

Explanation
Men with antisocial personality traits and paedophilic disorders are more likely to com-mit sexual acts with children and thus qualify for a diagnosis of paedophilic disorder. Antisocial traits were a particularly important predictor of violent non-sexual recidivism and general recidivism. Emotional congruence with children is related to both paedo-philic sexual interest and the likelihood of sexually reoffending among individuals who have been sexually offended. Certain clinical presentations (e.g., denial, lack of victim empathy, low motivation for treatment), were surprisingly unrelated to sexual recidivism risk [2].

Q3: B

Explanation

Paraphilic disorders are largely male conditions. More than 50% of all paraphilic disor-ders have their onset before age 18 [3]. In paedophilic disorder, because a child is a vic-tim, greater effort is spent tracking down the culprit than in other paraphilic disorders. Persons with fetishistic disorder rarely become involved in the legal system. Diagnosis of paraphilic disorders requires a minimum of 6 months of persistent symptoms.

References

1. Rape Abuse and Incest National Network (RAINN). Child sexual abuse statistics (2015). RAINN; 2015. Available from: www.rainn.org/articles/child-sexual-abuse

2. Hanson KR, Morton-Bourgo K. Predictors of sexual recidivism: an updated meta-analysis. Public Safety Canada; 2004. Available from: www.publicsafety.gc.ca/cnt/rsrcs/pblctns/2004-02-prdctrs-sxl-rcdvsm-pdtd/index-en.aspx

3. American Psychiatric Association. *Diagnostic and statistical manual of mental disorders*, 5th edition, text revision (DSM-5-TR). Washington, DC: American Psychiatric Association Publishing; 2022. Available from: www.psychiatry.org/psychiatrists/practice/dsm

Answers to Case 46

Q1: B

Explanation
People with paraphilias (as opposed to paraphilic disorders) do not experience any other distress and can achieve sexual satisfaction even without the use of paraphiliac stimuli. A paraphilic disorder is considered if the individual experiences distress or impairment or has a paraphilia whose satisfaction has entailed personal harm or risk of harm to others.

Q2: E

Explanation
The above-mentioned are all good prognostic factors for successful treatment of paraphilic disorders, of which substance abuse leads to poor prognosis for patients. Other poor prognostic factors include early age of onset, high frequency of acts and lack of shame or guilt concerning such acts.

Q3: C

Explanation
The listed specifiers in DSM-5-TR include body part(s), non-living object(s) and other. There is no such specifier as 'combined'.

Answers to Case 47

Q1: B

Explanation
Mood and anxiety disorders are the most common psychiatric co-morbidities.

Q2: B

Explanation
A strong preference for playmates of the other gender is typical in the presentation of children with gender dysphoria.

Q3: D

Explanation
In adults, more biological males seek gender-affirming treatment, with ratios ranging from 1:1 to 6.1:1 in most studies in the United States and Europe [1].

References

1. American Psychiatric Association. *Diagnostic and statistical manual of mental disorders*, 5th edition, text revision (DSM-5-TR). Washington, DC: American Psychiatric Association Publishing; 2022. Available from: www.psychiatry.org/psychiatrists/practice/dsm

Answers to Case 48

Q1: E

Explanation

Firesetting in pyromania is a compulsive act and not performed for monetary gain, as an expression of a sociopolitical ideology, to conceal crimes, etc. It should also not be better explained by conduct disorder, antisocial personality disorder or influenced by psychosis.

Q2: D

Explanation

Pyromania has co-morbidity with substance use disorder, affective disorders and other disruptive, impulse-control and gambling disorders.

Q3: D

Explanation

Pyromania most often begins in late adolescence.

Answers to Case 49

Q1: A

Explanation

Items stolen in kleptomania are typically of trivial value and not needed by the patient.

Q2: A

Explanation

Kleptomania most often begins in adolescence.

Answers to Case 50

Q1: C

Explanation

PANDAS occurs after a group A streptococcal infection and is a post-infectious auto-immune disorder characterised by the sudden onset of obsessions, compulsions and/or tics. Other neuropsychiatric symptoms include motoric hyperactivity (e.g., fidgeting, difficulty remaining seated) and choreiform movements.

Q2: E

Explanation
The above signs and symptoms are suggestive of child abuse and should prompt an escalation of the case to the appropriate seniors and relevant child protective services. Other signs and symptoms include but are not limited to frenulum tears, bruises in children who cannot cruise, long-bone fractures in children who cannot walk, rib fractures in children less than one year old and intracranial haemorrhages.

Q3: D

Explanation
Selective serotonin reuptake inhibitors (SSRIs) are suitable first-line treatment options except for paroxetine, which is avoided in children because of greater susceptibility to its side effects. Tricyclic acid antidepressants and venlafaxine are also avoided for similar reasons of increased susceptibility to side effects. Other antidepressants, such as mirtazapine, are typically used if SSRIs are not well tolerated or are not efficacious. Antipsychotics may be used to augment the management of treatment-resistant depression in children.

Answers to Case 51

Q1: C

Explanation
A family history of delirium is not significant in predisposing one to delirium.

Q2: B

Explanation
Mirtazapine has an antagonistic effect on serotonin type 2A, 2C, 3 and histamine H1 receptors, resulting in an anti-emetic and appetite-stimulating effect. The other antidepressants listed have greater gastrointestinal side effects.

Q3: B

Explanation
CBS is characterised by complex visual hallucinations in patients with visual impairments with a unique feature of retained insight that the imagery experiences are not real. There are no other features of psychosis in CBS. Balint syndrome is characterised by a triad of optic ataxia, oculomotor apraxia and simultagnosia. In simultagnosia, there is an inability to perceive more than a single object at any one point in time; it does not lead to visual hallucinations. While patients with LBD can present with complex visual hallucinations, insight is typically lost and it is accompanied by other features of parkinsonism and fluctuating cognitive impairment.

Q4: E

Explanation

The woman likely has LBD, and the most appropriate medication would be an acetylcholinesterase inhibitor such as rivastigmine. Patients with LBD who take antipsychotics can develop severe antipsychotic sensitivity reactions, which should be avoided. Antidepressants have no effect on the visual hallucinations.

Answers to Case 52

Q1: D

Explanation

Paroxetine has been specifically associated with cardiac malformations if taken during the first trimester.

Q2: D

Explanation

Quetiapine has the lowest placental passage rates amongst antipsychotics.

Q3: B

Explanation

One of the most concerning teratogenic effects of lithium exposure during pregnancy concerns the heart. Ebstein's anomaly describes malformation abnormalities of the tricuspid valve and right ventricle. First-trimester exposure to lithium increases the relative risk by 20 times [1]. The other listed malformations are closely associated with valproate *in utero* exposure.

Q4: B

Explanation

Clozapine should be continued, and breastfeeding stopped, given that patients are likely to be treatment-resistant before being started on clozapine, and a switch in antipsychotics post-partum is not advised. Clozapine is excreted in breast milk and carries adverse effects on the infant, such as sedation, agranulocytosis, seizures and cardiovascular instability.

Q5: B

Explanation

Breastfeeding while on lithium has been associated with early feeding problems, hypotonia, lethargy and lithium toxicity with raised creatinine. There is no significant association with increased susceptibility to infections.

References

1. Boland RJ, Verduin ML, Ruiz P, Shah A, Sadock BJ, editors. *Kaplan & Sadock's synopsis of psychiatry*, 12th edition. Philadelphia: Wolters Kluwer; 2022.

Answers to Case 53

Q1: E

Explanation
Given the significant history of liver impairment, an agent with the shortest half-life (lorazepam) would be most appropriate to avoid excessive sedation and respiratory depression from the poor metabolism of the chosen benzodiazepine.

Q2: A

Explanation
Amisulpride is predominantly renally excreted, and dose reduction is not required in patients with hepatic impairment. The other antipsychotics are hepatically metabolised.

Q3: A

Explanation
Agomelatine has been associated with liver impairment, especially in the first few months following initiation and requires regular liver function test monitoring in the first 24 weeks. The other listed antidepressants may be hepatically metabolised but are less likely to cause hepatic impairment compared to agomelatine.

Q4: C

Explanation
Lithium is not hepatically metabolised, and dosage reduction is not required. While topiramate is rarely known to cause liver injury, it is typically used as an adjunctive agent in the treatment of bipolar disorder. Carbamazepine, lamotrigine and valproate are hepatically metabolised and not advised for use in patients with advanced hepatic impairment.

Q5: A

Explanation
Hy's rule is defined as ALT > three times the upper limit of normal combined with serum bilirubin > two times the upper limit of normal.

Answers to Case 54

Q1: C

Explanation
Kidney impairment is a known side effect of lithium. The other medications do not typically cause kidney injury.

Q2: D

Explanation
Sulpiride is predominantly renally excreted and is best avoided in renal impairment.

571

Q3: C

Explanation

Pregabalin is removed during dialysis, and the serum concentration of other medications is not as significantly affected.

Q4: A

Explanation

While citalopram can be used in haemodialysis patients, it can cause dose-dependent QT interval prolongation, which can lead to arrhythmias and cardiac complications and hence is less preferable [1].

References

1.   US Food & Drug Administration (FDA). Clarification of dosing and warning recommendations for Celexa. FDA; 2016. Available from: www.fda.gov/Drugs/ResourcesForYou/SpecialFeatures/ucm297764.htm

Answers to Case 55

Q1: D

Explanation

Tarasoff I refers to the duty to warn the potential victim. Tarasoff II refers to the duty to take reasonable precautions to protect the victim from any significant danger posed by the patient. The ALI test is used to determine if a person is not responsible for their actions due to a mental disease or defect. The Durham rule guides the jury to determine that a defendant is not guilty by reason of insanity because a criminal act was the product of a mental disease. The M'Naughten rule determines legal responsibility where a defence of insanity has been made.

Q2: B

Explanation

The term *actus reus* refers to guilty act and *mens rea* refers to guilty intent.

Q3: D

Explanation

The Bolam test and the Montgomery test are the two common tests employed to determine if malpractice occurred. The other listed options do not exist.

Index

581

587

For EU product safety concerns, contact us at Calle de José Abascal, 56–1°,
28003 Madrid, Spain or eugpsr@cambridge.org.

www.ingramcontent.com/pod-product-compliance
Ingram Content Group UK Ltd.
Pitfield, Milton Keynes, MK11 3LW, UK
UKHW040951090126
466816UK00019B/355